Building a New Biocultural Synthesis

Linking Levels of Analysis
Emilio F. Moran, Series Editor

Building a New Biocultural Synthesis

Political-Economic Perspectives on Human Biology

Edited by
Alan H. Goodman
and Thomas L. Leatherman

Ann Arbor

THE UNIVERSITY OF MICHIGAN PRESS

2001   2000   1999   1998   4   3   2   1

A CIP catalog record for this book is available from the British Library.

Library of Congress Cataloging-in-Publication Data

Building a new biocultural synthesis : political-economic
     perspectives on human biology / edited by Alan H. Goodman and
     Thomas L. Leatherman.
        p.   cm. — (Linking levels of analysis)
     Includes bibliographical references.
     ISBN 0-472-09606-0 (cloth : acid-free paper)
     ISBN 0-472-06606-4 (pbk. : acid-free paper)
   1. Physical anthropology.   2. Social history.   3. Human remains
   (Archaeology)   4. Medical anthropology.   I. Goodman, Alan H.   II.
   Leatherman, Thomas L.   III. Series.
   GN62 .B85   1998
   306—dc21   98-25385
                                                              CIP

I think that the tendency of applied science is to magnify injustices until they become too intolerable to be borne, and the average man whom all the prophets and poets could not move, turns at least and extinguishes the evil at its source.

—JBS Haldane, 1923

Contents

Foreword

Richard Levins and Richard Lewontin

The struggle between biological and social explanations of human life is nowhere more pronounced than in anthropology. Indeed, the disciplinary distinction between biological anthropology and cultural anthropology, which manifests itself in departmental factions, in separate academic programs, and sometimes in residence in separate buildings, is a mirror of a fundamental epistemological disagreement. It is obvious to everyone that human beings are biological objects, distinguishable from other species in an immense array of anatomical, physiological, and behavioral manifestations, and that genetic differences between us and even our closest relatives among the primates are somehow involved in that manifest divergence. No chimpanzees will ever form a Department of Human Studies. On the other hand it is equally obvious, even to the most obdurate biological determinist, that the differences in food, dress, daily activity, language, rules of proper behavior, and unfounded beliefs between the Tupí-Mondé of the Amazon and the anthropologists who study them are not explicitly coded in their different genes, but are a consequence of their different historical experiences. So how are we to bring together the biological and the social in our understanding and explanation of what it is to be human?

Biological reductionists argue that we are "basically" articulate chimpanzees. Then, the more ancient an evolutionary origin, the more "fundamental" it is. Anything that has happened since the Pliocene is a veneer of socialization painted over the deep, dark, and ultimately determining forces of the hypothalamus. Cultural determinists, preoccupied with an opposition to vulgar biological determinism, urge that the development of symbolic language inserts us into a new universe where our biological heritage is merely an origin story of no relevance to our current state because it has been overruled by culture. A more liberal approach allows for both biology and society and then tries to assign numerical weights to the biological and the social. A more sophisticated interactionism abandons weighing of the relative contributions of the two domains because they obviously interact with each other on some third ground while each causal pathway remains distinct.

It is not possible to understand the ongoing struggles over the explanation of the nature of human beings without asking what work the explanations are supposed to do. The evolutionist's question of how *Homo sapiens* and *Pan troglodytes* diverged from a common ancestor and what difference has accumulated between them in the ensuing five to ten million years is a question to which a genetic answer can be given. But it is naive to suppose that the evolutionary question is what really motivates the struggle between biological and cultural determinism. The real issues are political: Could human life be other than it is? If so, are some social organizations more in accord with "human nature" than others? If so, can we get there from here? Is bourgeois society the final completion of a human historical trajectory, embodying the best that human biology allows? The confrontation between biological and social explanations and their various hybrids is, at bottom, a question of constraints and enablements. It should not surprise us that conservatives speak only of constraints while the liberals celebrate flexibility and the openness of possibilities. Either we are Richard Dawkin's "lumbering robots, created by our genes, body and mind" or we are, in Simone de Beauvoir's clever conundrum, "l'être dont l'être est de n'être pas," the being whose essence is in not having an essence. Yet, whether affirming or denying the importance of the biological or social, both sides accept the separate existence of these categories as distinguishable causal chains, differing only in what weight is to be assigned to them.

We, and the contributors to this book, begin by rejecting the categories themselves. But we are trapped by language into manipulating the very entities whose separate existence we reject. Our solution is to think in terms of the interpenetration of these categories, of the transformation of one by another, circling back in our analysis to find that the categories have become so transformed as to be something quite different than they were at the beginning. Such a view is more than simply a static interactionism. The most sophisticated developmental biology accounts for each organism as a unique outcome of a historical process of the transcription of particular genes at particular times in particular environments. But that answer is not helpful. First, it leaves entirely without specification what the array of outcomes of different genes in different environments may be, except to say, "it depends." Second, it takes environments as given, failing to take account of the historical change in the outer world produced by the activities of the organisms themselves. Third, it is a statement about individual organisms, taking as an unstated assumption that the individual is ontologically prior to the collectivity. No correct account of the world can ignore the way in which categories like "organism" and "environment" or "individual" and "collective," if they are to work at all, must be dynamically linked. What we label as a "dialectical" mode of thought is a mirror of the actual history of things in the world which in their historical actuality acquire their real, but ever changing properties in concrete, but ever changing contexts.

Our perspective, shared with the contributors to this book, is that biology is a socialized biology. It is our claim that social life is the major mode of evolution of our species including our biology, that our evolution continues on the basis of historically received but malleable biological constraints, that our biological constraints (already socialized) set the stage for further social process, and that these in turn change the significance of the constraints. Our biology as warm-blooded animals makes us eat a lot to keep up body temperature. Our biology as large animals means that we have to eat a few percent of our body weight per day, not the 30 to 40 percent or more that a hummingbird requires. Our biology as primates makes vision rather than smell our dominant sensory modality. Our biology as mammals makes touch an important part of social behavior and development. But the same touch may be sexually arousing, painful, ticklish, or abusive, or have other meanings depending on circumstance and history. It does not in any way negate the biological inheritance of the importance of touch to show that how it's important is socially determined. Our biology connects our adrenals with stress, but the subjective content of that stress may be frightening, exhilarating, or uproariously funny. We have to eat, and we do eat a wide range of different types of food that is further enlarged by our food preparation. But we are not simply omnivores but also productivores, consuming the products of our own labor.

However, the claim that society is the mode of evolutionary adaptation of the human species is also misleading. First, it seems to endorse the organism/environment dichotomy in which the environment sets a problem and the species adapts to it. This is clearly only one limb of the feedback loop: the environment that sets the problem has already been selected, transformed, and defined by the species that confronts it. While species do adapt to environments, they also change the problem rather than merely solve it. Second, it presumes a functionalism and a purposefulness that are not justified by our understanding of society. The notions of homeostasis and goal-seeking behavior of systems have been introduced into social science from engineering and from physiology. In the former, the goals and the "parts" of the system are known because the engineers put in the parts in order to pursue the goals set by their employers. In physiology, homeostasis is presumed to result from natural selection that strengthens those pathways and calibrates those parameters that keep fragile variables within tolerable bounds. We get on shakier ground when the "system" as a whole has no goal. While it is true that predators may increase when there is more available prey and that prey increase when the predators are reduced, neither species is pursuing the goal of balancing nature. In society this is even clearer: under capitalist conditions of nearly full employment, workers are sometimes in a stronger bargaining position and can force wages up. Employers, suffering relative losses of profits, may cut back on production and increase unemployment, which allows them to reduce wages. The apparent goal-seeking behavior of the feedback loop is the outcome of the opposing goal-seeking behaviors of the contending parties rather than a systemic striving for balance. With this insight, we can now look back on both homeostatic systems and see them as resultants of opposing processes at work.

This difference in approach determines how we see apparent failures: the failure of world agriculture to feed people, of industrial countries to stop pollution, of developing countries to save their forests. The functionalist viewpoint will look for failures in information flow, delays in responding, and other familiar kinds of failures of engineered systems. What they do not deal with is that the feedback loops are the result of conflict of interest and that ostensible goals are always subject to constraints hidden because of class interest. Therefore, agriculture fails to alleviate hunger not because of generic ineptitude but because food is mostly produced as a commodity response to commodity markets rather than human hunger. The pattern of knowledge and ignorance in medicine is not due to a problem of "information flow" but reflects the fact that some kinds of knowledge are more easily commodified than others and, as commodities, are allocated where there is "effective demand."

When we speak of human biology being a social biology, we recognize several interpenetrations of the biological and the social. First, the forms of basic biological functions become transformed socially. We must eat. But what we eat, with whom, on what occasions, on what occasions we must abstain from food, the amount and kinds of food that produce satiety are all socialized decisions. Second, the biological becomes transformed utterly into the social, losing entirely its original physiological meaning. When we invite a friend over for a "drink," it is not to adjust our electrolyte balance, nor are ritual eatings to be confused with the nutritive events from which they have historically grown. The cold lunch packed by the Israelites in their hurried escape into the desert was transformed into an annual ritual of the Passover Seder, a single occurrence of which—the Last Supper—became a founding event of a world-perturbing religion, finally to be enshrined as the central sacrament of that religion in the form of the unchewed wafer and the unsavored wine. Third, biological connections can be created by social history. Sticks and stones will break my bones, but names can never hurt me. Unless, of course, I belong to a society that believes in the efficacy of spells and curses, in which case I may easily waste away and die from a name pronounced backward. Fourth, a socialized biology creates new biological units, effective organs that arise only in a socialized context. It is enough to examine the limbs of a chimpanzee to know that it cannot fly, nor can any human being by flapping her arms. But human individuals do fly in consequence of a social interaction that has designed and produced airplanes, airports, fuel, and skilled labor forms. And these are the products of an integration of brains, eyes, ears, tongue, opposable thumbs, and delicate fingers, in addition to limbs, into an effective organ of invention and production.

Anthropology, properly construed, is not separable into the physical and the social. Anthropology is at the nexus of the biological and social, a biocultural synthesis spanning an enormous range of comparative, historical, and dynamic material. What holds this volume together is its challenging of the common sense of our sciences by seeing interpenetration rather than rigid dichotomies, historicity rather than static universals; and it is held together by a committed partisanship that hones objectivity.

Acknowledgments

The majority of the chapters in this book were originally presented during the Wenner-Gren International Symposium no. 115, "Political-Economic Perspectives in Biological Anthropology: Building a Biocultural Synthesis," held in Cabo San Lucas, Baja California Sur, Mexico in November 1992. The participants at the conference engaged in an informative, supportive, and unselfish exchange of ideas and information that made this book possible. We thank them all. We owe a special debt of thanks to R. Brooke Thomas who provided ideas and assistance from the planning of the symposium through publication of this volume. Moreover, Brooke's continued reflections on human adaptability theory, and his ability to expand and challenge his own ideas and assumptions, have been a constant inspiration to both of us. We are grateful to the Wenner-Gren Foundation both for supporting the conference and for providing a grant that enabled the publication of this book. Laurie Obbink and Mark Mahoney at Wenner-Gren expertly shepherded the conference and Susan Whitlock at the University of Michigan Press did the same for the book. We extend a special thanks to Sydel Silverman, President of the Wenner-Gren Foundation, for her constant guidance, support, and advice.

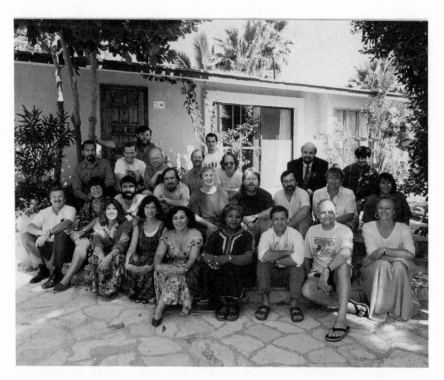

Participants in the 115th Wenner-Gren Conference (November 1992; Cabo San Lucas, Mexico): *bottom row (from left to right):* Billie DeWalt, Barbara Bender, Laurie Obbink, Lynn Morgan, Lourdes Márquez Morfín, Fatimah Linda Collier Jackson, Alan Goodman (co-organizer), Gavin Smith, and Ann Millard; *middle row (from left to right):* Dean Saitta, R. Brooke Thomas, Sydel Silverman, Thomas Leatherman (co-organizer), William Roseberry, Debra Martin, and Magalí Daltabuit; *top row (left to right):* Michael Blakey, Steven Kunitz, Merrill Singer, Pertti Pelto, Alan Swedlund, Ricardo Santos, Arturo Escobar, George Armelagos, and Mark Mahoney.

Series Introduction

The series Linking Levels of Analysis focuses on studies that deal with the relationships between local-level systems and larger, more inclusive systems. While we know a great deal about how local and larger systems operate, we know a great deal less about how these levels articulate with each other. It is this kind of research, in all its variety, that Linking Levels of Analysis is designed to publish. Works should contribute to the theoretical understanding of such articulations, create or refine methods appropriate to interlevel analysis, and represent substantive contributions to the social sciences.

The volume before you, *Building a New Biocultural Synthesis: Political-Economic Perspectives on Human Biology,* is the product of daring thinking at a Wenner-Gren Foundation–sponsored conference. The book breaks new ground by moving biological anthropology into the realm of the political. As such it is likely to be viewed years from now as a seminal contribution to biocultural research. The editors, Alan Goodman and Thomas Leatherman, have brought together an excellent mix of senior and junior colleagues who believe that the future of biological anthropology lies in bringing biological anthropology into closer touch with contemporary trends in cultural anthropology. We believe it may prove an important contribution to the reintegration of anthropology. If it succeeds in this regard, it will have made a major contribution to correcting years of fragmentation of the many subfields of anthropology, and to correcting the loss of the important focus on the holistic study of the human species that has been anthropology's distinct contribution to the human sciences.

The goal of the editors—to broaden the theoretical scope of explanations in biological anthropology toward consideration of political economy, political ecology, and critical theory—is ambitious. Such a change would represent a radical redirecting of a field that has been moving for years away from cultural anthropology toward the biological and medical sciences. It would also mean that biological anthropology would become more anthropological in its analysis—and force cultural anthropologists to begin to take biology more seriously than they have in recent years. As such, it could also help bring cultural anthropology back to a greater holism with fields such as archaeology and biological anthropology.

The book combines conceptual articles from biological anthropology, political economy, and critical medical anthropology with case studies that demonstrate the utility of integrative frameworks that do not overlook the political-economic dimensions of health and disease. As such, it will also provide a link with emerging literatures in the medical sciences that have tried to grapple with the distribution of disease and its economic and political spatial distributions. Contemporary research on the implications of global warming, sea level rise, the new viruses, and the return of diseases previously confined to distant rural areas cannot be effectively carried out without a sophisticated and integrative approach that has robust biological and sociopolitical components. An approach such as the one suggested by this volume will also make it more likely we will see a greater participation of biological and cultural anthropologists in the current work on the global spread of diseases brought about by the global economy, the international migration of labor, and the many other forces that are transforming our earth. People interested in the future of a reunified anthropology and a holistic approach to biological evolution and human health will welcome this volume.

Biological anthropology found a comfortable paradigm in the 1960s, with strong research support from the human adaptability section under the International Biological Program. Since then, there have not been many new approaches. Similar to that earlier initiative, research on the Human Genome Diversity Project has been one of the few exciting directions. By showing how a marriage of political economy and ecology can be productive, the authors in this volume have identified a direction for the field, one that is in touch with the awesome issues of our contemporary situation: global transformation of the earth and human communities with highly differentiated political and economic capacities to buffer themselves from the impact of global forces. By showing how local-level processes can buffer human communities from the forces of globalization (or not), the new biocultural synthesis represented by this volume makes itself a necessary partner in helping us understand how to cope and even thrive.

We hope this book inspires some readers to submit their work to the series. Please contact the series editor, or other members of the editorial board, to discuss your work.

PART 1

Historical Overview and Theoretical Developments

Chapter 1

Traversing the Chasm between Biology and Culture: An Introduction

Alan H. Goodman and Thomas L. Leatherman

As we approach the next millennium the cold war has ended and the threat of a nuclear holocaust may be diminished. Metaphors of a divided east and west, north and south, have been replaced by ones accentuating global unity and a "new world order." New international trade agreements such as GATT and NAFTA epitomize to some a blurring of national boundaries and the free exchange of goods and ideas. In Mexico, Indios, farm workers, and maquilladores respectively produce ethnic art, fruits, and industrial parts for distant markets. Like workers in other emerging countries, these individuals also enter the global community as consumers of foods and ideas; Mexicans drink an average of one Coca-Cola per day (Pendergrast 1993), and new ideas are absorbed from ubiquitous billboards and U.S. television programs.

Yet there is no blurring of relations of power. The poor emulate the rich, but the gap in wealth only widens. The wealth of 447 billionaires is greater than that of half of humanity. A sugary beverage might relieve pangs of hunger, perhaps an effective short-term solution to calm a crying infant, but persistent malnutrition and endemic disease remain unabated. Each year over ten million children die from the deadly synergy of malnutrition and disease, the equivalent of a jumbo jet full of passengers crashing every ten minutes of every day. Unlike the jet crash, these deaths are so much an everyday part of the background of life that this "silent violence" is accepted as inevitable, common, and even natural. The human toll commands little attention or action.

While the old scourges of malnutrition and infectious diseases persist, globalized capitalism has increased the pace of population displacement and environmental contaminations. Chronic "diseases of civilization" such as diabetes, heart disease, and obesity, as well as new and reemerging infectious diseases, also threaten survival. The new world order has also brought a crisis of disorder evidenced by an increase in ethnic conflicts, terrorism, racist attacks, and genocide.

These old and new challenges continue to deny many individuals access to a safe environment, basic productive resources, and the ability to meet basic needs. Peasants now often have the worst of both worlds. As parents and workers find their efforts insufficient to maintain the basic needs of their families, they begin to evade or alter the sociopolitical systems constraining them. Their strategies range from systems-altering reform to transformation—from resistance to revolution (Thomas, this vol., chap. 2).

Our ability to understand the social, environmental, and biological dimensions of these problems tests the relevance of anthropology. Understanding symbolic meanings or evolutionary implications, while important to some degree, is insufficient in the face of extreme poverty. Clearly, too, ethnographic and population description as closed, autonomous systems have little pertinence in addressing these complex changes. What is key, we think, is understanding local realities in global contexts. The infinite intersections of global economies and local ecologies, and of world history and local history, have made it equally critical to understand the local, and the global within the local. With its broadly holistic and biocultural approach, anthropology is seemingly well-positioned to help address these challenges.

Anthropology, unfortunately, has not been very helpful in these struggles. One key reason for this failing—the *biocultural split*—is addressed in this volume. Biocultural syntheses (or synthetic models of any type) have not been a central concern of anthropological theory in the past two decades. With the specialization and diversification of subdisciplines and perspectives, the chasm dividing biological and cultural anthropologies has deepened. Sociocultural anthropologists generally have been inattentive to the biological consequences of changing cultures and environments; biological anthropologists have not paid attention to how large-scale political-economic processes interrelate with local-level ecologies to shape biologies. Sociocultural anthropologists have perhaps been too introspective, and this has further muffled anthropological voices; biological anthropologists have not been reflexive enough. Thus, we see the need for synthetic approaches that incorporate the diversity of knowledge and approaches in anthropology and that provide an effective framework for analysis of how the processes of inequality and social change interact with human biologies.

Unfortunately, the biosocial perspective is most recognized for efforts to bridge biology and culture. Derived from evolutionary ecology and sociobiology, this approach aims to explain such behaviors as food gathering and fertility regulation as having evolved to maximize Darwinian fitness (see Betzig 1997). We say "unfortunately" because while this approach appeals to some cultural anthropologists, its lack of sensitivity to learned behavior and its strong genetic-evolutionary determinism have without doubt further distanced most cultural anthropologists from biologically oriented anthropologists.

We, and the contributors to this volume, propose a radically different science. Our dominant interest is in how sociocultural and political-economic processes affect human biologies, and then how compromised biologies further threaten the social fabric. Behaviors are not seen to maximize fertility due to genetic adaptations; rather biology and culture are dialectically intertwined (Levins and Lewontin 1985). As biological anthropologists our ultimate concern is with understanding the roots of human biological conditions, which are traced to the interaction of political-economic processes and local conditions. We surmised that integrating perspectives from anthropological political economy and ecology-adaptation is a logical place from which to begin building a biocultural synthesis.

In order to begin working toward such a synthesis we organized a Wenner-Gren International Symposium entitled "Political-Economic Perspectives in Biological Anthropology: Building a Biocultural Synthesis." Participants included biological anthropologists with diverse subfield specialties, archaeologists, a historian, and cultural anthropologists with specializations that included ecological, nutritional, medical, and political-economic anthropology.[1] The main goal of this conference was to consider fresh, new approaches in which human biologies are understood in broader historical, political-economic, ideological, and sociocultural contexts. We hoped that a more contextualized study of human biologies would, as Singer (this vol., chap. 4) discusses for medical anthropology, provide a disciplinary adhesive, thus reinvigorating communication across divided anthropological specialties. Moreover, better understanding of the biological dimension of economic and sociocultural changes broadens and deepens understanding of these changes. And framing biological studies in an analysis of history and large-scale political-economic processes illuminates the contexts and processes by which biological suffering and adaptation occur. It is one thing to know that limited access to food causes malnutrition. We know that it does. The questions we now wish to answer concern the processes by which food is limited, not least because the answer to these questions may point to solutions.

In a review of the political economy of demography, Susan Greenhalgh (1990) pays homage to Eric Wolf's *Europe and the People Without History* (1982), a masterpiece of anthropological political economy. She notes that "*People* is filled with people, their production, displacement, enslavement, and eradication," but goes on to comment, "How much stronger Wolf's forceful arguments could be were they systemically backed up and perhaps sharpened by quantitative assessments of the levels and trends of fertility, migration, mortality and population growth" (Greenhalgh 1990, 101).

We agree. In analyses seeking to capture the everyday realities of anthropological subjects, an understanding of human biology—from cumulative fertility and mortality to skinfolds, blood pressures, stress hormone levels, and rates of anemia—adds an integral layer of information that is too often missed. To paraphrase Duden (1991), histories are inscribed beneath the skin. A political-economic perspective that includes biologies should not merely integrate biological anthropology back into anthropology proper, but should sharpen and enrich the relevance of anthropology for understanding a wide variety of struggles to cope with and combat persistent human suffering.

The following chapters reflect their authors' ideas and efforts toward a new analysis of the relationship between sociocultural and biological domains. Because of the degree to which sociocultural anthropologists have not kept up with developments in biological anthropology, and vice versa, readers from different backgrounds may find various parts to be novel, old, or perhaps overly simplified. Given the bridging nature of the volume, we hope this introduction helps to bring readers onto a common ground. In the following sections we present background on the biocultural split in anthropology and our vision of common ground in bringing together perspectives from human adaptability/human ecology and political-economic anthropology. We illustrate themes and perspectives from anthropological political economy that we find particularly useful for building a new biocultural synthesis (see this vol., Roseberry, chap. 3, and Singer, chap. 4, for a more complete review of the roots of political economy and its merging with anthropology). We conclude by introducing the individual chapters and their particular contribution toward achieving this synthesis and with a parable on the need for biological anthropologists to look upstream.

The Biocultural Split: Forces of Fission and Common Ground

In a commentary in *Science* entitled "Failing to Cross the Biology-Culture Gap," Holden (1993) scolds anthropologists, trained to bridge gaps between cultures, for their inability to bridge the chasm between biology and culture. She characterizes the discipline as having broken down into two tribes, one oriented toward science and the other toward more humanistic and interpretive approaches. The tribes typically ignore each other, which is bad enough for a discipline that prides itself on its holism. At other times, wars break out at the most fundamental levels of worldview, ethics, and goals. According to Holden, there is a growing inability to find common language, concerns, and relevance. Biological anthropologists' interpretations of the human condition, too often empty of social content, and often reductionistic, appear irrelevant or simply wrong to many cultural anthropologists. Many of the recent theoretical directions in cultural anthropology are seen by biological anthropologists as excessively relativistic navel gazing, unimportant, and antiscientific.[2]

This crisis of excessive specialization and fragmentation is also recognized by anthropologists (Peacock 1995; Weiner 1995). In an editorial in the *Anthropology Newsletter* Brown and Yoffee ask, "Is anthropology coming apart at the seams? Is it breaking down into academic specialties that are unable and unwilling to talk to one another?" (1992, 1). The conclusion of a conference they organized at the School of American Research (Santa Fe, NM) on "Is Fission the Future of Anthropology?" as well as of subsequent commentators in the *Anthropology Newsletter* is that there are myriad signs of fission. Moreover, fission is welcomed by many who feel uncomfortably tied to individuals of different perspectives and methods. Historical critiques point out that biological and cultural anthropologists are members of the same discipline because anthropology was constructed to suggest that "primitive men" are more natural (biological) than men of civilization, an uncomfortable reminder of the colonialist project. Yet, most commentators recognize the dangers of fission: anthropology without biology loses much of its uniqueness, and a biological anthropology without anthropology becomes second-rate biology. The questions raised by Brown and Yoffee are critical. The points made by Holden ring true. How did we get here, and can we get out of this mess?

Of particular concern is that the forces of fission are reinforcing. A common opinion among biological anthropologists is that training should increasingly emphasize biomedical and physical sciences.[3] In the mid-1980s membership in the Biological Anthropology Section (BAS) of the American Anthropological Association was nearly on a par with membership in the American Association of Physical Anthropologists (AAPA), suggesting that biological anthropologists valued their dual connections to anthropology proper and to the subdiscipline. Not surprisingly, since the mid-1980s membership in the AAPA has gradually increased while membership in the BAS has declined by over 50 percent.

As biological anthropologists continue to separate themselves from current thinking in cultural anthropology, they remain uninformed about theoretical shifts and, not surprisingly, might view these changes as incomprehensible and foreign. Jokes about postmodernism have become standard fare at physical anthropology gatherings. When listening to these comments and jokes, one clearly senses a disdain along with fear and apprehension. Postmodernism jokes sound like ethnic jokes.

We are less privy to the unedited thoughts of cultural anthropologists, but similar signs of disdain are evident. Many of us have encountered cultural anthropologists who, having found out that we are biological anthropologists, fit us into a tired, old stereotype. They assume we have no interest in the living, we believe in "race," and we explain all human behaviors and differences as due to primordial genes. Saying that one is interested in culture and behavior, and, worse yet, biocultural interactions seems to conjure up the most stereotyped images of sociobiological reductionism. We sense that they have not read any biological anthropology since they were undergraduate students. Particularly disheartening is that this stereotyped view of biological anthropologists may be most strongly held by younger cultural anthropologists. Cultural anthropology doctoral students now study physical anthropologists as "the Other."

In summary, the gulf between biological and cultural anthropology is widening. Yet, there is a countertrend. In the last decade a sustained dialogue among biological, ecological, and political-economic anthropologies has emerged in specialties such as medical and nutritional anthropology (Baer 1996), and growing interest in "political ecology" as an interdisciplinary approach is attracting political economists, poststructuralists, and ecologists alike (e.g., this vol., Dewalt, chap. 12, and Hvalkof and Escobar, chap. 18). These movements give us hope in the possibility of developing a radical, biocultural middle ground.

Still, fragmentation is the rule, synthesis the exception. As a preface to presenting one version of a critical biocultural approach, we provide some historical perspective on how this chasm grew and on possible paths toward synthesis. Here we are concerned with the development of three approaches within materialist anthropology—ecology, human adaptability, and political economy. It is the diversion of paths that resulted in fragmentation and it is their reconnection that we see as a part of the solution. In the following section we aim to provide an outline or sense of the approaches that have influenced the synthesis attempted in this volume. Chapters 2, 3, and 4 in the first section, by Thomas (on human adaptability), Roseberry (on political economy), and Singer (on critical medical anthropology), elaborate on these themes.

Toward a New Biocultural Synthesis: History and Trends

Ecological Bioculturalism: A Golden Age?

In the 1960s ecological and evolutionary perspectives merged, and the concept of adaptation provided powerful means of understanding human biological diversity and evolution. Livingstone's (1958) work on the adaptiveness of sickle-cell trait to endemic malaria was influential in convincing biological anthropologists of the promise of finding genetic adaptations to specific environmental challenges. Throughout the 1960s and 1970s, research focused on adaptation in challenging environments such as arctic and high altitude regions. Investigators searched for genetic adaptations and, with insights from environmental physiology, nongenetic acclimatization responses. As research expanded into considerations of phenotypic plasticity, socially influenced factors such as nutrition, disease, energy flows, and migration emerged as research foci. These studies were framed in a general ecological approach that considered systemic interaction of cultural, physical, and biological environments as milieus of human biology and behavior. The breadth of these interactive systems, and the conceptual underpinnings of evolution and adaptation, seen as applicable to both biological and cultural phenomena, seemed to provide the holism that many anthropologists strived for (Baker 1996; Little 1982; Thomas, Gage, and Little 1979).

Similar approaches infused much of anthropology, and by the late 1960s the "ecological perspective" was dominant among materialist perspectives. In a way that had not existed before or since, it served to unify work in biological, archeological, and sociocultural anthropologies, and led to the formation of bridging fields such as medical and nutritional anthropology (Singer, this vol., chap. 4). Pioneering field studies such as those by Lee (1968) and Gross and Underwood (1971) focused on the flow of protein and calories, and the technological and social features (adaptations) that allowed people to extract resources from their environments. These studies, conducted during what might be called the golden age of biocultural and ecological anthropology, were resolutely materialist, ecological, and biocultural and also made important links to larger theoretical issues. Lee's (1968) work on San time allocation was critical to disrupting the discourse that capitalism represented the pinnacle of progress. Gross and Underwood's (1971) paper on sisal production in Brazil provided a devastatingly clear view of the nutritional costs of the shift from subsistence to market production. For many commentators, anthropology had found its theory and voice (Harris 1968).

Yet, there were problems in the application of 1960s-style ecological approaches—especially in applying biological metaphors to sociocultural systems. Critiques within evolutionary biology argued against progress as inherent to evolution, noting that the concept of adaptation as used in the "adaptationist program" was tautological, teleological, reductionist, progressive, and victim-blaming (Gould and Lewontin 1979; Levins and Lewontin 1985; Lewontin 1978). Rather, evolution and adaptation should be seen as less purposeful and progressive and as more historically contingent (Gould 1991). Sociocultural critiques targeted the functionalist view of systems as closed, homeostatic, and self-regulating (Orlove 1980; Ortner 1984; Wolf 1982, 17). As Singer (this vol., chap. 4) notes, "Ignored in this close-to-the-ground empiricism were the sweeping processes and broader social relations that transcended micro-populations historically uniting them with each other and with broader developments in capitalist development."

It is within these critiques and responses to critique that separate paths formed and unification became less evident. In sociocultural anthropology, critiques of ecological approaches came from emerging political-economic approaches and later from more humanistic, interpretive, and postmodern approaches. Within ecological anthropology, neoevolutionist and neofunctionalist studies persisted alongside a newer "processual ecology," which is in part a response to critiques from political economy.

Developments in Sociocultural Anthropology

Key to our project are insights from an anthropological political economy and a more sophisticated "processual ecology," providing a basis for current thinking in political ecology (Hvalkof and Escobar, this vol., chap. 18). These developments open up an essentially materialist perspective to ideology, politics, and outside influence.

　We also wish to break out of the separation of materialist-scientific from humanistic-interpretive approaches.[4] Of clear importance to the future of any human science are understandings of the social contexts of both subject and scientist, and how these contexts influence fact-gathering and the generation of knowledge. Also, increased attention to the more subtle uses of power in the "daily lives" of "real people," as well as to scientists generating knowledge (Foucault 1980), is a further "postmodern trend" in anthropological theory. There, sensibilities contribute to current perspectives in anthropological political economy and political ecology. Finally, attention to these issues aids us in understanding biologies: who becomes ill and what are the consequences, who gets fed when food is limited, and why is food limited in the first place.

Processual Ecology.　Processual ecology developed alongside neoevolutionist and neofunctionalist approaches which dominated cultural ecology in the 1970s and beyond. Key themes included a greater concern with the mechanisms of change (as opposed to homeostasis), a stronger focus on actor-based models, and the development of adaptive strategies (Bennett 1976). Conceptions of adaptation as "actors operating under a set of constraints allocating scarce resources to a hierarchical series of ends or goals" (Orlove 1980, 247) provided a strong link to human adaptability studies in biological anthropology (Thomas 1997; Thomas, Gage, and Little 1979). One influence from political-economic theory was the role of position and power in shaping decision making and adaptive strategies. As Orlove notes, "If adaptive strategies are seen as the outcome of decision making, or repeated allocation of scarce resources to a hierarchy of goals under conditions of constraints, then it is necessary to examine the pattern of resource distribution and the source of the goals and constraints" (1980, 252). The contribution of political economy to processual ecology was in specifying resource distribution and the source and goals of constraints. These perspectives were used to examine social responses to challenges such as famine and environmental disasters.

More sophisticated merging of macro-micro processes emerged in the processual ecology of the 1980s, which some even called political ecology (DeWalt and Pelto 1985; DeWalt, this vol., chap. 12). Many of these studies were in applied settings, and this, along with the perception that they were refinements rather than paradigm shifts, may be why they failed to receive much attention as advances in theory. Nevertheless, they provide a foundation for the recent emergence/resurgence of a variety of approaches labeled political ecology that share a focus on environment, macro-micro interaction, and power relations.

Political Economy.   With radical social movements, political-economic theories proliferated in the 1970s as challenges to anthropology's colonial past and current theoretical frameworks (Ortner 1984). Cultural ecology was criticized for its vision of closed and homeostatic systems, and modernization theory for its progressive evolutionism. While there are many "political economies," for the most part new approaches were reformulations and expansions of Marxism[5] (Roseberry 1988).

The related approaches of dependency theory and world systems theory were central to this resurgence within anthropology. Dependency theory emerged as a direct refutation of modernization theory, which held that the development process was ideologically neutral, that development occurred in stages, and that the Third World, which creates its own perpetual state of poverty, could only "modernize" by following the lead of the West. Dependency theory radically challenged this evolutionary and deterministic view. It highlighted how relations with capitalist/imperialist powers distorted third world economies; development and underdevelopment were, in fact, inextricably tethered. Development occurs at the expense of underdevelopment (Frank 1967; Williams 1966; also see Marable 1983 on the underdeveloped of Black America). World systems theory was developed from dependency theory by Immanuel Wallerstein (1976, 1977) and focused on the emergence of the modern world (capitalist) system as a process of shifting relationships between capitalist core areas and peripheries that supported the core.

Both theories (and sometimes the whole of political economy) have been criticized for their "capitalism-centered view of the world" (Ortner 1984, 142) and for providing too little attention to "real people doing real things" (Ortner 1984, 144; also see Morgan 1987 on the consumption of dependency theory in medical anthropology). The critiques highlight the concern for placing human agents at the center of analysis, as in a more anthropologically informed political-economic analysis.

An anthropological political economy can be traced to early proponents such as Wolf, Mintz, Leacock, and Nash. Wolf and Mintz developed a "cultural history" approach to political economy, a specific reaction to cultural ecology (Roseberry 1988). Themes carried on in their later works include a focus on the importance of history on a global scale and the struggles and conflicts that formed anthropological subjects, real people doing real things at the intersection of local histories and the larger processes of state and empire making. The goal of such analyses is a "unity of structure and agency, the activity of human subjects in structured contexts that are themselves the products of past activity but, as structured products, exert determinative pressures and set limits upon future activity" (Roseberry 1988, 172). These approaches were also more explicitly concerned with class, ethnicity, gender, culture, and politics. Wolf's *Europe and the People Without History* (1982) begins to consider both the big picture of historical development of capitalism and the significance of local variations that account for the actions and local realities of diverse populations outside of the capitalist core.

Themes that emerge in anthropological political economy include concerns with how global systems and history intersect with local systems and history in creating the contexts for understanding the actions of peoples. This approach is concerned with the social relations and institutions which control fundamental resources, including social labor, the exertion of this control being an expression of power. It locates actors wielding power in social fields and concentrates on the specificity of local constructions of power relations in these fields, including those that have their source outside of particular regions—that is, how "external" forces are "internalized." A concern with power as wielded by everyday people in everyday situations, and the recognition that cultural formations are grounded in unequal relations, also were central to "domination and resistance" studies (e.g., Scott 1985, 1990).

Merging Critical Perspectives into Anthropological Political Economy. Recent poststructuralist contributions expand upon anthropological political economy by providing a stronger sense of the contingency of social realities, and by showing how power and meaning are constructed in the specific contexts and moments of everyday action and discourse. For example, Emily Martin's (1987, 1990, 1994) work on the metaphors and tropes used to describe immunological and physiological processes has made us aware of the degree to which doctors and patients view health as a military-like battle and disease as an enemy. Escobar (1995) has similarly "unmasked" the ideology of the development enterprise, still rooted in modernization theory, to show how the practice of development validates existing relations of power. Smedley (1993) has shown how "race" developed as a Western worldview and became reified.[6] All of these works provide insights into the stakes involved in the control of knowledge, and all have clear relevance for biocultural and biological research.

Although theories of postmodernism are certainly assailable, there is no doubt that in this postmodern time scientist-researchers cannot assume shared ideologies or the obvious superiority of their explanations. This change is seen in recent challenges by Native Americans and other indigenous peoples to the ethics of research into human genomic diversity (Corpus 1996) and to the analysis of the skeletal remains of ancient peoples (see Martin, this vol., chap. 7). The debates over the study of archaeological remains have been simplified to one of science and freedom versus religion and uninformed antiscience (Clark 1996). Yet, possibilities for a new "collaborative science" are now emerging out of greater concern for the different positions (and sometimes variant interests) of archaeologists and the "subjects" of their research (Fine-Dare 1997). Skeletal biologists are now frequently consulting and working with Native Americans to answer questions of mutual interest (Martin, this vol., chap. 7). The title of Rose and co-workers' (1996) recent review, "NAGPRA Is Forever," is to the point. Few can doubt that there has been a strong "postmodern" shift away from viewing science and scientists as absolute authorities and problem solvers. The possibilities for collaborative knowledge and solutions make biocultural work more complex, more interesting, and more exciting.

The Position of Biological Anthropology

It is revealing that the developments of the last quarter century that come to mind on the biological side of anthropology are nearly entirely method-ological. Almost every area of inquiry has gotten better at measuring human biologies. For example, developments in endocrinology have made it much easier to measure stress (Flynn and England 1997) and reproduc-tive hormones (Ellison 1990) in the field. Chemical methods for the analy-sis of bones and teeth have led to more direct dietary interpretations in bioarchaeology (Armelagos et al. 1989; Klepinger 1993). The development of the polymerase chain reaction (PCR) has allowed biological anthropol-ogists to obtain detailed knowledge of the genetics of individuals, both liv-ing and past. These methods, borrowed and modified from other fields, collectively promise more precise answers to old questions and the possi-bility of addressing questions that formerly could not be scientifically stud-ied (note 3).

Less developed are models and theories, especially those that make central interactions between culture and biological systems.[7] This is par-ticularly surprising at a time when the social sciences and humanities have undergone deep and prolonged debates around fundamental issues of the-ory, practice, and ethics. What Martin (this vol., chap. 7) says for skeletal biology—that the laboratory blinds were pulled down to avoid contact with an external reality—generally applies to other areas of biological anthropology. Biological anthropologists, for the most part, became more attached to developments coming from biomedical sciences. They increas-ingly began to be employed in departments in professional health schools, where they could work alongside geneticists, cell biologists, and anatomists, rather than with linguists, archaeologists, and cultural anthro-pologists.[8]

It is understandable, though unfortunate, that biological anthropolo-gists have generally been reluctant to engage in dialogues over the origin and salience of theory and scientific practice (see note 3). As we hope this volume begins to show, insights from political-economy perspectives on relations of power, on the importance of historical contingency, and on local-regional-global interactions are pivotal to understanding human biologies. These realizations have been central to the concerns of a number of researchers in human adaptability. It is in this effort to integrate human adaptability with political-economic perspectives that we see promise for building a new biocultural synthesis.

Developments in Human Adaptability.   Following Livingstone's (1958) explication of the sickle cell trait–endemic malaria connection, nearly four decades of searching for similar genetic adaptations have not led to similar successes. There seem to be few situations in which human populations develop a genetic adaptation to a local and specific environmental challenge.[9] On the other hand, decades of research reaffirm that biological plasticity is a species-wide adaptive mechanism; evolutionary history has produced a species that is adept at rapid, plastic adjustments to a range of environmental conditions.

Less clearly understood at first were the limits to plasticity. At what point, for example, is short stature a sign of intolerable stress, rather than an adaptation to caloric limitations? Impoverishment takes its toll on the resilience of many populations and on their ability to cope. The underside of adaptation is seen in the realization that much of the biological variation measured is attributable to malnutrition and disease (Thomas, this vol., chap. 2). Labeling this an "adaptation" seems to be perverse and vulgar (Goodman 1994).

Research in the 1980s increasingly became oriented to documenting biological dysfunction in impoverished environments and the biological consequences of ubiquitous social change. In this work, biological anthropologists have excelled at relating a range of proximate social indicators (household demographics and socioeconomic status, parental education and occupation) to nutrition and disease, and in effect mirroring a social epidemiological approach.[10] They also have provided rich detail on the costs of intolerable conditions on adaptive domains (Mazess 1975) such as disease resistance and work capacity.

Most research, however, still fails to assess the roots of socioeconomic variation or historical forces of change. While adept at relating proximate conditions (such as lack of available food and exposure to stressors) to biological suffering, researchers have not addressed well the reasons for variation in exposure to these conditions. In characterizing social and historical change by generic terms such as traditional versus modern, we learn almost nothing about why and how people experience change differently. Thus, the childhood deaths noted in the prologue are viewed as natural and even inevitable, rather than as products of human interaction. In many ways, our use of a telescopic evolutionary lens obscures the historical specificity needed to understand changing patterns of human-environment interactions.

Toward a Political Economy of Human Biology

The ascent of political-economic and critical approaches in the social sciences led to the development of complementary approaches in archaeology and medical anthropology (critical and postprocessual archaeology and critical and political-economic medical anthropology). These approaches all foregrounded perspectives from political economy and adopted a self-critical stance on the social context of praxis and theory in their related disciplines. Adherents of the critical/political-economic medical anthropology see their approach as a much needed "corrective for the disciplinary fragmentation of social science that obscures the relationship among economic systems, political power, and ideologies" (Morsy 1990, 27; also see Singer 1989b; Singer and Baer 1995). Archaeologists turned their attention to social relations in shifting modes of production as a corrective to "stage" analyses common to neoevolutionary approaches, and to documenting social inequalities in prehistoric and historic contexts (Paynter 1989; Cobb 1993; Maguire 1992, 1993; Saitta 1988 and this vol., chap. 5).

As noted before, critiques by evolutionary biologists showed the tautology and functionalism in the "adaptationist program" (Gould and Lewontin 1979). Variations in traits, by their mere existence, are assumed to have functional import and to have arisen to meet that function via natural selection. Adaptation to fill niches is particularly problematic since niches are created through organism–environment interactions. Looking back through evolutionary time provides a false sense of inevitability and progress (Gould and Lewontin 1979). This view tends to "naturalize" social processes.

Applied to human biocultural studies, Blakey, in his historical research on the roots and continuities of American physical anthropology, shows a history of naturalizing social processes, which rather than being based on good science, tends to maintain existing socioeconomic inequalities (Blakey 1987, 1991; also see Haraway 1989, 1990).

At about the same time, human adaptability studies increasingly focused on adaptive responses to "multiple stress" environments. Researchers found that responses to one stressor could influence (and often constrain) responses to another (Baker 1984; Thomas, Gage, and Little 1979). As well, while stress and response occur at several levels (cellular, individual, population, etc.), responses at one level cannot be directly extrapolated to other levels; what serves the individual phenotype might not benefit larger social groups (Mazess 1975). These insights challenged the understanding that the environment simply selected the best-fit phenotype.

The history of Andean research provides a relevant example because so much has been written about Andean "adaptations" from an ecological and evolutionary perspective (see Leatherman, this vol., chap. 10, for a more detailed discussion). Early expectations were that broad adaptive patterns would be discerned through comparisons of human biobehavioral adjustments to Andean, Himalayan, and Ethiopian high mountain systems. However, less similarity than expected was found, and in spite of the constancy of hypobaric hypoxia, relatively little evidence has been found of any genetic adaptation. Taking histories into account, particularly the frequent population movement between low and high altitude ecosystems (e.g., Murra 1984), helps to explain this result.

Issues raised by the "small but healthy" hypothesis illustrates deeper problems with the notion of cost-free adaptations. The small-but-healthy hypothesis, as developed by economist David Seckler (1980), asserted that short stature is an adaptation to mild-to-moderate malnutrition (MMM). Seckler suggested that small body size ought to be interpreted as an appropriate and effective biological adaptation to marginal food supplies. Hence, national economic/food resources should be directed at those who most clearly suffer from severe malnutrition, and not at the moderately malnourished. They were small, yes, but healthy and adapted to their conditions of life.

This "insight" into the adaptiveness of small body size came from the writing of biological anthropologists and international nutritionists who had estimated caloric savings of smaller bodies. Anthropologists and others responded and soon began to explore the biobehavioral and sociocultural contexts of smallness (Martorell 1989; Messer 1986; Pelto and Pelto 1989). Whereas smaller people require fewer calories (beneficial in low energy contexts), their "smallness" entailed substantial cost to their biology and behavior. In context, smallness could also signal a plethora of functional deficits (Allen 1984; Martorell 1989), thus Pelto and Pelto (1989, 14) conclude that "the concept of a 'no-cost' adaptation makes virtually no sense." Perhaps more important, the small-but-healthy hypothesis alerted us to the political implications of research findings and theorizing. In this case Sekler was writing to advise the Indian government on its food relief policies.

These realizations and trends led some biological anthropologists in the 1980s to begin integrating perspectives from anthropological political economy and human adaptability. These developments were influenced by similar developments in medical anthropology and archaeology and were applied to examples of how social inequalities shape human biology in prehistoric, historical, and contemporary contexts (Goodman et al. 1988; Goodman and Armelagos 1985; Leatherman et al. 1986; Thomas et al. 1988). This work was variably labeled as "biology of poverty" (Goodman et al. 1988; Leatherman and Goodman 1997; Thomas, this vol., chap. 2), "critical bioculturalism" (Leatherman 1996), "critical biological anthropology" (Crooks 1996), "dialectical biological anthropology" (Leatherman et al. 1986), "political ecology of human biology" (Goodman, Leatherman, and Thomas 1996; Leatherman and Thomas 1996), "political economy of human biology" (Blakey 1985), and "humanistic biological anthropology" (Blakey, this vol., chap. 16).[11]

Political Economy and Its Relevance to Biocultural Analyses

The developments previously noted provided a framework and context for biological anthropologists to search for perspectives that complement evolution, ecology, and adaptation, particularly ones that direct attention to global contexts, history, and social relations that shape local environments. Because human biologies are affected by and reciprocally influence such factors as the control, production, and distribution of material resources, ideology, and power, we find a political-economic perspective to be an invaluable and necessary complement. In outline, political-economic perspectives contribute to biocultural anthropology by emphasizing five interrelated issues.

The importance of examining biological variation in terms of *social relations* through which individuals gain access to basic resources and labor. Simply stated, these social relations are key to resource production and distribution (that is, they are relations of power) and are thus key to forming proximate environments—what individuals eat; their exposure to pathogens, temperature stress, and toxic substances; and what resources may be brought to bear to adjust to these stressors and constraints. Political-economic analysis calls for the analysis of social processes, rather than just indicators such as socioeconomic status. As Saitta notes (this vol., chap. 5), these social processes, although full of complexity and contradiction, are key to a deeper understanding of who becomes ill and other biocultural processes.

The importance of *links between the local and the global* (macro-micro interconnections). Threats and benefits to health and nutrition are invariably linked to regional and international processes, and how they intersect with local conditions to shape the microenvironment of adaptation. To not consider how these processes affect biologies in this interlinked world is clearly limiting, and the same may be true for ancient populations (Goodman, this vol., chap. 6).

History and historical contingency are critical to understanding the direction of social change and the biological consequences of change (and by extrapolation, evolutionary change; cf. Gould 1991). As suggested by the example of Andean research, understanding biological responses often requires understanding local history.

Humans are *active agents in constructing their environments.* Part of this constructing entails resistance and revolution, as well as accommodation and adjustment; and these system-challenging responses need to be more fully integrated into our understandings of coping and adaptation. Humans create their environment and at the same time are created by their environment, an insight that goes back to Frederick Douglass (Blakey, this vol., chap. 16). The environment takes on meaning only in relationship to the subject (Levins and Lewontin 1985).

Ideology and knowledge, of subjects and scientists alike, are key to understanding human action. While both adaptation and political economy are materialist perspectives, it is increasingly clear how power and resources are maintained by control of knowledge.

Hence, a bioanthropological political economy seeks to understand how particular local histories shape everyday realities of anthropological subjects, and moreover, how separate communities are connected through larger historical political-economic processes that affect human biologies. Understanding humans "under the skin" can enrich our understanding of the link between global change and the everyday struggles of human groups. After all, *what is more real about the human condition than people's biology?*

Directions and Implications for Biological Analyses

The development of a political-economic perspective has a variety of implications for biological anthropology theory and practice. In the following sections we outline some possible implications for: (1) human-environment interaction and adaptation, (2) the expanded context of research, (3) dialectics and the conceptualization of the adaptive process, and (4) the politics and practice of bioanthropology.

Human-Environment Interaction and Adaptation

Both ecological and political-economic approaches are concerned with how people transform nature into human resources. This economic act of transformation, whether by direct extraction or through production, is carried out by social groups. The nature of this social organization (who makes decisions over how labor is allocated in production and who controls the product) is key to descriptions of economy.

Ecological perspectives tend to treat these acts as processes in which homogeneous social formations operating with a given technology and social organization (e.g., hunter-gatherers, horticulturalists, industrial agriculture) work toward a particular end that serves the group. In contrast, a political-economic perspective highlights the social relations involved in the allocation and control of labor. These relations of power underlie inequalities and exploitation, exposure to risks, who eats what, and so on, all of which have biological consequences. Biological anthropologists often study the process of transforming environment in light of adaptive decision making about resource and labor allocations, whereas those taking a political-economic approach study environmental transformations in terms of social and power relationships. Central to both perspectives is control over resources and labor. In adaptation studies, autonomous control by the individual, group, or population is central. Key is their ability to read the environment and act to achieve best outcomes (or, in the face of unpredictability, to minimize costs by hedging bets). Over the long run those strategies that enhance survival, reproduction, and prosperity will be perpetuated through time, biologically via natural selection and/or culturally as "adaptive strategies."

A political-economic perspective views individuals and groups as acting in what Roseberry refers to as social fields of power (chap. 3). These webs of relationships structure what responses are appropriate, available, and allowed. The content of these relationships is power: over who owns what, who works where, for how long, and with what return. Thus, human responses, what one might label as adaptations (if successful) or maladaptations (if not), are fraught with conflict and contradiction. Individuals try to balance these conflicting inputs and imperfect knowledge using personal experience, local cultural knowledge, and available resources to meet specific goals. The adaptation perspective implies that if it works more than it fails, then the response is adaptive. A political-economic perspective implies that responses and their consequences differ depending on their contexts and individuals' positions within social webs. "Logical" and "appropriate" behaviors may differ by class, gender, and ethnicity. What works for one group might work against another. Moreover, humans have imperfect knowledge and structural constraints on their actions, and they necessarily respond in ways that have unintended consequences, which are just as critical to understand as those that are intended.

A political-economic perspective is particularly useful for biological anthropology because it addresses our attention to problems people must confront and their capacity to cope, both of which are conditioned by available material and social resources. Biological anthropologists have made great strides in detailing variation in biology (such as growth, morbidity, mortality, nutritional status), but have paid less attention to variation in coping capacity. A political-economic perspective adds a potential to go beyond static measures of social status and class to examine the factors that perpetuate poverty such as lack of land and education, high rents, illness, and so forth. The list goes on; the point is that underlying causes of material and social conditions vary, and they vary with different effects and solutions.

Expanding Contexts

A major goal of a political economy of human biology is to frame questions in broader environmental and sociopolitical contexts. How, for example, in an increasingly delocalized and interlinked world, do the flows of information, resources, peoples, and their genes move from nested regional, national, and global systems to new local systems? Hence, the changing use and meaning of sugar in English food systems, the colonization of the Caribbean, and the creation of plantation economies in the Dominican Republic are interconnected and part of the same history (Mintz 1985). The marginal Andean environment is as much a product of four centuries of domination and recent capitalist penetration as of low oxygen pressure and irregular rainfall (Leatherman, this vol., chap. 10). The environmental context of disease and evolution in the Amazon is largely a context of conquest and colonization (Santos and Coimbra, this vol., chap. 11). Even in antiquity, the health and nutritional status of individuals living in Sudanese Nubia and west-central Illinois is more fully understood in relationship to seats of political power and changes in political autonomy (Goodman, Leatherman, and Thomas 1996, chap. 8).[12] By framing local problems within broader contexts, different questions are asked, questions about deeper roots of exposure to stress. Without consideration of these broader contexts, the preferential feeding of adult males to the detriment of child growth among sisal farm workers in Brazil could be seen as a case of maladaptive intrahousehold food allocation. Rather, it can be seen as a product of horticulturalists abandoning subsistence farming for cash cropping sisal, at the insistence of development efforts (Gross and Underwood 1971). To see the malnutrition of Brazilian children as a product of their own adaptive failures rather than of maldevelopment suggests a variant of victim blaming.

Rethinking Adaptation: The Dialectics of Adaptation

Merging a political-economic perspective into human adaptability leads to a rethinking of the concept of adaptation. First, it leads us to see adaptation as an ongoing process rather than a collection of measures. Speaking of problems inherent in the comparative analysis of cultures, Eric Wolf (1981, 42) notes that "we often take the data observed or recorded as realities in and of themselves, rather than as more or less tangible results of underlying process operating in historical time." In adaptation studies, the tendency is to apply a cost–benefit analysis and cite a measure or behavior as an adaptation, forgetting the caveats raised by Mazess (1975) that what is adaptive at one level or domain is not necessarily so at another, that what is adaptive now is not necessarily so in the future, and that what is adaptive for one person is not always so for another. Thus, it is always relevant to ask, "adaptive in what context, adaptive for whom, at what level, at what point in time?"

A variety of biobehavioral responses may satisfy an immediate set of problems. The danger is that labeling them as adaptations suggests that an adequate or acceptable solution has been reached; the potential costs of the response are of little importance. One solution is to focus on adaptation as a process with tangible outcomes one can measure and record, but not end points in and of themselves, thus avoiding reifying responses as adaptations or maladaptations. In turn, by considering a range of outcomes, one sees costs and conflicts along with benefits. It is critical to recognize that costs are not negated by benefits, but often create future binds and limitations. Thus, the context for future response is altered by the responses themselves; the adaptive process operates dialectically, contributing to ongoing change in the human condition and the nature of human-environment interactions (Leatherman 1996; Levins and Lewontin 1985).

Biology, Politics, and Praxis

The "small but healthy" debate, NAGPRA, and indigenous responses to the Human Genome Diversity Project (HGDP) all highlight the need to foreground the politics and ethics of bioanthropological research. The key lesson from the "small but healthy" hypothesis is that the reporting and interpretation of biological information is unavoidably a political act. Discussions of adaptations are not abstractions, but potentially consequential for real peoples. NAGPRA and indigenous concerns over the HGDP show clearly that a hidden and unapproachable ivory tower no longer exists.[13] Increasingly, research can no longer be justified for the sake of knowledge alone. It is no longer possible for biological anthropologists to measure and probe biologies with only vague notions of consent. Rather than see these developments as attacks on science, they are calls to make science ethically accountable and to debate what is at stake.

It may come to be that the anthropology of the twenty-first century will be an anthropology of praxis—of collaboration and applied work—and if so, a new ethics of practice is needed. In many places biological suffering is witnessed and ignored, or explained with reference to genetics and evolutionary theory or static notions of maladaptive cultures and naturalized class divisions. A new ethics of practice mandates that we examine the human condition with an eye to the complex social relations that shape lives and biologies, and with a commitment that our analysis should be relevant to relieving persistent suffering. As noted before and by Martin (this vol., chap. 7), NAGPRA has led to collaborative efforts involving researchers and descendant communities (also see Blakey's discussion of collaboration around the African Burial Grounds Project, chap. 16).

These collaborative efforts make clear that science can be done in many ways, and there is no natural division between science and human rights. In fact, the science we stand for should be "for the people" and on the side of human rights.

Goals and Structure of the Book

It is our hope that this volume points to a new biocultural anthropology, one that is nearly 180 degrees different from a biosocial perspective. The goal of this volume is to consider the possibility for a biocultural synthesis that takes into account the complexities and contradictions of social life and how they influence biologies. Following the goals of the original Wenner-Gren conference, for which most of these papers were originally written, the chapters focus on a wide range of biocultural topics. As well, all of the papers from the original conference focus on the Americas, although their implications are global.

The conference generated great excitement and optimism for the future of biocultural perspectives in anthropology in which the "realness" of biology and biological well-being are brought back into anthropology. We hope this excitement is conveyed in this volume. There is a healthy diversity of ideas and opinions, and even some serious trepidation over the merging of metatheories with such obvious differences. Can ecological and evolutionary theory, with the central concept of adaptation, merge with a political-economic theory of power and social relations? Is a reformulating of the adaptation concept simply pouring new wine into an old and worn-out wineskin (Singer 1996), or are we creating a more socially informed and relevant adaptation theory? The authors of the chapters to follow suggest a wealth of responses to these questions, and a diversity of foci in building a new biocultural anthropology. We hope the diversity provides food for rethinking theory and practice and that this volume, as a whole, is a step toward building a biocultural approach that is of greater relevance to the human condition.

Historical Overview and Theoretical Development

The first section further develops the historical and theoretical themes introduced in this chapter. In the following chapter R. Brooke Thomas outlines the historical development of the human adaptability perspective.

He delineates a series of key phases and human-environment models that document an increased focus on the importance of sociopolitical conditions, ending with a discussion of an emerging "biology of poverty."

In parallel fashion, William Roseberry presents an overview of the development of political-economic perspectives in anthropology (chap. 3). Of particular note for biological inquiry is Roseberry's development of the notion of "fields of power" and the problematization of commonly held concepts such as region and household.

One purpose of including a wide range of participants from cultural anthropology and archaeology is to gain perspective on the development of critical and political-economic perspectives in other areas of anthropology. As a key example, Merrill Singer outlines the development of critical medical anthropology. This perspective foregrounds the political-economic roots of (dis)ease and suffering as well as the significance of power in medical care and research, in the process of medicalization, and in defining normality and disease.

Case Studies from Prehistoric and Historical Contexts

The second and third parts of the volume focus on case studies and applications. Rather than show a uniformity in method and vision of what a political economy of human biology ought to look like, which would not be sensitive to local conditions and problems, these five papers illustrate a wealth of issues for consideration.

Dean Saitta (chap. 5) brings the perspective of a critical archaeologist to the task of linking political economy and human biology in North American antiquity. He argues that a class perspective has utility in precapitalist societies and focuses on labor as a key variable in political-economic analyses, linking the social and the biological. Yet he also provides an important cautionary note by showing how simplified notions of class might break down in studies of precapitalist, past populations.

Alan Goodman follows by considering the health consequences of relations of power in antiquity. He first looks at evidence for class or rank-type variation in biological health and provides two different examples of class-based difference in health. Goodman then focuses on precapitalist regional systems of exchange and exploitation, and suggests that such systems had biological consequences for diet, nutritional status, and health.

Debra Martin begins with a critical history of bioarchaeology in the

American Southwest (chap. 7). For Martin, a political-economic approach includes concern for power relations in the research process, as well as attention to the role of political-economic factors in the lives of past peoples. Although the Southwest was used as a training ground for biological anthropologists, she contends that they ignored the needs and problems of the descendants' communities. In her analysis of the evidence for violence directed against women she considers how larger political-economic processes such as raiding and migration articulated with gender relations.

Moving to historical populations, Alan Swedlund and Helen Ball focus on current and past explanations for childhood mortality in Massachusetts from 1830 through 1920 (chap. 8). Their innovative approach simultaneously considers current statistical models to explain mortality and explanations of experts of that period. Their historical research shows how public health workers framed problems such as the relationship between mothers' work and child mortality, and it provides insights into the use of previously collected demographic data.

In an example of how ethnicity, migration, and class affect health, Lourdes Márquez Morfín focuses on the typhus epidemic in Mexico City in 1813. She shows how the epidemic differentially affected individuals depending on their geographic location within the city. Migration to the city to find employment led to crowding and swamped public resources, leading to poor sanitation and increased exposure to infectious agents. Thus, Márquez is able to draw connections between larger historical processes and how they affected local conditions, which ultimately affected morbidity and mortality. She also situates her work within the historical development of Marxian biological anthropology that developed in Mexico at about the same time that ecological perspectives developed in the United States.

Case Studies of Contemporary Groups

These five chapters approach a variety of human biological problems faced by peasants and impoverished populations in the Americas. Leatherman (chap. 10) begins this section by comparing bioanthropological research in the Andean Highlands in the 1960s and 1980s. This chapter provides a grounded example of developments in human adaptability that mirror theoretical issues discussed previously and by Thomas (chap. 2).

The case study, which examines relationships between health and household economy in three Andean communities, is an explicit attempt to merge adaptability and political economy.

The three chapters that follow all focus on aspects of economy and health in local systems framed in larger and historical, political-economic contexts. In a provocative paper on the "(un)natural history" of the Tupí-Mondé Indians of the Brazilian Amazon, Ricardo Santos and Carlos Coimbra show how contact with the West, the "un-natural history," nearly destroyed the Tupí-Mondé (chap. 11). Although physiological stress, as measured by enamel hypoplastic defects and other means, was clearly evident before sustained contact, stress increased dramatically at this time.

Billie DeWalt examines a similar point of articulation of contact between the West and peasants (chapter 12). Working in southern Honduras, he focuses on the larger context of population increase and its association with malnutrition. DeWalt labels his approach "political ecology," which he defines as a blending of human ecology and political-economic perspectives. DeWalt shows how development efforts often fail to consider either the locations of peasant farmers in political-economic systems or local ecological constraints, resulting in ecological and social destruction, rather than revitalization.

Daltabuit and Leatherman (chap. 13) focus on a third type of contact—tourism. They show how tourism-led development is having unpredicted effects among Mayan communities in the Yucatán, Mexico. Because men are most likely to be employed for wages, and frequently migrate on a weekly basis for work, tourism differentially affects men and women. A particular effect examined here concerns shifting aspects of women's work, health, and reproduction. Also, diets are changing to the point where soft drinks and junk foods are the third leading source of calories, and the stage is set for a paradoxical combination of micronutrient undernutrition and obesity.

The final paper in this section, by Debra Crooks, focuses on policy developments and research into child malnutrition in the United States. Crooks uses studies of human growth to highlight the problems of persistent malnutrition in eastern Kentucky and shows how individuals are given mixed messages about what to eat (and what they can afford to eat). This paper is particularly important in that it provides an example of the biological problems and the possibility for practice-oriented research among the hidden poor in the United States.

Toward a Critical Biocultural Anthropology

By raising a number of issues, the papers in the final section suggest key elements and possible directions toward the further development of a critical biocultural anthropology. Armelagos and Goodman (chap. 15) provide a historical review of the concept of race in biological anthropology. They suggest that race has long outlived its scientific utility; its persistence is an example of the power of politics in our science, a power that has long been ignored. They call for a focus on the biological consequences of racism, a new and vital area of biocultural inquiry.

Michael Blakey calls for a humanistic approach that is reflexive, considers the role of the researcher and the subjects of research, and pays explicit attention to embedded politics and hidden assumptions (chap. 16). He questions the historic politics of positivism and naturalism, and provides examples of alternative approaches. For example, Blakey and colleagues' work on the New York African Burial Ground illustrates the involvement of the descendant community in research decision making.

In her paper "Latin American Social Medicine and the Politics of Theory" (chap. 17), Lynn Morgan continues the theme of reflexivity. She focuses attention on the contexts in which a critical theory has already developed. Like Saitta's chapter on archaeology and Singer's chapter on critical medical anthropology, Morgan's provides important lessons for the development of a critical biocultural theory and praxis. More than the others, Morgan emphasizes efforts to be explicit about the role of the researchers in their work.

The last chapter, by Søren Hvalkof and Arturo Escobar, illustrates that some anthropological concerns and theories are coming full circle and also suggests the possibility for a radical and praxis-oriented biocultural-ism. These authors elaborate upon the development of a political-ecological approach, as noted earlier by DeWalt. They provide a brief history of the development of ecological and materialist approaches in anthropology and the way they were critiqued for excessive materialism, closed-systems perspective, and functionalism. In their example of the rain forest–human relationship, it becomes very clear that, as they paraphrase Raymond Williams, there is a lot of culture in nature.

The final commentary brings together Gavin Alden Smith, a political-economics–oriented anthropologist, and R. Brooke Thomas, a leading theorist in human adaptability. They provide some cautions around the pitfalls of ill-defined concepts, for example. However, the basic thrust echoes the introduction in suggesting the need for a new and radical synthesis, and the great promise of merging perspectives for a new generation of anthropologists.

Conclusion

As we approach the next millennium, the U.S. economy has entered a phase of bullish growth and there is optimism in continued economic expansion. Multinational corporations are extending markets and going global. Peasant farmers in Tezonteopan, Mexico, grow peanuts for foreign markets, while their children suffer from protein-energy malnutrition. Pastas, which cook quickly and require less fuel, are replacing beans in diets. (However, the amino acid complementarity with maize is diminished, and the biological costs are unknown.) Further south, Mayan villages are replete with advertisements on tienda walls proclaiming the excellent flavor and healthiness of Fanta, Crystal, Pepsi, and Coca-Cola. Yet it is little understood how drinking a "harmless cola" might affect a Mayan peasant family's economics and the nutritional status of infants. Hannerz writes that "the people in my favorite Nigerian town drink Coca-Cola, but they also drink *burukutu* too; and they can watch *Charlie's Angels* as well as Hausa drummers on the television sets" (cited in Clifford 1988, 17).

Ours is a time of both great optimism and widespread criticism of the production and use of scientific knowledge, and even of the privileged position of science itself. On one hand, the promise of science is greater than ever, but so too is distrust and lack of faith in science. Newspapers report on a daily basis advances in genetic research that promise better crop production and the elimination of defective traits—from AIDS cures to increased agricultural productivity, from designer drugs to designer genes. But the promise has not yet improved the human condition. Scientific and biomedical advances are heralded; the public grows weary. The Human Genome Project is equated with the Holy Grail, like reading the book of life (Gilbert 1992). Yet the chronic diseases that kill most individuals are still exacting their toll and are joined by new and emergent infectious diseases, most notably AIDS, further decreasing the triumph of science "over nature."

Indeed, there is great public confusion over the very nature of human nature, and over the relationship between culture and nature. What, for example, do genes actually do and control? As reported in the popular press, are there really "risk-taking" and "jigsaw-puzzle solving" genes? Are intelligence and violence in our genes, and more prevalent in the genes of individuals from certain "races"?

While starvation is a daily event in much of the world, in the United States an abdominal exerciser was the number-one selling gift of the 1996 Christmas season. New nonfat products appear on a daily basis; a potato chip made with the synthetic compound olestra mimics the taste of fat. Yet restaurants serve bigger and bigger proportions, and obesity rates increase.

Despite advances in predicting the weather, better and more varied systems of communication, the development of the information super-highway, and unprecedented knowledge of the human genome, not every-one has shared equally in the benefits or been positively affected by these changes. Poverty, class divisions, exposure to toxic substances, and star-vation persist in many places. As cultures, peoples, and ideas come into contact, the fabric of daily life can do little more than unweave. Some indi-viduals benefit, but many more suffer socially, economically, and biologi-cally.

As scientists and citizens, we look ahead with both excitement and some skepticism. The last decades have witnessed increasing fragmenta-tion and specialization, especially between biological and cultural analy-ses, scientific approaches, and humanistic approaches. Our overriding optimism is that the divide between approaches can be bridged, and that bridging, rather than diminishing the parts, leads to better understand-ings—of real people doing real things with real consequences. Finally, we hope that these stronger analyses will lead to improvements in the lives of individuals in the real world.

Epilogue: Refocusing Upstream—The Making Social
of Biology

An often repeated parable is germane to our efforts. The first version we are aware of is from McKinley's (1986) "A Case for Refocusing Upstream: The Political Economy of Illness" and is credited to Irving Zola.[14] In the original version a physician on the shore of a swiftly flowing river hears the cries of a drowning man. He jumps into the river, pulls the man to safety, and successfully applies artificial respiration. Just when the man recovers, there is another cry from the river. The physician jumps back in, pulls the second man out, resuscitates him, and then hears another cry, another body to resuscitate. He finally realizes that he is so busy with rescue that he has no time to see "who the hell is upstream pushing them all in" (McKinley 1986, 613). The point of this tale is that resources and activities in health are excessively devoted to downstream endeavors that are often inefficient, expensive, and superficial; efforts are sometimes heroic but ultimately inefficient. Because they do not solve any deeper or more systemic problems, McKinley suggests that biomedicine ought to cease excessive preoccupation with short-term tinkering and begin to refocus upstream to the origins of the problem.

In our version the physician goes about rescuing the drowning victims while the biological anthropologists huddle at the riverside discussing who will get to measure and probe the bodies as they are laid on the side of the river. One, trained in forensics, measures the bodies in order to establish sex, age, and "race." Another, trained in demography and epidemiology, records the numbers of dying and surviving in order to establish the incidence and prevalence of morbidity and mortality. A third, trained in environmental physiology, measures skin temperatures to establish the thresholds of adaptive responses to hypothermia. A fourth, with a stress perspective, obtains saliva samples in order to measure hormones, concluding that almost dying of hypothermia is a stressful event. A fifth, biomedically trained, asks the now resuscitated individuals about their education, SES, family size and structure, and activity patterns to isolate proximate determinants of near-drowning. A sixth biological anthropologist, trained in nutritional anthropology, measures skinfolds and conducts a dietary interview to establish the role of diet and nutrition in the etiology of drowning. A seventh, an anthropological geneticist, takes blood samples in order to establish genetic risk factors for falling into rivers. A session on the biology of exposure to cold water is organized for next year's annual meetings.

The main point of this parable is that nobody hikes upstream or questions what is going on. Biological anthropology has a long tradition of describing and documenting biological status—stunting and wasting in children, disease, birth and death rates, changes in working capacity, and so on. We are good at reading signs from the body. It is also common for us to be involved with individuals in dire situations (although their thoughts and sufferings infrequently appear in our writings). However, we have rarely "focused upstream" to the larger factors shaping shorter height, reduced working capacity, or high mortality rates. For example, while it has become relatively common to associate biological variation with socioeconomic variation, it is rare that the context or roots of the socioeconomic variation are addressed. It is not trivial whether the poverty associated with undernutrition and illness in much of the Third World stems from marginal physical environments, drought, feudal arrangements with wealthy landowners, or low wages and constrained subsistence production often associated with capital penetration. Too often, we view undernutrition and illness as regrettable but inevitable consequences of an impoverished environment, as if poverty were a component of a natural environment and not a product of social relations and inequality. The point is that people don't just end up rich or poor, sick or healthy, landed or landless. These all happen for reasons, and those reasons frequently lie upstream. If there is a single overarching theme to a political-economic perspective it is in focusing upstream on the intersection of forces which place people by the river and push them in.

In various ways the authors of the papers that follow have tried to leave the safe banks of the river, and, with apologies for mixed metaphors, have tried to bridge the chasm between biology and culture.

NOTES

We owe a great debt of thanks to R. Brooke Thomas, who commented on drafts of this paper. More important, Brooke's continued reflections on human adaptability theory, and his ability to expand and challenge his own ideas and assumptions, have been a constant inspiration to both of us. Ann Kingsolver, Debra Martin, Lynn Morgan, Sydel Silverman, and Alan Swedlund provided a wealth of helpful comments on a prior draft. Finally, we wish to express our gratitude to Sydel Silverman for her constant support, advice, and direction of this project.

1. Participants in the 115th Wenner-Gren Conference (November 1992; Cabo San Lucas, Mexico) included George Armelagos, Barbara Bender, Michael Blakey, Magalí Daltabuit Godas, Billie DeWalt, Fatimah Linda Collier Jackson, Arturo Escobar, Alan Goodman (co-organizer), Steven Kunitz, Thomas Leatherman (co-organizer), Lourdes Márquez Morfín, Debra Martin, Ann Millard, Lynn Morgan, Pertti Pelto, William Roseberry, Dean Saitta, Ricardo Santos, Merrill Singer, Gavin Smith, Alan Swedlund, and R. Brooke Thomas. Sydel Silverman, Laurie Obbink, and Mark Mahoney provided intellectual guidance and assistance at all levels.

2. Cartmill (1994) is one of just a few biological anthropologists to write about the effects of the postmodern turn in anthropology on biological anthropology. As a primatologist and evolutionary theorist Cartmill apparently cannot easily envision a biological anthropology that is not solidly based on evolutionary theory. Conversely, he recognizes the danger of evolutionary metaphors and modes of

inquiry in cultural anthropology and agrees with the trend wherein many cultural anthropologists have stopped trying to explain sociocultural phenomena as evolutions. We agree in part. In some places where humans suffer biologically, evolutionary theory is of little utility, at least at the level of practice, yet we strongly believe that our work, for example, in exploring the relationship between food, nutrients, and growth, is biological anthropology. Second, we are more enthusiastic about the potential contribution to biological inquiry of current developments in sociocultural anthropology. Cartmill misses entirely the development of political-economic anthropology and sees little more than some minor correctives to excessive positivism in the postmodern turn. We see more, and this too is likely due to our political commitments and our position as human biologists/ecologists.

3. At a recent plenary symposium on the future of physical anthropology at the 1996 annual meetings of the American Association of Physical Anthropologists, leaders in the field commented on the future of their subfield or specialization. With one exception all commentators saw a bright future based on improved methods and technological developments. Theory was not in question; it is fair to say many simply see no need for theoretical revision or infusion. A sign of this thinking is that some major departments such as at Duke University now have split biological and sociocultural anthropology.

4. An example of the separation of what we here characterize as materialist-scientific versus humanistic-interpretive approaches developed within medical anthropology, where both a political-economic and an interpretive/critical perspective developed as separate responses to the ecologically and clinically dominant perspectives. Soheir Morsy (1990), talking of the more political-economic perspective, has aptly said that medical anthropologists need to switch focus from what is in people's heads to what is on their backs. While we agree, we hope to go further to consider the relationship between what is in people's heads and what is on their backs.

5. This discussion on developments in political-economic theory and practice is necessarily brief. The contribution of structural marxists, modes of production theories and debates, and a host of other important themes are left out. Included are references to dependency and world systems approaches and the legacy of a cultural historical approach in political economy. The ideas and approaches of these latter schools of thought we feel have more direct relevance to the problems focused upon in this volume. The anthropological political economy we are advocating here was developed at least in part in response to the lack of agency in these macro-system models.

6. There is great consternation over the importance of the history of ideas in biological anthropology. In her review of Barkan's *The Retreat of Scientific Racism,* a book that emphasizes how politics affects scientific ideas about race, Alice Brues (1992, 52) states that it is "unlikely that physical anthropologists will find this book of much interest" as it is a study in "the sociology of knowledge." Armelagos (1994) responded to the contrary.

7. There are still many debates over the interpretation of the fossil record, highlighted by the long-standing debate between the "multiregional" and "Eve" hypotheses. The most relevant theoretical development of the last decade is the

development of evolutionary or Darwinian medicine (Lappé 1994; Nesse and Williams 1994), which, unfortunately, in its popularized version comes off as evolutionary just-so stories.

8. Many others who discerned the importance of maintaining anthropological connections have begun to affiliate with bridge fields such as nutritional, medical, and applied anthropology. The depth of their continued commitment to biological anthropology remains to be seen.

9. It is interesting that what is remembered and reproduced in Livingstone's work is how the sickle cell trait provided a case of natural selection. Less emphasized is that the context for endemic malaria was a social construction, what Singer (this vol., chap. 4) and Santos and Coimbra (this vol., chap. 11) call "un-natural selection." In retrospect, while we may have been misguided in so readily accepting this genetic mode of adaptation as typical of human populations, it set the agenda for much subsequent research on human adaptation.

10. This led one participant at the conference to speak of the "epidemiology wannabes" among biological anthropologists. More to the point, it is interesting that as biological anthropology has expanded perspectives into the social arena of health and nutrition they have by and large sought guidance and legitimacy from the more reductionistic epidemiology and biomedical sciences—rather than from social anthropology.

11. Many of us involved in this endeavor were students or professors at the University of Massachusetts, Amherst during the 1980s. The department's rich tradition of biocultural research and strong political-economic perspectives within social anthropology and archeology provided an encouraging environment for these efforts.

12. While these broad historical contexts are often recognized by biological anthropologists, they are typically left to others (archaeologists, historians, social anthropologists) to explore. Although this follows a presumed more efficient and pleasing division of labor in science, unless the analyses are linked back to biology, the biology remains disconnected, and the power of analysis is diminished.

13. The negative publicity received by the HGDP is perhaps summarized by the fact that it is labeled the "vampire project" by many indigenous groups. This project, which involves immortalizing bloods (genes) of indigenous peoples from around the globe, highlights the problems of doing anthropological research in a world of widespread communications. The increased political awareness of indigenous peoples, along with their development of computer networks (Lock 1994), makes very public any case of possible ethical violation.

14. Another version was adapted to medical anthropology by Scheper-Hughes (1990). The use of masculine pronouns is from the original.

REFERENCES

Allen, L. H. 1984. Functional Indicators of Nutritional Status of the Whole Individual or the Community. *Clinical Nutrition* 3:169–75.

Armelagos, George J. 1994. Racism and Physical Anthropology: Brues's Review of Barkan's *The Retreat of Scientific Racism. American Journal of Physical Anthropology* 93:381–83.

Armelagos, George J., B. Brenton, M. Alcorn, D. Martin, and D. Van Gerven. 1989. Factors Affecting Elemental and Isotopic Variation in Prehistoric Skeletons. In *The Chemistry of Prehistoric Human Bone,* ed. D. Price, 230–44. Cambridge: Cambridge University Press.

Baer, Hans. 1996. Toward a Political Ecology of Health in Medical Anthropology. *Medical Anthropology Quarterly* 10:451–54.

Baker, Paul. 1984. The Adaptive Limits of Human Populations. *Man* 19:1–14.

Baker, Paul. 1996. Adventures in Human Population Biology. *Annual Review of Anthropology* 25:1–18.

Barkan, Elazar. 1992. *The Retreat of Scientific Racism: Changing Concepts of Race in Britain and the United States between the World Wars.* Cambridge, MA: Cambridge University Press.

Bennett, John 1976. *The Ecological Transition: Cultural Anthropology and Human Adaptation.* New York: Pergamon Press.

Betzig, Laura, ed. 1997. *Human Nature: A Critical Reader.* New York: Oxford University Press.

Blakey, Michael. 1985. Stress, Social Equality, and Culture Change: An Anthropological Approach to Human Psychophysiology. Ph.D. diss., University of Massachusetts.

Blakey, Michael. 1987. Skull Doctors: Intrinsic Social and Political Bias in the History of American Physical Anthropology with Special Reference to the Work of Ales Hrdlicka. *Critique of Anthropology* 7 (2): 7–35.

Blakey, Michael. 1991. Man and Nature: White and Other. In *Decolonizing Anthropology,* ed. F. Harrison, 8–16. Washington, DC: American Anthropological Association.

Brown, Peter J., and Norman Yoffee. 1992. Is Fission the Future of Anthropology? *Anthropology Newsletter* 33 (7): 1, 21.

Brues, Alice. 1992. Review of Elazar Barkan's *Retreat of Scientific Racism. American Journal of Physical Anthropology* 89:52.

Cartmill, Matt. 1994. Reinventing Anthropology: American Association of Physical Anthropologists Annual Luncheon Address, April 1, 1994. *Yearbook of Physical Anthropology* 37:1–9.

Clark, Geoff. 1996. NAGPRA and the Demon-Haunted World. *Society for American Archaeology Bulletin* 14 (5): 2.

Clifford, James. 1988. *The Predicament of Culture.* Cambridge: Harvard University Press.

Cobb, Charles R. 1993. Archaeological Approaches to the Political Economy of Nonstratified Societies. In *Archaeological Method and Theory,* vol. 5, ed. M. B. Schiffer, 43–100. Tucson: University of Arizona Press.

Corpus, V. T. 1996. Indigenous People's Reactions to the HGDP. In *The Life Industry: Biodiversity, People and Profits,* ed. M. Baumann, J. Bell, F. Koechin, and M. Pimbert, 147–48. London: Intermediate Technology Publications.

Crooks, Deborah L. 1996. American Children at Risk: Poverty and Its Consequences for Children's Health, Growth, and School Performance. *Yearbook
of Physical Anthropology* 38:57–86.

DeWalt, Billie R., and Pertti J. Pelto, eds. 1985. *Micro and Macro Levels of Analysis in Anthropology: Issues in Theory and Research.* Boulder, CO: Westview
Press.

Douglass, Frederick. [1854] 1950. The Claims of the Negro Ethnologically Considered. In *The Life and Writings of Frederick Douglass,* ed. P. S. Foner. New
York: International.

Dressler, William W., and James R. Bindon. 1997. Social Status, Social Context,
and Arterial Blood Pressure. *American Journal of Physical Anthropology* 102
(1): 55–66.

Duden, Barbara. 1991. *The Woman beneath the Skin: A Doctor's Patients in Eighteenth-Century Germany,* trans. Thomas Dunlap. Cambridge, MA: Harvard
University Press.

Ellison, Peter. 1990. Advances in Human Reproductive Ecology. *Annual Review of
Anthropology* 23:255–75.

Escobar, Arturo. 1995. *Encountering Development: The Making and Unmaking of
the Third World.* Princeton, NJ: Princeton University Press.

Fine-Dare, Kathleen. 1997. Disciplinary Renewal Out of National Disgrace:
Native American Graves Protection and Repatriation Act Compliance in the
Academy. *Radical History* 68:25–33.

Flynn, Mark, and Barry England. 1997. Social Economics of Childhood Gluco-
corticoid Stress Response and Health. *American Journal of Physical Anthropology* 102 (1): 33–53.

Foucault, M. 1980. *Power/Knowledge: Selected Interviews and Other Writings,
1972–1977.* New York: Pantheon.

Frank, Andre Gunder. 1967. *Capitalism and Underdevelopment in Latin America.*
New York: Monthly Review Press.

Giddens, A. 1987. *Sociology: A Brief But Critical Introduction.* San Diego, CA:
Harcourt Brace Jovanovich.

Gilbert, Walter. 1992. A Vision of the Grail. In *The Code of Codes,* ed. D. J. Kevles
and L. Hood, 83–97. Cambridge, MA: Harvard University Press.

Goodman, Alan. 1994. Cartesian Reductionism and Vulgar Adaptationism: Issues
in the Interpretation of Nutritional Status in Prehistory. In *Paleonutrition:
The Diet of Prehistoric Americans,* ed. K. Sobolik, 163–77. Carbondale:
Southern Illinois University Press.

Goodman, Alan, and George J. Armelagos. 1985. Death and Disease at Dr. Dickson's Mounds. *Natural History* (Sept.): 12–18.

Goodman, Alan, Thomas Leatherman, and R. Brooke Thomas. 1996. Does
Human Adaptability Plus Political Economy Equal Political Ecology? Paper
presented at the Annual Meetings of the American Anthropological Association.

Goodman, Alan., R. B. Thomas, A. Swedlund, and G. J. Armelagos. 1988. Biocultural Perspectives on Stress in Prehistoric, Historical and Contemporary
Population Research. *Yearbook of Physical Anthropology* 31:169–202.

Gould, S. J. 1991. *Wonderful Life: The Burgess Shale and the Nature of History.* New York: W. W. Norton.

Gould, S. J., and R. Lewontin. 1979. The Spandrels of San Marcos and the Panglossian Paradigm: A Critique of the Adaptationist Programme. *Proceedings of the Royal Society of London, Series B,* 205:581–98.

Gramsci, Antonio. 1957. *The Modern Prince and Other Writings,* trans. Louis Marks. New York: International.

Greenhalgh, Susan. 1990. Toward a Political Economy of Fertility: Anthropological Contributions. *Population and Development Review* 16:85–106.

Gross, Daniel, and Jane Underwood. 1971. Technological Change and Caloric Costs: Sisal Agriculture in Northeastern Brazil. *American Anthropologist* 73 (3): 725–40.

Haraway, Donna. 1989. *Primate Visions: Gender, Race and Nature in the World of Modern Science.* New York: Routledge.

Haraway, Donna. 1990. *Simians, Cyborgs, and Women: The Reinvention of Nature.* London: Free Association Books.

Harris, Marvin. 1968. *The Rise of Anthropological Theory.* New York: T. Y. Crowell.

Holden, Constance. 1993. Failing to Cross the Biology-Culture Gap. *Science* 262:1641–42.

Klepinger, Linda. 1993. Culture, Health and Chemistry: A Technological Approach to Discovery. In *Investigations of Ancient Human Tissues,* ed. M. K. Sanford, 167–80. New York: Gordon and Breach.

Lappé, Marc. 1994. *Evolutionary Medicine: Rethinking the Origins of Disease.* San Francisco: Sierra Club.

Leatherman, Thomas L. 1996. A Biocultural Perspective on Health and Household Economy in Southern Peru. *Medical Anthropology Quarterly* 10 (4): 476–95.

Leatherman, Thomas L., J. Carey, and R. B. Thomas. 1995. Socioeconomic Changes and Patterns of Growth in the Andes. *American Journal of Physical Anthropology* 97:307–21.

Leatherman, Thomas, and A. H. Goodman. 1997. Expanding the Biocultural Synthesis Toward a Biology of Poverty. *American Journal of Physical Anthropology* 102:1–3.

Leatherman, Thomas., J. S. Luerssen, L. Markowitz, and R. B. Thomas. 1986. Illness and Political Economy: An Andean Dialectic. *Cultural Survival Quarterly* 10 (3): 19–21.

Lee, Richard. 1968. What Hunters Do for a Living or How to Make Out on Scarce Resources. In *Man the Hunter,* ed. R. Lee and I. DeVore, 30–48. Chicago: Aldine.

Levins, Richard, and Richard Lewontin. 1985. *The Dialectical Biologist.* Cambridge, MA: Harvard University Press.

Lewontin, Richard. 1978. Adaptation. *Scientific American* 239 (3): 156–69.

Little, Michael. 1982. Development of Ideas on Human Ecology and Adaptation. In *History of American Physical Anthropology, 1930–1980,* ed. F. Spencer, 405–33. New York: Academic Press.

Livingstone, Frank B. 1958. Anthropological Implications of Sickle Cell Gene Distribution in West Africa. *American Anthropologist* 60:533–62.

Lock, Margaret. 1994. Interrogating the Human Genome Diversity Project. *Social Science and Medicine* 39:603–6.

Maguire, Randall H. 1992. *A Marxist Archaeology.* Orlando: Academic Press.

Maguire, Randall H. 1993. Archaeology and Marxism. In *Advances in Archaeological Method and Theory,* vol. 5, ed. M. B. Schiffer, 101–57. Tucson: University of Arizona Press.

Marable, Manning. 1983. *How Capitalism Underdeveloped Black America.* New York: Monthly Review Press.

Martin, Emily. 1987. *The Woman in the Body: A Cultural Analysis of Reproduction.* Boston: Beacon Press.

Martin, Emily. 1990. Toward an Anthropology of Immunology: The Body as Nation State. *Medical Anthropology Quarterly* 4 (4): 410–26.

Martin, Emily. 1994. *Flexible Bodies.* Boston: Beacon Press.

Martorell, Reynaldo. 1989. Body Size, Adaptation, and Function. *Human Organization* 48:15–20.

Mazess, Richard B. 1975. Biological Adaptation: Aptitudes and Acclimatization. In *Biosocial Interactions in Population Adaptation,* ed. E. S. Watts, F. E. Johnston, and G. W. Lasker, 9–18. The Hague: Mouton.

McKinley, John B. 1986. A Case for Refocussing Upstream: The Political Economy of Illness. In *The Sociology of Health and Illness,* ed. P. Conrad and R. Kerr, 613–33. New York: St. Martin's Press.

Messer, E. 1986. The "Small but Healthy" Hypothesis: Historical, Political, and Ecological Influences on Nutritional Standards. *Human Ecology* 14:57–75.

Mintz, Sidney. 1985. *Sweetness and Power: The Place of Sugar in Modern History.* New York: Viking.

Morgan, Lynn. 1987. Dependency Theory in the Political Economy of Health: An Anthropological Critique. *Medical Anthropology Quarterly* 1 (2): 131–54.

Morsy, Soheir. 1990. Political Economy in Medical Anthropology. In *Medical Anthropology: Contemporary Theory and Method,* ed. T. Johnson and C. Sargent, 26–36. New York: Praeger.

Murra, John. 1984. Andean Societies. *Annual Review of Anthropology* 13:119–41.

Nesse, Randolph, and George Williams. 1994. *Why We Get Sick: The New Science of Darwinian Medicine.* New York: Times Books.

Orlove, Benjamin. 1980. Ecological Anthropology. *Annual Review of Anthropology* 9:235–73.

Ortner, Sherry B. 1984. Theory in Anthropology Since the Sixties. *Comparative Studies in Social History* 26:126–66.

Paynter, Robert. 1989. The Archaeology of Equality and Inequality. *Annual Review of Anthropology* 18:369–99.

Peacock, James. 1995. Claiming Common Ground. *Anthropology Newsletter* 4: 1, 3.

Pelto, Gretel H., and Pertti J. Pelto. 1989. Small but Healthy? An Anthropological Perspective. *Human Organization* 48 (1): 11–15.

Pendergrast, David. 1993. *For God, Country and Coca-Cola: The Unauthorized*

History of the Great American Soft Drink and the Company that Makes It. New York: Scribner's.

Rappaport, Roy A. 1967. *Pigs for the Ancestors.* New Haven: Yale University Press.

Rose, Jerome C., Thomas J. Green, and Victoria D. Green. 1996. NAGPRA Is Forever: Osteology and the Repatriation of Skeletons. *Annual Review of Anthropology* 25:81–103.

Roseberry, William. 1988. Political Economy. *Annual Review of Anthropology* 17:161–85.

Roseberry, William. 1989. *Anthropologies and Histories.* New Brunswick: Rutgers University Press.

Saitta, Dean. 1988. Marxism, Prehistory and Primitive Communism. *Rethinking Marxism* 1:145–68.

Scheper-Hughes, Nancy. 1990. Three Propositions for a Critically Applied Medical Anthropology. *Social Science and Medicine* 30 (2): 189–97.

Scott, James C. 1985. *Weapons of the Weak: Everyday Forms of Resistance.* New Haven: Yale University Press.

Scott, James C. 1990. *Domination and the Arts of Resistance: Hidden Transcripts.* New Haven: Yale University Press.

Seckler, David. 1980. "Malnutrition": An Intellectual Odyssey. *Western Journal of Agricultural Economics* 5 (2): 219–27 (December).

Singer, M. 1989a. The Limitations of Medical Ecology: The Concept of Adaptation in the Context of Social Stratification and Social Transformation. *Medical Anthropology* 10:218–29.

Singer, Merrill. 1989b. The Coming of Age of Critical Medical Anthropology. *Social Science and Medicine* 28:1193–1204.

Singer, M. 1992. The Application of Theory in Medical Anthropology. *Medical Anthropology* 14 (1) (special issue).

Singer, M. 1993. A Rejoinder to Wiley's Critique of Critical Medical Anthropology. *Medical Anthropology Quarterly* 7 (2): 185–91.

Singer, M. 1995. Beyond the Ivory Tower: Critical Praxis in Medical Anthropology. *Medical Anthropology Quarterly* 9 (1): 80–106.

Singer, M. 1996. Farewell to Adaptationism: Unnatural Selection and the Politics of Biology. *Medical Anthropology Quarterly* 10 (4): 496–515.

Singer, M., and H. Baer. 1995. *Critical Medical Anthropology.* Amityville, NY: Baywood.

Smedley, Audrey. 1993. *Race in North America: Origins and Evolution of a Worldview.* Boulder, CO: Westview Press.

Thomas, R. Brooke. 1997. Wandering toward the Edge of Adaptability: Adjustments of Andean People to Change. In *Human Adaptability Past, Present, and Future,* ed. R. S. J. Ulijaszek and R. Huss-Ashmore, 183–232. New York: Oxford University Press.

Thomas, R. Brooke, T. B. Gage, and M. A. Little. 1979. Reflections on Adaptive and Ecological Models. In *Human Population Biology: A Transdisciplinary Perspective,* ed. M. Little and J. Haas, 296–319. Oxford: Oxford University Press.

Thomas, R. B., T. Leatherman, J. Carey, and J. D. Haas. 1988. Biosocial Consequences of Illness Among Small Scale Farmers: A Research Design. In *Capacity for Work in the Tropics,* ed. K. J. Collins and D. E. Roberts, 249–76. New York: Cambridge University Press.

Thomas, R. Brooke, B. Winterhalder, and S. D. McRae. 1979. An Anthropological Approach to Human Ecology and Adaptive Dynamics. *Yearbook of Phys. Anthropol.* 22:1–46.

Van Gerven, Dennis P., Mary K. Sandford, and James R. Hummert. 1981. Mortality and Culture Change in Nubia's Batn el Hajar. *J. Hum. Evol.* 10:395–408.

Van Gerven, Dennis P., Susan G. Sheridan, and William Y. Adams. 1995. The Health and Nutrition of a Medieval Nubian Population. *American Anthropologist* 97:468–80.

Wallerstein, Immanuel. 1976. *The Modern World System: Capitalism, Agriculture and the Origin of the European World Economy in the Sixteenth Century.* New York: Academic Press.

Wallerstein, Immanuel. 1977. Rural Economy in Modern World-Society. *Studies in Comparative International Development* 12 (1): 29–40.

Weiner, Annette B. 1995. Culture and Our Discontents. *American Anthropologist* 97:14–21.

Wiley, Andrea. 1992. Adaptation and the Biocultural Paradigm in Medical Anthropology: A Critical Review. *Medical Anthropology Quarterly* 6:216–36.

Williams, Eric. 1966. *Capitalism and Slavery.* New York: Capricorn Books.

Wolf, Eric. 1981. The Mills of Inequality. In *Social Inequality: Comparative and Developmental Perspectives,* ed. G. Berreman, 41–58. New York: Academic Press.

Wolf, Eric. 1982. *Europe and the People Without History.* Berkeley: University of California Press.

Chapter 2

The Evolution of Human Adaptability Paradigms: Toward a Biology of Poverty

R. Brooke Thomas

As stated in the introductory chapter, the goal of this volume is to expand the scope of research in physical anthropology by explicitly incorporating political-economic analyses into the assessment of human biological well-being.

The goal is twofold. First is to explore a reformulation of the adaptation concept, which constitutes the theoretical core of biological anthropology. By broadening the scope of adaptive theory and adopting a perspective that more accurately acknowledges social and political realities, physical anthropologists can more comprehensively address a set of prevalent problems compromising the human condition. Such a perspective would provide valuable insights, for instance, into why so many people suffer the consequences of stress despite their best efforts to adapt to environmental conditions.

The second goal is to construct methodological linkages between human adaptability and political economy. This seems particularly feasible in examining problems related to the biology of poverty, where the two perspectives converge and offer much potential for a complementary approach. Here, human adaptability research has developed considerable expertise in describing the dynamics between environmental constraints and human biological responses associated with impoverishment. Such a perspective is of obvious necessity in a world where environments change rapidly and can have significant impacts on human health and behavior. Similarly, political economy has shown how social relations construct both environmental exposure and response opportunities, leaving the poor at a distinct disadvantage in their adaptive repertoire.

The issues at stake are considerably broader than the academic construction of theory and method. In a world where most anthropologists are dismayed at the worsening conditions among large segments of humanity, a discipline which entertains pluralistic approaches, considers the range of human diversity, and accepts as valid non-Western systems of knowledge is desperately needed to address the complex issues that will arise in the next century.

Thus, a complementary political-economy/human adaptability perspective that acknowledges the dialectic between adjustment and exploitation would seem to offer much in addressing a reality where hope and human action are entangled with oppression and marginality. The need to understand this dialectic seems to have intensified in recent decades as political-economic relationships constrain adaptive capacity, and people attempt to circumvent or counter the social conditions that cause them.

It would seem, then, that the potential of this endeavor lies in "enriching our understanding of interregional and global processes" (Goodman and Leatherman, this vol., chap. 1) in a manner that not only interprets but provides a more comprehensive means of addressing relevant problems of the next century. In order to be effective such a complementary approach would need to cover the following.

1. The historical conditions and political-economic processes that structure local social relations, environmental use, and human health.
2. Local environmental conditions that provide opportunity and constraint to human action and health. Here, the multiple environmental and social stressors that challenge the health of the poor deserve detailed examination.
3. Biological, social, cultural, and psychological adjustments to the array of local conditions need to be identified and assessed for their effectiveness.
4. Both short- and long-term consequences of people's attempt to adjust—however successful or unsuccessful—on household relations, social interactions, and environments should be especially considered.
5. Having assessed the broad processes that contribute to the formation of local conditions, how people respond to these conditions, and how the consequences of such responses feed back on the conditions of life, the aim is to generate solutions that can prevent or break the cycle of poverty.

In addressing these points, this chapter will briefly review the broad processes of the last half century that have contributed to the impoverishment of peoples. These have set the agenda for problems anthropologists will have to confront in the foreseeable future. I will then summarize the analytical strengths and weaknesses of human adaptability and political-economic perspectives in an effort to find methodological complementarity. Next, a set of models used in human adaptability are developed which lead to the inclusion of a political-economic perspective. Finally, the dialectical nature of the two perspectives as they are intertwined in the impoverishment process is explored. Here, focus is upon the extraction of surplus, adaptive disintegration, and the accumulation of biocultural contradictions which promote action and change.

The Fifty Years Before and After 2000 A.D.

The waning years of the twentieth century have prompted many to reflect on the consequences that this period of unprecedented change has had on the human condition (Boyden 1987, 1991). One is particularly drawn to the pervasive social, economic, and environmental transformations of the last half century which have drastically altered lives throughout the world. Since the sequence of what has happened during these fifty years has often been told, a brief review will suffice in order to place concerns for the next fifty years in context (Gaul and Thomas 1991, 74–75).

As independent nations budded off from colonial empires at the end of World War II, the promise was held out that they might also share in "profits" from an international commoditization of environment and labor. Guided by policies of economic progress, plans to make the Third World "developed or modernized" commenced. But this was more than a set of policies that bound nations of the world together and remote populations to their national economies and capitals. Instead, over the course of the last four decades a system of knowledge based on Western scientific management, economic evaluation, and individualized consumerism has permeated most societies. As such it has become a dominant system of categorizing, prioritizing, and creating rules that govern relationships between insiders and outsiders, elites and workers, urban and rural, families and community, humans and nature (Marglin 1990).

In essence, policies of modernization have created a cosmology that has actively stifled other systems of knowledge, labeling them as irrational, backward, and irrelevant. In doing so, a reality has been constructed which has facilitated the marginalization of a large part of the world's people and pauperized one-sixth of humanity (Brown 1988). The relevance that these remarks hold for the human biological condition and the need to synthesize human adaptability with political economy are clarified later.

Increasingly, natural resources, agricultural produce, and human labor were transformed into commodities as local economies of self-production were reorganized to encourage market participation and consumerism. And as capitalist ideology permeated the villages and hamlets of most nations, groups were expected to shed "traditional" values and acquire "modern" ones. In an effort to create new revenues in order to fulfill the promises of economic progress—or to pay off debt—third world countries have placed much of their best agricultural lands into the production of export-oriented crops. This, generally, has reduced their potential to feed themselves, especially the poor. Displaced rural peoples who once supported themselves from these lands have migrated to urban slums or been pushed onto marginal lands where their impact continues to cause desertification, soil erosion, and general impoverishment.

Communities that once emphasized reciprocity and redistribution of wealth now hire one another. And when wage labor is not available locally, men leave their families in search of work, placing an added burden on women and the elderly left behind. Meanwhile industrial wastes from the First and the former Second World have tainted the air and water quality within their boundaries and beyond, and are compromising both human health and ecological well-being from by-products of overconsumption. There is every indication that the Third World will replicate this pattern in the next century as the new global economy expands the scope of consumption and commodification. Again, the poor are most exposed to the adverse consequences of these trends.

Thus, in a matter of half a century we have undoubtedly witnessed one of the most rapid and massive transformations in human history. Building on the inertia of an exploitative past, advances in extractive technologies and transportation have become capable of turning useful flora, fauna, and minerals into commodities almost anywhere on earth, when they exist in sufficient concentrations. At immediate risk are the last great tropical forests, the productivity of heretofore rich coastal fisheries, the numerous endangered species, and the knowledge systems built upon for millennia by cultural groups who are being assimilated into "Western" values and modernity.

As the century ends, the adverse consequences of this transformation on so many people and habitats have become common knowledge. Even many political scientists and economists who advanced modernization and development are showing less confidence in their theories (Gudeman 1992). Yet, trends set in motion are not easily halted, and many consequences of a global economy will undoubtedly intensify well into the first half of the twenty-first century. As anthropologists, many of us have witnessed the disruption of groups we studied in the past to the extent that our ethnographic conclusions are unrecognizable today. In short, we have seen our anthropological world turned upside down and with it the problems we address and the methods and theory we employ to help understand these changes.

Whereas adaptation theory has been helpful in explaining how groups adjusted to local and relatively stable conditions, such conditions have increasingly become the exception. In fact, the state of adaptiveness as well as adaptability (flexibility in adjusting) of many groups can be seriously questioned as peoples have become severed from their lands, communities, knowledge systems, languages, and customs. By the late 1970s human adaptation and human ecological theory fell under increased criticism as being too narrowly constructed to sufficiently explain the pervasive realities of change, where much was initiated from outside the immediate environment by forces poorly understood by local residents.

Conversely, political economy offers powerful insights into how capitalist penetration fosters social inequalities and fuels the marginalization process. Thus, in anthropology and other social sciences it became the dominant materialist theory of the 1980s. In forming the foundation of critical and feminist theory, and linked to poststructural interpretation, it has provided a rich perspective from which to comprehend both the material conditions and ideological constructs of exploitative social relationships.

The main point is that a reformulation of human adaptability and human ecology concepts could considerably complement the scope of political-economic inquiry. The necessity of emphasizing a better understanding of the full range of human biobehavioral adjustment (including agency), within the context of environmental dynamics and resource availability, stems from the following broad trends which will surely impact and create the poor in the next fifty years.

1. As environmental degradation spreads and intensifies, this will increasingly deny substantial segments of local populations access

     to basic needs, forcing them to further abuse their homelands and/or to migrate from them.

2. Population growth and the concentration of migrants in urban slums, refugee camps, and sites of migrant labor, coupled with inequities in access to and distribution of resources, will exacerbate these conditions. Human health and security will be put at greater risk, and social, cultural, and psychological measures of well-being will decline in a growing number of groups.

3. Expansion of world capitalism into local economies will further erode the capacity of self-production and exaggerate present inequities between rich and poor, north and south.

4. As noted in the first chapter, individuals will find ways to circumvent or change social systems when they are unable to make ends meet.

It is out of these trends that a new set of anthropological problems will be forged. Our ability to accurately understand the social, biological, and environmental dimensions of these complex problems—that is, to encompass this new reality—and to offer solutions based on this comprehensive understanding will test our anthropological abilities and imagination.

Human Adaptability Evolving

The timing of this volume is underscored and necessitated by the success of a paradigmatic shift in the study of human adaptability that began in physical anthropology over forty years ago (Coon, Garn, and Birdsell 1950). In 1964 at the symposium on "The Biology of Human Populations of Anthropological Importance," the research agenda of the human adaptability perspective coalesced. The symposium was organized jointly by the Wenner-Gren Foundation and the International Biological Programme. It brought together a group of physical anthropologists, anatomists, geneticists, pediatricians, physicians, and physiologists who had begun to study the biology of contemporary human populations from an adaptive perspective.

     Similar to that of the conference upon which this book is based, their goal was to report on a set of preliminary studies which showed the possibilities of the new paradigm and to identify a set of promising research paths. *The Biology of Human Adaptability* (Baker and Weiner 1966), which resulted from the symposium proceedings, was indeed an exciting text for young graduate students like myself. In providing an initial synthesis of ideas, it begged for further inquiry into how adaptive processes operated in human groups exposed to a diversity of environmental conditions around the world.

Heretofore, the study of living populations had largely emphasized description and classification based on shared morphological characteristics. As the synthetic theory of organic evolution became widely accepted throughout the biological sciences in the 1950s and early 1960s, the concept of adaptation provided a powerful means for understanding human biological diversity and change. Like other theories of change, adaptation simplified the real world through a set of assumptions in order to make it analytically tractable. Thus, in its formulation the adaptive process juxtaposed the environment and organism as independent and dependent variables, identified challenges from the environment, and reduced the organism to a set of discrete traits responsive to these challenges. It then sought adaptive functions for these traits by linking beneficial function to reproductive fitness, thereby explaining genetic change within populations.

In their critique of adaptation theory, Levins and Lewontin (1985, 71–76) maintain that many of these reductionistic assumptions have remained unchallenged in evolutionary biological research. Consequently, they limit our understanding as to how traits interact with the organism, and how organisms interact with and affect their environment. If correct, such criticisms would particularly constrain the interpretation of human adaptation, since biological and behavioral traits are seen as interacting in complex ways, and human groups are continuously altering their environments. The degree to which human adaptability models have addressed and brought understanding to these issues, therefore, serves as an assessment of their utility.

In essence, the adaptive perspective laid out a process whereby demographic, morphological, physiological, and genetic differences between populations could be investigated as possible beneficial adjustments to past and/or present environmental conditions. Similarly, behavioral and cultural characteristics could be examined as adaptive responses facilitating the formation of a biocultural approach and its extension to human ecology. The study of human adaptation, therefore, has become largely and appropriately an anthropological endeavor that has attempted to understand why our species is so adept at adjusting to change. This question is one of obvious relevance, not only for unraveling our evolutionary past and factors leading to present human diversity, but in trying to comprehend the limits of our biological capacity to adapt to rapid change.

The answers to such a question have not been derived from narrow inquiry within a single area of biology. If adaptation is broadly concerned with identifying adjustments aiding in biological function, then assessment must include an integration of responses that facilitate a population's health, nutritional status, behavioral functional capacity, and reproductive performance (Baker 1984, 2). Nor has inquiry remained isolated within biology. To ignore the rich diversity of behavioral responses to constraints, and the consequences these have in both a positive and negative sense for human biology, is to ignore the dynamics of human adaptability. Human behavior is strongly molded by culture and subject to socioeconomic and political constraints as well as ecological conditions. Therefore, although behavior serves as our primary means of adapting, it is guided by cultural and social agendas which do not always support biological well-being. Together these points emphasize the complexity in trying to comprehend processes of human adaptability, and the necessity of multiple approaches to the problem (see Thomas 1997; Huss-Ashmore and Thomas 1997).

Undoubtedly the major conclusion to come out of research in human biological adaptability has been that humans respond to environmental problems primarily through phenotypic acclimatization (morphological responses, and/or physiological responses made in the course of one's lifetime) rather than by genetic adaptation. This is not to suggest that genetic adaptation has been unimportant in human evolution, but rather that it has generally selected for individuals who have been able to adjust to environmental constraints without recourse to directed genetic change. As Slobodkin (1968, 204) states: "In well adapted organisms there is a strong correlation between the probability of environmental events occurring and the probability of responding to these events without any genetic change. That is, gene frequency changes are a type of last resort in the process of adjusting to environmental change." Indeed it would seem that the human species, which has evolved during a period of unprecedented change, and which is continuously reordering its natural and social environments, has become a specialist in adjusting to rapidly changing conditions. Thus, when referring to the adaptive process of contemporary groups the term *human adaptability* rather than *human adaptation* is preferentially used denoting this phenotypic flexibility.

A similar conclusion regarding human genetic adaptation—as a type of last resort response—might be extended to the comparison between behavioral and biological adjustments. We have tended to find the clearest examples of phenotypic acclimatization in individuals living under extremely harsh conditions. These are conditions such as high altitude, cold, or heat, where behavioral or technological solutions offer inadequate protection. Under such conditions, developmental acclimatizations are frequently observed. They are laid down in the early years of life and confer an increased capacity to resist stress throughout the life cycle. Yet, even in these cases, social, economic, and political conditions have been seen to exert even greater pressures on human biology (see Leatherman, this vol., chap. 10).

Thus, in a species which emphasizes techno-behavioral responses to problems, biological adjustments may serve principally as backup responses. Stated differently, whereas genetic adaptation may be the response of last resort at the population level, phenotypic acclimatization may serve similarly for individuals. This generalization has an important bearing on the interpretation of the biology of poverty since a high emphasis on biological adaptation may suggest that other means of adjustment have already become eroded. Where the threshold lies between effective acclimatization and growing dysfunction is most important to understand. Clearly the biological well-being of many groups defined as poor has slipped beneath an adaptive level. This indicates that despite a considerable capacity for phenotypic plasticity, conditions have exceeded even their biological capacity to effectively respond.

Tracing developments which have contributed to the human adaptability paradigm illustrates the scope of inquiry into how different biological adjustment processes operate. Livingston's (1958) early work on the adaptiveness of sickle cell anemia to malaria amply demonstrated the utility of a combined evolutionary and human ecological approach, one which accounted for biological and cultural change in both historical and contemporary contexts. While we might have been misguided into so readily accepting this genetic mode of adaptation as typical of human populations, it set the agenda for much of the human adaptation research to come.

Over three decades later Smith (1993, 44–46) reviewed research accomplishments in human genetic adaptation and builds on this critical point. "Malaria stands out as a beacon and a siren. We navigate by it, yet it drags us on the rocks. There is no question that malaria is the agent responsible for the most profound and fascinating occurrences of selection and adaptation in man. And yet we are tired of it . . . nothing else has been able to measure up. I think we can safely say that malaria is not a good model for explaining other polymorphisms. If there are other agents exerting this kind of influence they would now surely be found." He concludes in noting: "At present, if we are asked what constitutes the evidence that genetic variation within mankind is adaptive, we have to answer cautiously . . . from this survey of research into human genetic variation the evidence of selection's scrutiny is to be found more in what we have in common than in our differences."

Interest in human morphological and physiological differences broadened into a study of their adaptability to environmental conditions. At the same time that anthropologists were concentrating on climatic adaptation through body morphology and composition, environmental physiologists were investigating acclimatization among native peoples residing in harsh climates (Little 1983). Such work led naturally to the mechanisms of adaptability, placing emphasis on phenotypic adjustments (both short-term and developmental acclimatization) that would obviate the need for genetic adaptation.

The initial focus on the adaptation of native peoples to climatic stress was expanded to include aspects of the biotic environment such as undernutrition and disease. This opened up the possibility of studying a wide range of human populations constrained by food intake and compromised by not being able to maintain adequate biological function (e.g., dysfunction, disease, death). Primary attention was placed on the identification of factors disrupting the growth processes of children, and how developmental adaptations laid down during childhood increased plasticity and hence buffered these consequences throughout life (Lasker 1969; Baker 1991; Frisancho 1993; Harrison and Brush 1991).

Obviously, socioeconomic status (SES) was seen as an important correlate of food intake and nutritional status; however the majority of the investigations in human biology have not probed much beyond this rather amorphous indicator of social relations (Carey 1990). Effects of the social environment on human biology have been primarily approached through concepts of psychosocial stress: a broad class of actions, real or imagined, which are perceived as threatening. Such threats activate endocrinological substances which act throughout the body in initiation of alarm and resistance. Under conditions of real threat, the response is generally adaptive if both the threat and response are short-lived. However, chronic or repeated activation of the stress may lead to a variety of functional disorders including cardiovascular disease, ulcers, hypertension, and immune suppression (see Goodman et al. 1988).

Thus, nonspecific, persistent psychosocial factors, such as unpredictability, loss of control, and suppressed hostility appear to have a causal role in disease (Kagan and Levi 1974). Conversely, the study of social support systems that provide social, economic, and emotional assistance have been shown to buffer psychosocial stress and the consequences of illness. Work in this area has been undertaken by both cultural anthropologists (Dressler 1995; Jacobsen 1987) and biological anthropologists (Bindon et al. 1994; Brown 1981; Blakey 1994; Carey 1990; Flinn and England 1996; Hanna, James, and Martz 1986; Harrison 1993; James et al. 1987; Jenner, Reynolds, and Harrison 1980; McGarvey and Schendel 1986). Because this area of research binds social environment, biological consequence, and social response, the concepts of psychosocial stress and social support provide a comprehensive means of investigating the biology of poverty.

A final human adaptability perspective links phenotypic responses occurring at the individual level to household and population outcomes in morbidity and mortality (see Little 1983). The latter constitutes the ultimate consequence of failure to rally from stressful conditions, and infant mortality rates serve as an excellent comparative indicator of adaptiveness between groups (see Swedlund and Ball, this vol., chap. 8). Here, demographic research within physical anthropology has been able to track changes in marriage patterns, resource use, and socioeconomic practices as they influence vital statistics.

The Potential of Human Adaptability

In summarizing research trends in human adaptability that have provided important insights into the biology of poverty, four approaches emerge:

> Environmental physiology with its attention to: (a) both short-term and developmental acclimatization of individuals in their maintenance of homeostasis and homeorhesis, and (b) the characteristics of specific environmental conditions which produce these responses.

Growth and development studies which focus on factors such as undernutrition and disease, capable of disrupting normal maturation processes.

Psychosocial stress research which links biological function to: (a) an individual's perception of control over events, and (b) the ability of social support to counteract a sense of helplessness.

Demographic approaches that can evaluate the aggregate and long-term ability of population units to adjust to the conditions around them through measures of morbidity and mortality.

The central, juxtaposed variables that reappear in these four complementary approaches are *adaptive response* and *stress*. Stress, as a condition capable of leading to functional impairment and disease, draws attention to the biological costs of environmental stressors. In studying adaptation, we have been oriented to finding positive and functional responses to environmental constraints where stress is largely overcome (Boyden 1970). However, it is clear that under conditions such as persistent poverty, where multiple environmental stressors result in unresolved levels of stress, adaptive solutions may be minimal. The difference between the two variables is only one of focus. While adaptation concentrates on beneficial responses to conditions of the physical, biotic, and social environment, stress emphasizes the adaptive costs and limitations of the adaptative process (Goodman et al. 1988, 192). In essence, when conditions of marginality are increased the fine line between what might be called adaptive response and stress becomes increasingly blurred (Leatherman 1996).

Biological anthropologists appear to be in a position to contribute substantially to understanding the interrelated conditions of poverty if integrative concepts such as stress are viewed from a broadened human adaptive perspective. In attempting such an integration, Alan Goodman, Brooke Thomas, Alan Swedlund, and George Armelagos proposed the following framework for examining "Biocultural Perspectives on Stress in Prehistoric, Historical, and Contemporary Population Research" (Goodman et al. 1988, 192–95). This entails the linking of four components in the response continuum: causation, impact, response, and consequence (fig. 1).

Endeavoring to understand *causation* is first an effort to identify the relevant stressors imposing on human groups. At one level this may be seen as a rather simplistic effort of measuring environmental conditions. It involves, however, identifying the specific characteristics of the stressors

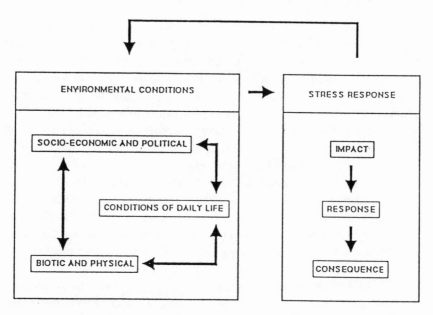

Fig. 1.   Model of the stress process, showing the cyclical nature of the relationship between environmental conditions and stress response. (Reproduced from Goodman et al. 1988, 192.)

such as their onset rate, frequency of occurrence, regularity and predictability, intensity, duration, and spatial and temporal distribution. Also, stressors tend to interact with one another, sometimes in unpredictable ways, and most stressors have perceived components necessitating analysis of the dialectical nature of individual–environmental interactions.

While it is easiest to focus on measurement of the proximate or immediate environment, what is of primary interest are the antecedent, sustaining conditions. Poverty, for example, is a multicomponent stressor which causes increased perception of vulnerability and increased exposure to "tangible" stressors such as undernutrition, infectious pathogens, toxic materials, and environmental extremes. These proximate conditions, in turn, are frequently downstream manifestations of sociopolitical and economic processes whose origins might be displaced in time and space. Thus, if human adaptability is to be viewed from a wide anthropological lens, making our findings relevant to colleagues in other subdisciplines, these connections need to be made explicit.

Impact relates to the disruption of homeostasis in some critical biological variable. This implies that a physiological strain (or stress) has been placed on the organism which, if sustained, is capable of disrupting biobehavioral functioning. Clearly an accurate definition of homeostatic normalcy is essential for the determination of impact, and we are cautioned against uncritically accepting Western standards to establish such norms in diverse populations. Given the array of possible impacts, selection of appropriate measures is dependent upon an understanding of intra- and interindividual variability for a given indicator as this relates to different levels of exposure. Elevated catecholamine levels, high blood pressure, low weight for height, infectious disease rates, and infant mortality constitute commonly used impact indicators. If our frequently reported findings of associations between environmental variables and impact indicators are to have biocultural significance, we will need to show how compromised biological functioning does, in fact, affect individual behavior and social interaction. For example, Leatherman (see this vol., chap. 10) shows how the frequency and severity of illness in Andean populations decreases household agricultural production and influences the ability of poorer families to remain in farming.

Response to impact assumes that the individual senses or perceives a deviation from normalcy and initiates actions to cope with the assault. Here, one is interested in assessing the success of the response as measured not only in the effectiveness of restoring homeostasis but the costs—that is, how efficiently limited resources (e.g., calories or calcium) are utilized, and what other functions are compromised. Effectiveness can be measured in terms of time it takes to engage the response, how long it can be sustained, its rate of action, and reliability. Reversibility is a measure of fixity of response once initiated, or alternatively how difficult it is to disengage. Such a measure becomes relevant in assessing the adaptive flexibility of a response since irreversible changes may compromise the ability of the individual to adjust to environmental shifts where the response is inappropriate. Many developmental acclimatizations fall into this category where morphological structures, once laid down in early years, are relatively unalterable. What becomes apparent in assessing the adaptive repertoire of impoverished peoples is that the costs of adjusting are high and flexibility is decreased. As mentioned with regard to causation, a biocultural orientation seeks to determine how responses of the poor are constructed and constrained by social relations.

Consequence refers to the effects of both impacts and responses on the biobehavioral functioning of individuals within populations. Relevant areas of functional assessment include physical performance, nervous system functioning, physical growth and behavioral development, disease resistance, and reproductive performance. These have been referred to as "adaptive domains" (Mazess 1975) or "areas of functional competence" (NAS 1977). As Mazess notes, the interpretation of benefits in any single domain can be temporally, spatially, and population specific depending on patterns of historical exposure to stressors, including length of exposure as well as the order and combination of stressors encountered. Rather than being a list of independent adaptive domains against which to evaluate the relative benefits of responses, it is the interactive effects of these domains on one another which is of primary concern. Thus, we are ultimately interested in functional interrelationships such as how lowered immunological competence influences growth and development, and in turn affects adult working capacity and/or fertility (see Haas 1983 and Allen 1984 for reviews of functional indicators of nutritional status).

Finally, assessment of consequences should not end with a review of the preceding areas of functional competence, for they provide few insights into how life-style is actually affected. In order to become accessible to anthropological interpretation we will need to know how impairment or improvement influences productive behavior at the individual, household, and population levels. What, for example, are the consequences of growth faltering during childhood, respiratory disease, or lowered working capacity on a household's ability to attain basic needs? And at what point does impairment within a number of households compromise productive capacity and health status of the entire community?

Unfortunately, most biological anthropologists stop short of providing answers to these more socioeconomic-oriented questions. By so doing, we leave our data in a form that is inaccessible or uninteresting to most social anthropologists and deny ourselves a glimpse of the real consequences of biological dysfunction. Finally, causation and consequence do not constitute two discrete ends of an elaborate linear progression. Instead, they form a continuum whereby consequences feed back on causation, helping to shape its subsequent characteristics. This is clearly the case in situations of progressive poverty where problems of nutrition and health become intensified with each cycle and further compromise adaptive potential.

In concluding this review of human adaptability, the following points characterize the perspective.

1. In the course of human evolution, individuals who have been able to adjust to environmental constraints without genetic solutions have been increasingly selected for. Thus, humans have emphasized phenotypic plasticity over genetic adaptation in biologically adjusting to rapidly changing conditions. This, of course, means that the conditions under which individuals live can have a profound effect in molding their biology, both in beneficial and dysfunctional ways.

2. Developmental acclimatization and dysfunction, laid down in the early years of life when stress is most intense, are extremely important in understanding human adaptive capacity and flexibility in later years.

3. Biological adaptations are difficult to understand without a knowledge of cultural (i.e., material, behavioral, social, and mental) solutions which can both complement and interfere with their effectiveness. Likewise, it is difficult to determine what is an appropriate biocultural response without a detailed knowledge of the conditions that cause it, and the consequences of the response on several levels of biobehavioral functioning. All responses have their costs, and appropriate responses of one group do not necessarily serve others (e.g., class divisions).

4. While adaptation is frequently researched in a reductionist mode as specific cause-and-effect responses between the environment and the adaptive unit (e.g., individual, household, community), in reality it is an ongoing and rarely linear process of response to multiple problems and opportunities. Thus, optimal or ideal solutions are not likely to be present for this and historical reasons.

5. The rapid changes that have occurred in the last half century have fueled the process of worldwide impoverishment. This means that a large segment of humanity will continue to live under conditions of multiple stress with inadequate techno-behavioral means to buffer these constraints. As a consequence, they will increasingly engage their biological responses to compensate, and these may be insufficient in the long run. Clearly, it seems from morbidity and mortality data that even the limits of biological plasticity have been exceeded in many groups. This calls for an approach that can look beyond the limits of human adaptability into the broader causes of impoverished conditions.

Adaptive Models and Political Economy

Since the study of human adaptability draws on a broad information base from human biology, social science, and environmental science, and emphasizes the interconnectivity between multiple variables operating in complex systems, the reduction of complexity to a consideration of critical variables has made problems analytically tractable. Models serve as an entry point in this endeavor since they represent aspects of reality deemed important to particular objectives. As Levins (1968) has noted, they provide degrees of generality, realism, and precision appropriate to their purpose and ignore irrelevant features. Models are, therefore, based on a series of assumptions concerning what are important components of the system and how these relate to one another.

Having contributed so much to the formulation of adaptive concepts in biology, Levins and Lewontin in *The Dialectical Biologist* (1985, 267–68) lay bare the underlying assumptions of the approach and its base in Cartesian reductionism. Separating "internal and external, cause and effect, subject and object, independent and dependent variable, variable and constant, part and whole limits our construction of reality." Such analysis facilitates the conclusion that these interactions constitute separate systems with autonomous properties, and that "parts exist in isolation and come together to make wholes." In essence, their critique is that the analysis of adaptation is a "mechanistic, reductionistic, positivist ideology which pervades our academic development and intellectual development."

As will be apparent, much of this critique applies to the adaptive models reviewed later. However, rather than narrowing inquiry, the models have built on one another, expanding our appreciation for the scope, complexity, and dialectics of adaptive processes. Ultimately, they have taken us to the very limits of the adaptive framework's ability to explain reality and urged us to adopt a political-economic framework in order to probe further (Thomas 1997). The three adaptive models that follow illustrate a conceptual progression which has led us to recognize the need for a political-economic perspective in studying the biology of poverty.

The first and earliest model (fig. 2) is derived from work in environmental physiology with a behavioral component added. This is the simple cause-and-effect design referred to before. It analyzes how environmental stressors and the potential physiological strain on homeostasis are buffered by complementary biological and behavioral responses. Here the purpose is to review multiple stressors in the local environment, select out those capable of having the most serious biological impact, evaluate their exposure pattern and the subgroups at greatest risk, and determine the relative effectiveness of biobehavioral responses. As mentioned, behavioral and technological adjustments are assumed to form the first line of response. When these are inadequate, biological adjustments serve as backup responses. Poverty, clearly, erodes the capacity of the former and with time challenges even biological adaptability.

The second model (fig. 3) builds on the first and addresses human ecological relations surrounding the acquisition of basic needs. It assumes that of the many resources needed by groups, some become scarce, and there are no other alternatives. While the shortage of food poses a direct stressor, the lack of other resources such as adequate clothing or shelter interferes with responses to existing stressors. Similar to the first model, the objective of the analysis is to identify a series of essential resources, determine factors affecting their production and access, and identify those biological, social, and demographic strategies that allow for sufficient acquisition of basic needs. Whereas density dependent models from population biology suggest that growing population pressure limits access to resources, insufficient access to basic needs arising from social inequalities has a similar effect.

The third model (fig. 4) addresses the impact of psychosocial stress on biological function and the biobehavioral responses to other stressors. As has been noted, when conditions critical to sustaining an individual (i.e., housing, employment, physical harm) are perceived as excessive, increasingly unpredictable, and threatening to one's sense of control, psychosocial stress results. When such stress persists for prolonged periods it can lead to impairment of biological responses, such as immunological suppression. Similarly, it can erode the confidence in one's behavioral responses and diminish exploratory behavior. Among the poor, extraction of surplus eats into a household's ability to get by, and contradictions concerning access to basic needs come to affect most decisions. Also, responses may take on a higher cost, become less certain, and may be accompanied by suppressed hostility.

A final model (fig. 5) builds on but looks beyond relationships of human adaptation and inquires into broader political-economic structures that create and perpetuate significant stressors. Specifically it focuses on the formation of social inequalities based on class, gender, and race, and

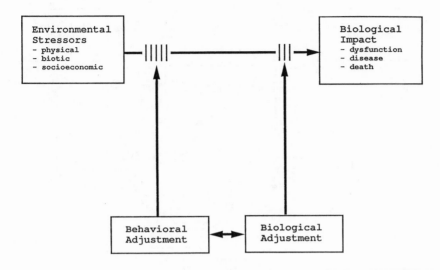

Fig. 2.   A biobehavioral model of adjustment to environmental stress

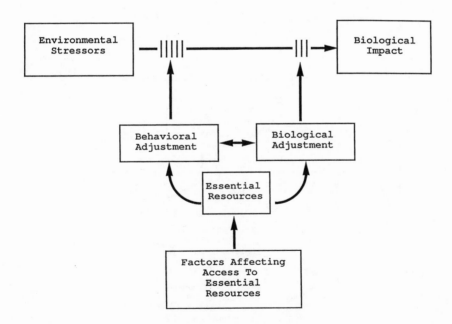

Fig. 3.   A limiting resource model of adjustment to
environmental stress

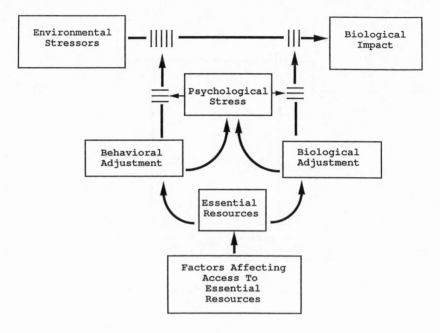

Fig. 4.   A psychological stress model

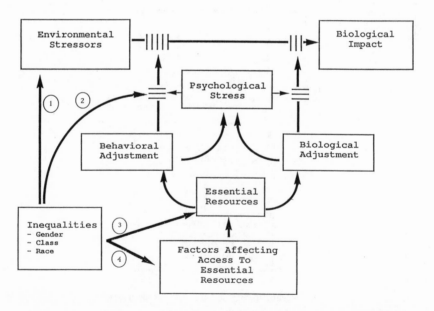

Fig. 5.   A political-economy model added to a human adaptation model. The numbers represent processes by which inequalities might affect adaptation.

how these conditions influence both the intensity of stress and the inability to respond. Discrimination in opportunity and exposure to more difficult working and living conditions multiply both the range of stressors one is exposed to as well as their strength.

Thus, in the high altitude region of the Andes where I have worked, the poor work harder under hypoxic conditions and are more exposed to cold because of work patterns and inadequacies of clothing and shelter. In addition, they take greater risks and live in areas where sanitary conditions pose more health problems (Carey 1990; Carey and Thomas 1987; Luerssen 1994; Leatherman 1996 and this vol., chap. 10). They have less access to fuel, fertilizer, labor, money, and other essential needs. Furthermore, although not studied, the range of degrading contradictions and exploitative interactions faced in daily life suggests psychosocial stress would be an important factor as well. This is especially true among the poorest (female-headed, indigenous households), where social support is frequently absent.

It is, therefore, not surprising that the Andean poor are more poorly nourished, are more retarded in their growth, perceive themselves as sicker, and have higher rates of morbidity and mortality (see Carey 1990; Leatherman et al. 1986; Leonard et al. 1990; Leonard and Thomas 1988). Were just an adaptive perspective to be applied to these indicators of impairment, the story would end with evidence that the biobehavioral responses were not very effective for this group, hence they are at high risk. Such a conclusion is hardly very revealing. Other than telling us where the holes in the adaptive system may be, such characteristics are generally shared among the poor wherever they live.

By adding a political-economic perspective to the analysis, the scope of the inquiry opens to a broader set of questions about the conditions and processes that structure much of the adaptive agenda. For example, how these conditions of biological functional impairment feed back on the initial stressors—intensifying them and further eroding social responses—is explained by Leatherman (1992, 1996) through a sequence of adaptive disintegration associated with chronic illness.

Likewise the perspective prompts us to ask, why should a population which has had such long-term exposure to high Andean conditions, and which in the past has developed such successful adaptations to this environment, express such marginal responses today? Where does all the surplus go? Why have conditions not substantially improved since the introduction of agrarian reform and the "modernization package" of the 1970s? Why is most of the meat, which is produced in abundance locally, sold outside the area, and why does imported rice sell for less than local potatoes in the local market? Why does the health clinic not adequately service the illnesses most frequently reported? Finally, and probably most importantly, why has terrorism spread across this region where the adaptive fabric has worn so thin?

Whereas most biological anthropologists acknowledge the relevancy of such questions, they would defer to social scientists for both the analysis and answers. Yet each question has a direct bearing on the conditions that affect the biological well-being of poorer individuals in the region. By asking these biocultural questions and becoming engaged in the analysis, one is led to a better understanding of how market penetration has altered socioeconomic conditions. Thus, as locally produced basic needs become commercialized and sold outside the region, there arises an increased need to engage in wage labor in order to buy what was formerly available through redistribution. Wage labor, especially when individuals leave the region to seek work, interferes with the access to social support that is much needed to produce these basic needs and assist in illness. In the end, access to nutrition and health care is compromised, biological functional capacity is lowered, and one's capacity to participate in productive activities is affected.

These relationships are depicted in figure 6. Methodologically, the variables in the diagram are not difficult to measure and, therefore, not beyond the data collection abilities of biological anthropologists. More importantly, however, such information allows one to see more clearly the erosion of adaptive flexibility, and the political-economic processes that perpetuate unequal adaptive potential. When adaptive analyses are taken to this point, the information becomes both accessible and interesting to social anthropologists. They, in turn, can link the findings to more detailed analyses of social dynamics and ideology, thus binding biology, social relations, and systems of knowledge.

In summary, when findings from the first three models (figs. 2–4) are put together into a synthesis of adaptive responses, we begin to address the criticism of relying on reductionist approaches. And when a political-economic model (fig. 5) is then added to this body of information, a route is provided whereby biological anthropologists can push beyond their so-called alienating perspective into one of adaptive dialectics.

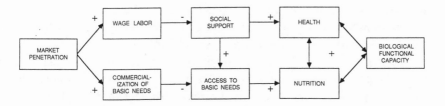

Fig. 6.   A schematic representation of a political economic approach to the relationships among health, nutrition, and biological/functional capacity in the Andes.

Methodological Complementarity

The epistemological and ideological differences that separate the adaptivist and political-economic perspectives have been reviewed by Levins and Lewontin (1985, 269–76) and are summarized later. In essence their position states that systems of knowledge are socially constructed and set the agenda for theoretical constructions. Theory, in turn, guides the selection of research problems, which tends to reinforce existing social relations and ways of thinking about them.

In this sense reductionism and dialectics are placed in opposition: one seeks explanations for existing balance in societal relations while the other stresses disharmony and transformation. Reductionism assumes that higher order phenomena can be understood by reducing complexity to a delimited set of independent causal pathways affecting internally homogeneous units. In the case of adaptation, the environment serves as the causal variable and is depicted as an external world over which one has relatively little control. It is then subdivided into the physical, biotic, and social environments. The latter categories seem to be particularly inadequate in construction since they reduce the rich variability of social relations that cause and assist human action into a set of social stressors.

Human adaptive units normally considered are the individual, household, and group or population; and the biological, behavioral, and technological adjustments of these units are compared as to their relative efficacy. As information accumulates on various adjustments to different constraints making up the local system, an overall adaptive pattern emerges. Thus, from analytical pieces acquired by posing a similarly formatted question about human-environment relationships, a whole is created. This was the intent of putting together the various adaptive models.

At question is how accurately and comprehensively the structure of the analysis represents actual relations and contemporary reality. What perspectives are precluded when taking this point of view? For instance, while the goal of adaptation is the study of responses to changing conditions, analysis most frequently emphasizes adjustment that maintains stability and continuity. Thus, the human adaptive approach has been criticized as having a passive orientation in that analysis focuses on responses to conditions rather than on their alteration. As Levins and Lewontin (1985, 275) maintain, stability and continuity "become positive virtues in society—and therefore objects of intellectual interest."

A dialectical perspective challenges the reality elicited from reductionistic approaches. Rather than assuming a correct division of the whole or primacy of certain relationships and homogeneous units of analysis, meaningful heterogeneity pervades every level of organization. Wholes do not exist in organizational harmony. Instead, they are composed of opposing processes held in balance, only temporarily. Under such conditions cause and effect, subject and object, and independent and dependent variables become interchangeable. Change results from a dynamic instability between internal and external tensions and internal heterogeneity. Thus, "systems destroy the conditions which brought them about and create possibilities for new transformations" (Levins and Lewontin 1985, 277).

In viewing human adaptability from a dialectical perspective new avenues of inquiry open up concerning contradiction, conflict, more active forms of adaptation, and adaptive transformation. Table 1 depicts major differences between a human ecology/adaptability and political-economic perspective, and suggests the promise of a complementary methodological approach.

Adaptive Dialectics

Just as reductionism and dialectics have been placed in opposition to one another as perspectives for analyzing reality, so have the processes of adaptation and exploitation in explaining material relationships. In the groups we study these are the oppositional forces which are in continuous contest: in a sense they become the dialectic of anthropological interpretation.

The adaptation perspective evaluates how well people respond to adverse conditions as well as their potential for recovery once their principal responses have been disrupted. People caught in systems of exploitation attempt to adapt within the constraints placed upon them. But they also try to find solutions that circumvent and challenge these systems, and sometimes they succeed. Because the adaptation perspective fails to inquire beyond the immediate conditions causing constraints, the processes influencing their perpetuation and exacerbation are ignored. Thus, a critical aspect of the dynamic is missing.

In contrast to focusing on processes of adjustment or self-organization, the political-economic paradigm takes a quite different approach. Historical precedence and external political-economic relationships are assumed to impact heavily, not only on the structure of local social relations but on how people use their resources and environment. Emphasis is placed on processes of social differentiation, as opposed to social cohesion, and on different capabilities of people to overcome constraints.

Throughout this paper the utility of expanding the scope of the human adaptability perspective by incorporating both concepts and methods of political economy has been proposed. The urgency of synthesizing these two materialist perspectives is underwritten by the types of problems we

TABLE 1. Major Differences between Human Ecological and Political-Economic Perspectives

	Human Ecological Perspective	Political-Economic Perspective
1. Units of Analysis	Human groups and critical aspects of the environment	Social class (Marxism) Core and periphery (World Systems)
2. Spatial Organization	Local and regional	Regional, national, international
3. Problems of Interest	Resource utilization practices, especially those of sustained control over the environment	Strategies and consequences of exploitation by more powerful groups
4. Prime Mover(s) of Change	Environmental (including social) conditions initiate human responses	Contradictions and differential power relationships between social groups
5. Process of Change	Adaptations or beneficial responses maintain biological and cultural well-being to changing environment; cooperative solutions emphasized	Exploitation of labor and resources by dominant groups in order to gain or maintain control over a human system, and responses to this exploitation; conflict, emphasized

are likely to face in the future, and the combined solutions that need to be forged in environmental quality, human health, and social justice. In this context, the biosocial dynamics surrounding growing impoverishment will undoubtedly be a central concern to anthropologists.

Since gaining an understanding of the biology of poverty will necessitate guidance from both perspectives, a series of recommendations is proposed that can lead biological anthropologists toward a more dialectical approach.

1. Human adaptability needs to establish a broader base of inquiry into the processes directly impacting the environmental constraints and adaptive units. This includes defining: (a) the historical context of political-economic processes that structure local conditions, (b) the local stressors and limited resources associated with meeting basic needs, (c) the array of biosocial responses to these conditions, and (d) the consequences of engaging these responses as they feed back and alter the system.

2. While the adaptive approach uncovers how people adjust to constraints, it is apparent that for many neither their actions nor biology can provide sufficient solutions in the long run. Thus, the poor enter into a process of "adaptive disintegration" where responses elicited in order to socially reproduce and biologically maintain themselves become progressively more risky, more costly, and more irreversible. This process is not well studied in its biosocial dimensions. Further work could define how biological and social compromise influence one another, and how inadequate responses exacerbate existing conditions.

3. Central to adaptive dialectics is the principle of contradictions. As the process of impoverishment intensifies, limited options surrounding social reproduction and biological maintenance pervade decision making. And ultimately these two factors are thrown into contradiction with one another. Thus, women worn down from having had too many children must decide whether to give birth once more, risking their own biology, with the hope that their offspring will provide needed household labor. Identifying these contradictions, and the thresholds beyond which people can no longer tolerate the conditions that cause them, will help us understand linkages between adaptive disintegration and agency.

4. Measuring socioeconomic status and its correlates with biological

well-being is but a first step in understanding how social differentiation molds the biology of the poor. In probing further into the social relations of production it is important to empirically analyze the patterns of surplus extraction. These include unpaid labor services, rent in kind (sharecropping), rent in cash, extraction of surplus value (low wages), and extraction via terms of trade, usury, and taxes (Deere and de Janvry 1979; Deere 1987). In attempting to measure the multiple paths whereby surplus flows from poor producers, the biological anthropologist is forced to confront the social dynamics lying behind socioeconomic categorization.

5. Because growing contradictions may be associated with psychosocial stress and its capacity to cause biological impairment, special attention should be given to the efficacy of social support systems in buffering these effects. This should be particularly relevant among the poor where social support is widely relied upon, yet concepts of individualism and conditions of wage labor often weaken its potential. Understanding the interaction between psychological stress and social support provides important insights into health by combining ethnomedical and biomedical perspectives. Likewise, it serves as a focal point for examining how social support may shift from facilitating adjustment to the system, to system reforming (better health care or wages) and system transformation (ideological confrontation and rebellion).

6. In collecting the sort of information suggested above, biological anthropologists will have to go beyond our traditional biological and environmental measures, beyond our structured questionnaires, and start talking with people about their concerns and aspirations. Here we must try, much better than we have, to understand the complex reality people construct around them, for this is where decisions affecting their biology and behavior will come from. Ultimately, we must come to understand how dominant systems of knowledge structure this construction of reality—but this is probably asking too much too soon.

In summary, the expanded scope of human adaptability, and particularly the biology of poverty, is one which attempts to understand the dynamics of how people adjust to the constraints around them using their biology and behavior, social organization, and ideology. While some of these constraints may be attributed to natural conditions, most are structured by social relations that deny access to resources and options, extract surplus, and generate contradictions in everyday life. Thus, the poor are left with greater exposure levels and a narrower range of adaptive solutions.

As processes of exploitation intensify, a slip into adaptive disintegration generates the morbidity and mortality statistics that we have come to associate with conditions of poverty. By themselves, these statistics are no longer particularly revealing except to track the spread and level of poverty. Likewise, we are fairly certain that we will find poverty and ill health associated with lower levels of education, employment, and ownership of productive assets.

Therefore, it seems the challenge for biological anthropologists is to move beyond this kind of reporting and beyond a narrow adaptive orientation which is primarily concerned with how people just barely get by— sometimes relying on their biological reserves. The expanded scope advocated here is one that understands the broader political-economic context in which adjustment is being attempted, that follows the process of adaptive disintegration into its biosocial consequences, and that inquires into avenues of adaptive reformulation whereby people are able to escape this downward slide and reorder the conditions around them. In conclusion, *adaptation should be a concept of hope!*

REFERENCES

Allen, L. H. 1984. Functional Indicators of Nutritional Status of the Whole Individual or the Community. *Clin. Nutr.* 3:169–75.

Baker, P. T. 1984. The Adaptive Limits of Human Populations. *Man* 19:1–14.

Baker, P. T. 1991. Human Adaptation Theory: Successes, Failures and Prospects. *J. Hum. Ecol.* 1:39–48 (special issue).

Baker, P. T., and J. S. Weiner, eds. 1966. *The Biology of Human Adaptability.* Oxford: Clarendon.

Bindon, J. R., A. L. Knight, W. W. Dressler, and D. E. Crews. 1994. Stress, Gender, and Household Employment Influences on Blood Pressure of Samoan Adults. *Amer. J. of Hum. Biol.* 6:116.

Blakey, M. L. 1994. Psychophysiological Stress Disorders of Industrial Society: A Critical Theoretical Formulation of Biocultural Research. In *Diagnosing America: Anthropology and Public Engagement,* ed. S. Forman, 149–92. Ann Arbor: University of Michigan Press.

Boyden, S. V. 1970. Cultural Adaptation to Biological Maladjustment. In *The Impact of Civilization on the Biology of Man,* ed. S. V. Boyden, 190–209. Canberra: Australian National University Press.

Boyden, S. V. 1987. *Western Civilization in Biological Perspective.* Oxford: Clarendon Press.

Boyden, S. V. 1991. Facing Up to Ecological Realities: A Biohistorical Perspective. *J. Hum. Ecol.* 1:89–96 (special issue).

Brown, D. E. 1981. General Stress in Anthropological Fieldwork. *Amer. Anthro.* 83:74–91.

Brown, L. R. 1988. *The Changing World Food Prospect: The Nineties and Beyond.* Worldwatch Paper 85, Washington, DC: Worldwatch Institute.

Carey, J. W. 1990. Social System Effects on Local Level Morbidity and Adaptation in the Rural Peruvian Andes. *Med. Anthro. Quart.* 4 (3): 266–95.

Carey, J. W., and R. B. Thomas. 1987. Social Influences on Morbidity and Mortality Patterns: A Case from Peru. *Am. J. Phys. Anthro.* 73:186–87.

Coon, C. S., S. M. Garn, and J. B. Birdsell. 1950. *Races.* Springfield, IL: C. C. Thomas.

Deere, C. D., and A. de Janvry. 1979. A Conceptual Framework for the Empirical Analysis of Peasants. *Amer. J. of Agricultural Economics* 61 (4): 601–11.

Deere, C. D. 1987. *The Peasantry in Political Economy: Trends in the 1980s.* Program in Latin American Studies Occasional Papers Series No. 19. University of Massachusetts, Amherst.

Dressler, W. W. 1995. Modeling Biocultural Interactions: Examples from Studies of Stress and Cardiovascular Disease. *Yearbook of Phys. Anthro.* 38:27–56.

Flinn, M., and B. England. 1996. Childhood Stress and Family Environment. *Current Anthropology* 36 (5): 854–66.

Frisancho, A. R. 1993. *Human Adaptation and Accommodation.* Ann Arbor: University of Michigan Press.

Gaul, K. K., and R. B. Thomas. 1991. Indigenous Perspectives: Ecology, Economy and Ethics. *J. Hum. Ecol.* 1:73–88 (special issue).

Goodman, A. H., R. B. Thomas, A. C. Swedlund, and G. A. Armelagos. 1988. Biocultural Perspectives on Stress in Prehistoric, Historical, and Contemporary Population Research. *Yearbook of Phys. Anthro.* 31:169–202.

Gudeman, S. 1992. Remodeling the House of Economics: Culture and Innovation. *Amer. Ethnol.* 19 (1): 141–54.

Haas, J. D. 1983. Nutrition and High Altitude Adaptation: An Example of Human Adaptability in a Multistress Environment. In *Rethinking Human Adaptation: Biological and Cutural Models,* ed. R. Dyson-Hudson and M. A. Little, 41–56. Boulder, CO: Westview Press.

Hanna, J. M., G. D. James, and J. M. Martz. 1986. Hormonal Measures of Stress. In *The Changing Samoans: Behavior and Health in Transition,* ed. P. T. Baker, J. M. Hanna, and T. S. Baker, 203–21. New York: Oxford University Press.

Harrison, G. A. 1993. Physiological Adaptation. In *Human Adaptation,* ed. G. A. Harrison. New York: Oxford University Press.

Harrison, G. A., and G. Brush. 1991. Environmental Quality as Expressed in Child Growth. *J. Hum. Ecol.* 1:49–54 (special issue).

Huss-Ashmore, R., and R. B. Thomas. 1997. The Future of Human Adaptability Research. In *Human Adaptability Past, Present, and Future,* ed. S. J. Ulijaszek and R. Huss-Ashmore, 295–319. New York: Oxford University Press.

Jacobson, D. 1987. The Cultural Context of Social Support and Support Networks. *Med. Anthro. Quart.* 1:42–67.

James, G. D., P. T. Baker, D. A. Jenner, and G. A. Harrison. 1987. Variation in Lifestyle Characteristics and Catecholamine Excretion Rates Among Young Western Samoan Men. *Soc. Sci. Med.* 25:981–86.

Jenner, D. A., V. Reynolds, and G. A. Harrison. 1980. Catecholamine Excretion Rates and Occupation. *Ergonomics* 23:237–46.

Kagan, A., and L. Levi. 1974. Health and Environment-Psychosocial Stimuli: A Review. *Soc. Sci. Med.* 13A:25–36.

Lasker, G. W. 1969. Human Biological Adaptability. *Science* 166:1480–86.

Leatherman, T. L. 1987. *Illness, Work and Social Relations in the Southern Peruvian Highlands.* Ph.D. diss., Anthropology, University of Massachusetts, Amherst.

Leatherman, T. L. 1992. Illness as Lifestyle Change. In *Health and Lifestyle Changes.* MASCA Research Papers in Science and Archeology, vol. 9, ed. R. Huss-Ashmore, J. Schall, and M. Hediger, 83–89. University Museum, University of Pennsylvania, Philadelphia.

Leatherman, T. L. 1996. A Biocultural Perspective on Health and Household Economy in Southern Peru. *Med. Anthro. Quart.* 10 (4): 476–95.

Leatherman, T. L., J. S. Luerssen, L. B. Markowitz, and R. B.Thomas. 1986. Illness and Political Economy: An Andean Dialectic. *Cultural Survival Quart.* 10:19–21.

Leonard, W. R., T. L. Leatherman, J. W. Carey, and R. B. Thomas. 1990. Contributions of Nutrition versus Hypoxia to Growth in Rural Andean Populations. *Amer. J. Hum. Biol.* 2 (4): 613–26.

Leonard, W. R., and R. B. Thomas. 1988. Changing Dietary Patterns in the Peruvian Andes. *Ecol. of Food and Nutr.* 21:245–63.

Levins, R. 1968. *Evolution in Changing Environments.* Princeton, NJ: Princeton University Press.

Levins, R., and R. Lewontin. 1985. *The Dialectical Biologist.* Cambridge, MA: Harvard University Press.

Little, M. A. 1983. An Overview of Adaptation. In *Rethinking Human Adaptation: Biological and Cultural Models,* ed. R. Dyson-Hudson and M. A. Little, 137–47. Boulder, CO: Westview Press.

Livingston, F. B. 1958. Anthropological Investigations of Sickle Cell Distribution in West Africa. *Amer. Anthro.* 60:533–62.

Luerssen, J. S. 1994. Landlessness, Health and the Failure of Reform in the Peruvian Highlands. *Human Organization* 53 (4): 380–87.

Marglin, S. 1990. Sustainable Development: A System of Knowledge Approach. *TOES: The Other Economic Summit/North America* 6:5–8.

Mazess, R. B. 1975. Biological Adaptation: Aptitudes and Acclimatization. In *Biosocial Interrelations in Population Adaptation,* ed. E. S. Watts, F. E. Johnson, and G. Lasker, 9–18. The Hague: Mouton.

McGarvey, S. T., and D. E. Schendel. 1986. Blood Pressure of Samoans. In *The Changing Samoans: Behavior and Health in Transition,* ed. P. T. Baker, J. M. Hanna, and T. S. Baker, 350–93. New York: Oxford University Press.

NAS. 1977. *World Food and Nutrition Survey.* Report to the U.S. Senate Select Committee on Nutrition and Human Needs. National Academy of Science, Washington, DC.

Singer, M. 1989. The Limitations of Medical Anthropology: The Concept of Adaptation in the Context of Social Stratification and Social Transformation. *Med. Anthro.* 10:223–34.

Singer, M. 1996. Farewell to Adaptationalism: Unnatural Selection and the Politics of Biology. *Med. Anthro. Quart.* 10 (4): 496–515.

Slobodkin, L. 1968. Toward a Predictive Theory of Evolution. In *Population Biology and Evolution,* ed. R. C. Lewontin, 185–205. Syracuse, NY: Syracuse University Press.

Smith, Malcolm. 1993. Genetic Adaptation. In *Human Adaptation,* ed. G. A. Harrison, 1–54. New York: Oxford University Press.

Swedlund, A. C. 1978. Historical Demography as Population Ecology. *Ann. Rev. Anthropol.* 7:137–73.

Thomas, R. B. 1997. Wandering toward the Edge of Adaptability: Adjustments of Andean Peoples to Change. In *Human Adaptability Past, Present, and Future,* ed. S. J. Ulijaszek and R. Huss-Ashmore, 183–232. New York: Oxford University Press.

Thomas, R. B., T. B. Gage, and M. A. Little. 1989. Reflections on Adaptive and Ecological Models. In *Human Population Biology: A Transdisciplinary Science,* 296–319. New York: Oxford University Press.

Wiley, A. S. 1992. Adaptation and the Biocultural Paradigm in Medical Anthropology: A Critical Review. *Med. Anthro. Quart.* 6 (3): 216–36.

Chapter 3

Political Economy and Social Fields

William Roseberry

This essay outlines an approach to anthropological political economy that is concerned with:

(a) the social relations and institutions through which control over fundamental resources is controlled and expressed;
(b) the relations and institutions through which social labor is mobilized and appropriated; and
(c) the location of these points of control within specific social fields.

This approach differs from world-systems theories in that it is, from one vantage, broader and, from another vantage, more specific. It is broader in that its concern for control of resources and labor is not limited to capitalism. It is more specific in that it rejects the attempts of world-systems theories to explain local processes and relations in terms of the dynamics and needs of global capitalism. Instead, it concentrates on the specifically local construction and shaping of power relations, including those that have their source outside of particular regions. A central concern, here, is how "external" forces are "internalized."

The concept of "social field" is central to this effort, and I begin by discussing an intersection between the anthropological literature on political economy with an older anthropological discussion of fields.

Basic Concepts

An Apparent Detour

In a recent review essay, Irene Silverblatt (1991) examines the literature on women and state formation. Criticizing Engels-inspired feminist literature that sought the "origins" of gender hierarchies in the formation of tributary states or the institution of private property (e.g., Leacock 1972, 1978; Sacks 1974, 1982; Gailey 1987), Silverblatt draws our attention to specific historical contexts, particularly processes of state formation and relations of gender. She claims further:

> New studies in "culture and political economy" question the implications of evolutionary laws and functionalist explanations, along with the utility of global typologies of humankind. Not only is the validity of categories like "state" and "status" up for review, not only do we question "origins" frameworks that have subtly, or not so subtly, shaped anthropological investigations into gender, but we are querying the nature, limitations, and possibilities of theorizing itself, of understanding and explaining social process. . . .
>
> As we place historical explanation in historical process, we can better perceive analytical problems tied to origin quests. As many contemporary debunkers have pointed out, origin-oriented research ends up distorting historical process by envisioning history as the unfolding of prepackaged essences. The equation of change with the "origin's" unfolding takes for granted a kind of global homogenization of historical experience. Whatever is essentialized (in our case, the "subordination of women") is rendered an assumed fact of life. Its basic, fundamental form—associated with its "origin" in simpler social arrangements (the tributary as opposed to bourgeois industrial state)—is presumed to underlie its manifestations in more complex configurations. Consequently, what should be accounted for is instead "naturalized," removed from historical investigation. As an "essential" thing, the "origin," much like the social type, is conceptualized apart from its historical form and experienced context. (1991, 153–54)

It might at first appear that Silverblatt's essay is another entry in a long-standing anthropological debate between history and evolution, the idiographic and the nomothetic, the local and the general. Such an interpretation would represent a profound misreading, however. Though she is clearly signaling the importance of historical context and specific or particular relationships, experiences, and meanings, her criticism of conceptual categories and essentialist assumptions is based on an understanding of history and evolution that can transcend the oppositions through which the issues are commonly discussed. In this essay, I wish to explore certain aspects of this understanding, especially the "culture and political economy" approach to which Silverblatt alludes. Although Silverblatt (1991, 142) points to two recent intellectual movements (postmodernism and Marxist cultural studies) that have questioned basic categories and inspired her own reconsiderations, I examine an older anthropological tradition in cultural history—one that has been ignored in both postmodernist and cultural studies intellectual genealogies. Unlike most of the essays in this volume, this essay does not specifically address biological questions or biocultural syntheses, but it reviews an approach to political economy that is necessary for such a synthesis.

Social Fields

We can begin with two important papers by Alexander Lesser (both republished in Mintz 1985). In the first ("Evolution in Social Anthropology," written in 1939 and published in 1952), Lesser, a student of Boas, attempted to draw a balance sheet at the conclusion of several decades of Boasian antievolutionism. Asserting overoptimistically that "social evolution, in the form given it by Morgan, Tylor, Spencer, and other 'classical evolutionists,' is today as dead as a doornail in social anthropology" (in Mintz 1985, 78), he nonetheless sought to avoid "the nihilistic tendencies of the anti-evolutionists" (78). Compiling a list of "dead as a doornail" evolutionary assumptions, he suggested that they include: the unilinear developmental assumption, the postulation of orderly, cause-and-effect, lawlike development, notions of inevitability, the presumed unfolding of social forms from simple to complex, the assertion of moral or cultural progress, and the assumption of parallel historical sequences in distinct social and cultural contexts. He suggested, however, that social anthropologists nonetheless work with certain basic, if implicit, evolutionary assumptions (often drawn from biological analogues): of historical continuity, sequence, differentiation, and development (the understanding that civilizations develop within and from earlier contexts). He then suggested a number of sequential, developmental processes—involving the division of labor, kinship and political organization, and the like—and claimed that they present important problems for "historical" and "chronological" analysis, problems that had been ignored because of the "over-dogmatic tendencies" and "complete nihilism as regards problems of cultural sequence and development" that had characterized the writings of his fellow Boasians.

Unfortunately, as evolutionism reemerged in the second half of the twentieth century, it did not take the contextualized and historical form that Lesser envisioned. Instead, a much more aggressively scientific evolutionism was triumphant, full of assumptions about lawlike sequences of cause and effect, notions of parallel processes of development, and—most importantly—of concepts (like *the* state, *the* tribe, *the* household, *the* subordination of women) that could be applied unproblematically to processes of history and evolution. With it came the reproduction of the antinomies Lesser was happy to set aside—evolutionism versus historicism or relativism, the general versus the local or particular, and so on. Such antinomies were immanent in the very structure of evolutionist discourse and have, in turn and in response, produced a new nihilism.

A quiet but important dissent, again by Lesser, suggested a more interesting path, which has been taken up by political economy. In "Social Fields and the Evolution of Society" (originally published in 1961, republished in Mintz 1985), Lesser drew attention to the phenomena of "borrowing" and "diffusion" and suggested that we should not think of such contacts as accidental or random. In an earlier antievolutionist literature, such phenomena had been taken as central to a historicist interpretation, emphasizing the importance of "accidents" and "contingency." Lesser suggested that we need to think of such phenomena in *relational* terms. For him, borrowing and diffusion emerge from regular (and irregular), patterned relations among communities and societies, and the ordinary way of conceiving of social wholes by evolutionists and their critics was too quick to draw boundaries around and between particular social aggregates—"societies." In contrast, he observed:

> I propose to ask what difference it makes if we adopt as a working hypothesis the universality of human contact and influence—as a fundamental feature of the socio-historical process; if we conceive of human societies—prehistoric, primitive, or modern—not as closed systems, but as open systems; if we think of any social aggregate not as isolated, separated by some kind of wall, from others, but as inextricably involved with other aggregates, near and far, in weblike, netlike connections. (In Mintz 1985, 95)

Lesser then suggested a number of ways in which concentration on social fields redefines and reconfigures evolutionary processes and concluded:

The field concept, I suggest, is particularly useful in understanding social evolutionary change that has taken place in human history. It unites into one field the study of those patterned interpersonal relations usually considered external, or merely a matter of historical accident, and those that are an integral part of a particular social aggregate. It breaks down the notion that history involves mere happenstance which interferes with analysis of social process in systems of relations, or order and regularity in events. (99)

Once again, Lesser had suggested a path between and beyond evolutionist and antievolutionist antinomies. Both the evolutionists and their critics had converged in a reification of social wholes or cultures. For the former, social wholes were the fundamental units in their statistical exercises demonstrating correlations in societal development; for the latter, they offered the essential disproof of evolutionary formulations (not in this valley; not at this time).

Anthropological Political Economy

This application of the social field concept as "weblike, netlike connections" has been most carefully developed by anthropological political economy. One of the central features of a political economic approach is, of course, its understanding of power, not as socially diffuse or "capillary" but as structured by and in terms of the control of social labor (see Wolf 1982, 73–100). In this, political economy remains indebted to Marx's double emphasis on *labor*. First, labor was an essentially human, transforming capacity. The labor process, broadly conceived, was the basis for his materialism, in that the "material," for Marx, was fundamentally *social*. Through the labor process, humans entered into relations with each other and with nature through which both humans and nature were changed. It was this structured process of alteration and transformation, even as a population was attempting to maintain or reproduce a particular mode of life, that attracted his attention. Second, he contended that the structural relationship between nonproducers and producers, and the means by which surplus labor is "pumped out of direct producers" (here one might say, more neutrally and academically, "appropriated") "reveals the secret of . . . the entire social structure" (1967, 791–92).

This particular formulation has often served (in the work of Marx, among others) as the basis for an evolutionary typology that would organize a sequence of societal types in terms of the dominant type or "mode" of labor extraction. Yet this procedure is vulnerable to the same criticism Lesser made of other evolutionary models. Here Marx's modest claim that the appropriation of social labor "reveals the secret" of the social structure can, in conjunction with an examination of social fields, lead to fresh insights. In a discussion that explicitly criticizes the reification of social units within evolutionary (and other) typologies, Eric Wolf observes:

> Anthropologists normally attempt a task of cross-cultural comparison by first assembling "cases," models of societies or cultures constructed from observed or reported data. These models are then either compared synchronically or seriated with respect to each other, using one or more diagnostic criteria to order the cases in question. On occasion, the synchronic or seriated sequence is given a diachronic interpretation and placed in a frame of elapsed time to arrive at statements of process (e.g., "adaptation" or "development"). We are all familiar with these procedures, and probably have employed them ourselves at some time. We know that it can be done and is done, often with scientifically and aesthetically pleasing results.
>
> I would, however, raise a number of objections to this procedure. First, we often take the data observed or recorded as realities in and of themselves, rather than as more or less tangible results of underlying processes operating in historical time. What we then see and compare are these tangible and observable (and indeed often temporary) precipitates of processes, not the processes themselves. Second, we have known at least since the diffusionists that no society or culture is an island. There are always interchanges and interrelationships with other societies and cultures. What seems less obvious, however, is that these interrelated "cases" appeared in the ken of Europocentric anthropology only because Europeans or Euro-Americans visited them, and these visitors did so because they were propelled by forces that were the outcome of something we call capitalism. Thus, what we explore and observe in the locations anthropologists visit around the world stands in a specific relationship to this process of expansion, which in turn responds to the workings out of a particular structure or relational set. (1981, 41, 42)

Because political economy is usually caricatured as a kind of world systems theory, or its principal assertions are glossed as an emphasis on the determining influence of "larger" or "wider" systems (generally understood as capitalist) on "local" societies, the radical reconfiguration suggested by Wolf's claim (and by Lesser's earlier suggestions) is often overlooked. To be sure, this understanding of political economy stresses the importance of connections and world historic processes and therefore unsettles all attempts to draw boundaries around presumed social units. What is less frequently emphasized, however, is this perspective's insistent focus on the particular and specific—indeed, the local—understood "not as isolated, separated by some kind of wall" but in terms of specific relationships (seen as "webs" or "nets") and particular social and political positions or connections within them. The social field places the local within larger networks and therefore requires a knowledge of those networks. But the networks themselves are uniquely configured, socially and historically, in particular places at particular times. The local is global, in this view, but the global can only be understood as always and necessarily local. Let us return to Wolf's claim and emphasize, here, the words "specific" and "particular": "What we explore and observe in the locations anthropologists visit around the world stands in a *specific* relationship to this process of expansion, which in turn responds to the workings out of a *particular* structure or relational set."

But, of course, anthropological political economy does not simply assert the universality of human connections. Here the two central features must be conjoined: social fields are fields of power, and the flows of resources, goods, people, ideas, ideologies, armies, weapons, and the like are structured in terms of the control of social labor. Political economy, then, takes as its point of departure a particular arena. The description of that arena begins with a delineation of the relevant actors—seen as groups, clusters, and classes of people—and their interrelations (again, structured primarily through the control of social labor); the analysis of the actors and their interrelations *necessarily* involves a variety of historical dimensions. The description of a group of merchants requires a study of the expansion and contraction of markets for certain kinds of products in and beyond the arena; the description of landlords requires a study of land tenure and the expansion and contraction of particular estates; and so on. All of the relevant groups may be bearers of distinct historical "moments," but in their interrelations within a particular arena, or a particular field of power, each constitutes a unique social, cultural, and political configuration. In the process, the very definitions and boundaries of local units are situated.

Implications for Social Analysis

The linkage of anthropological political economy with the analysis of social fields carries certain implications for social analysis. I explore some of these by discussing, first, some general problems of comparative analysis and, second, two areas of comparative work that have attracted anthropological and historical attention: the analysis of social *classes* and the comparative examination of *households.* These are, of course, differently located objects of inquiry. The problem of social classes and class relations is necessarily implicated in any attempt to make political economy more local and specific. The study of households, however, is a more specialized object of inquiry, taken as one among many possible examples for theoretical reflection.

Comparative Analysis

If social units are no longer available for taxonomic comparison or evolutionary schema, certain basic concepts (e.g., household, community, social class, state, even mode of production) with which anthropologists have analyzed those social units are also unavailable for ordinary comparative purposes. This does not mean that anthropologists must limit themselves to "experience near" concepts and forswear comparison altogether. Such a stance would return us to and reproduce the idiographic/nomothetic or local/general opposition that we are attempting to transcend. Nor does it mean that we must reject concepts of household, community, class, state, or mode of production altogether. All of these concepts remain essential for comparative work as long as they are not stripped of historical and sociological content. The kind of comparative work that is possible, however, is *relational.* For both social units and social types, the attempt must be to locate specific and particular configurations within social fields.

In contrast, the more usual procedure is to outline social concepts that can be *abstracted from* historical context and social field, to identify those formal features or elements that can be considered essential to or distinctive of the "type," to identify societies in which the type can be found, and to place the type within a variety of comparative and/or evolutionary schemes. For example, the "peasant" concept may be linked to such features as agricultural production, small-scale, household-based decision-making units, the action of small producers within social milieus that include nonpeasants, the production of a surplus, the payment of a portion of that surplus (as "rent") to nonpeasants, the existence of the state, and so on. A "proletariat" may be defined by its relation to the means of production. A particular "mode of production" may be defined by its characteristic mode of surplus extraction, and so on.

The fact that I have selected concepts that figure within Marxist analysis is, in this case, irrelevant to the central point. I could have chosen concepts from anthropological evolutionism, such as "foraging," "pastoralist," "horticultural," "agricultural," and "industrial" societies, or bands, tribes, chiefdoms, and states. Or I could have supplied non-Marxist definitions for each of the previous categories. My central argument concerns a mode of sociological abstraction and its role within comparative historical or anthropological work. With this mode of analysis, the primary *relational* figures concern relations between types, each of which is defined in terms of the presence or absence of specific formal features.

Yet this procedure is vulnerable to precisely the sort of criticism Irene Silverblatt raised against origin quests or Eric Wolf directed against the reification of societies in the passage quoted above. It takes "the data observed or recorded as realities in and of themselves, rather than as more or less tangible results of underlying processes." And it sees and compares "these tangible and observable . . . precipitates of processes, not the processes themselves." The kind of comparative analysis I am suggesting here is one that concentrates on the relational features suggested in some of our most common sociological concepts and places those features back within an analysis of power-laden social fields. If, for example, our concept of peasantry suggests the importance of the production by peasants of a surplus and the payment of part of that surplus to nonpeasants, we may examine a variety of asymmetrical social relations between specific groups of surplus producers and surplus appropriators, in specific historical contexts and social fields. If our concept of peasantry also stresses the centrality of the household, we need to examine specific relations of gender and generation within households, and specific relations of household and community, and/or household and state, and/or household and church— again in specifiable historical contexts and social fields. Such comparative analyses preclude the construction of certain kinds of evolutionary schemes, but they serve as methodological guides to more satisfying analyses of "the processes themselves."

Class Analysis

This, in turn, carries implications for our understanding of class relations. Let us begin with the classic Marxian analysis of the division of society into classes defined in terms of their relation to the means of production—for capitalism: bourgeoisie and proletariat, with intermediate class locations; for feudalism: landlords and peasants; and so on. For certain kinds of analysis, this basic structural opposition might be sufficient. For most analyses, however, the opposition might serve as a necessary starting point, but it lacks the sociological and historical content necessary for comprehension and understanding. Indeed, in Marx's own historical and political analyses, he did not detain himself with simple structural oppositions. In *The Eighteenth Brumaire of Louis Bonaparte,* for example, he clearly had in mind the structure of society and struggle as one marked by class, but he spent much of his time writing about divisions and factions within the French bourgeoisie, about artisans and shopkeepers in the petit bourgeoisie, about peasants, about the structure and history of the French state, about previous experience of revolution in France, about Bonaparte, about the symbolic relationship between Paris and the countryside and the ways in which Bonaparte was able to exploit that relationship—and so on.

Where *class,* as a first specification, marks what we might call a two-dimensional field—a set of relationships that can be mapped on a single plane, like a sheet of paper—the analysis Marx attempted in *The Eighteenth Brumaire* was necessarily multidimensional. By this I do not simply mean that class is too often understood at an "economic" level and that one also needs to examine "cultural," "social," and "political" relations and forces. The understanding of class in economic terms *also* needs to be made multidimensional—not just capitalism or feudalism or inclusion within "the world system," but a more precise analysis of spatial and social organization of production and marketing, of the temporal and spatial ebb and flow of product markets, of the relationship between food and commodity production, of the forms and relations through which "labor" is mobilized, compensated, and reproduced, and so on. How are manors organized in this parish or region? Through what kinds of field systems is cultivation practiced? At what distance from major towns or cities are manors and villages in this parish? From ports? From roads or rivers? What commodities are marketed in towns, cities, and ports, and how is this changing over time? Are urban merchants expanding their activities in rural regions, entering into "putting out" relations with artisans, cottars, and rural laborers? How do all of these relations and processes affect the character and quality of relations between lords and peasants in particular times and places? A similar set of detailed questions, again paying attention to space and time, needs to be posed about "noneconomic" dimensions—of church and chapel, of the density of presence of a variety of state institutions and agencies, and so on.

These are, in my view, "field" questions. They are ways of analyzing the social and political consequences of the emergence of human populations in "weblike, netlike connections," or of seeing how a population "stands in a specific relationship to this process of expansion, which in turn responds to the workings out of a particular structure or relational set." "The concrete is concrete," wrote Marx in another context, "because it is the concentration of many determinations, hence unity of the diverse. It appears in the process of thinking, therefore, as a process of concentration, as a result, not as a point of departure, even though it is the point of departure in reality and hence also the point of departure for observation and conception."

Household Analysis

A similar set of questions and specifications can be applied to the anthropological analysis of households. I am presently engaged in a comparative, historical study on the formation of household economies in particular fields of power. I began the study out of dissatisfaction with the formulaic assertion of the centrality of "the household" in most definitions of peasantries, but as the project has developed it has become clear that the problem is much more pervasive. Let us briefly consider some of the anthropological literatures in which "the household" figures as a formal and ahistorical social type.

In peasant studies, we are familiar with the Chayanovian postulation of the household as the primary economic and social unit of peasant life, inspiring a large literature on peasant and artisan householding. Interestingly, Chayanov drew on implicit and sometimes explicit evolutionary assumptions: the peasant farm was presented as a model of "our economic past," characterized by natural economy, in which

> human economic activity is dominated by the requirement of satisfy-
> ing the needs of each single production unit, which is, at the same
> time, a consumer unit. Therefore, budgeting here is to a high degree
> qualitative: for each family need, there has to be provided in each eco-
> nomic unit the qualitative corresponding product *in natura.* (Chaya-
> nov 1966, 4; see also Medick 1981, 40)

These evolutionary assumptions and associations have been developed in cultural anthropology, most provocatively in Sahlins's model of
the domestic mode of production. In his view:

> For the domestic groups of primitive society have not yet suffered
> demotion to a mere consumption status, their labor power detached
> from the familial circle and, employed in an external realm, made sub-
> ject to an alien organization and purpose. The household is as such
> charged with production, with the deployment and use of labor-
> power, with the determination of the economic objective. Its own
> inner relations, as between husband and wife, parent and child, are the
> principal relations of production in society. The built-in etiquette of
> kinship statuses, the dominance and subordination of domestic life,
> the reciprocity and cooperation, here make the "economic" a modal-
> ity of the intimate. How labor is expended, the terms and products of
> its activity, are in the main domestic decisions. And these decisions are
> taken primarily with a view toward domestic contentment. Produc-
> tion is geared to the family's customary requirements. Production is
> for the benefit of the producers. (Sahlins 1972, 76–77)

Sahlins is here making a political point (a criticism of modern or capitalist notions of affluence, in contrast to primitive or "Zen" models) and
a theoretical argument (a narrow conception of the economic, limiting it
to householding, as opposed to the more inclusive and wider social and
political bonds of kinship), basing both in an evolutionism. The domestic
mode is defined by a series of contrasts with Sahlins's model of the present;
present and past are then linked by the contrasts themselves, by the presence or absence of certain features, here defined within a critical but no less

evolutionistic anthropology (see O'Brien and Roseberry 1991). That is, in the time-honored fashion of classical social theory, the primitive is defined by what it is *not:* it is not Western, business-oriented, etc. That a positive valuation is placed on the primitive ("Zen") in contrast to the Western does not alter the basic contrastive or oppositional work the model is made to do. Other scholars may reject Sahlins's political reading of the domestic mode but may nonetheless begin with a concept of householding and the centrality of the household as a primordial social form or comparative starting point.

More recently, social anthropologists have also begun to concentrate on "the household" as a formal unit for comparative social analysis. In their 1984 volume *Households,* Netting, Wilk, and Arnould began with the assumption that "the household is sufficiently universal and recognizable for use in cross-cultural and historical comparison" (xix). While recognizing a variety of approaches to household analysis and a multiplicity of formal definitions, they suggested a mode of analysis that concentrated on what households "do," seeing domestic groups as "activity groups" that may or may not include such activities as production, distribution, resource transmission, reproduction, and coresidence. Although this framework is admirably flexible in examining a wide variety of social forms and activities within and among "households," it does not really address the criticisms of scholars like Guyer (1981), Yanagisako (1979), or Rapp (1978) because it maintains an assumption that the household—whatever its variation in form and multifunctionality—is a universal building block. More importantly, while it seems to avoid the sort of abstraction criticized above by remaining close to ethnographic and historical sources, it ignores relational questions that should be central, such as the relative "boundedness" of households, the historical and social shaping of inequalities of gender and generation, and the placement of household units within different kinds of power domains.

In each of these areas of inquiry, household analysis has been subjected to criticisms, the most important of which have been inspired and informed by feminist scholarship, from early criticisms of unequal relations within households to more recent work on waged and unwaged labor in a variety of settings (see, for example, Rapp 1978 on family and household ideologies; Yanagisako 1979 on models of domestic groups; Guyer 1981 on the predication of the household in Africa; Harris 1981 on the assumption of households as natural units; Fox-Genovese 1982 on the emergence of "domestic economy" in relation to "political economy";

Collins 1990 on the separate but related literatures on domestic labor and peasantries).

We can mention two well-developed lines of criticism. One concerns the position of household units within a wider set of social relations. In peasant studies, this has sometimes involved attention to a "hidden economy" of kinship and community. Orvar Lofgren (1984), for example, notes that the household was the basic unit of assessment on feudal estates and has therefore been recorded and taken as a basic unit of evidence by latter day historians. Taking these units, scholars can easily assert that the household was the basic unit of production without considering a range of social relations, practices, and rituals of kinship and community that may have been central to the organization of peasant life and livelihood but marginal to the keeping of feudal accounts.

Along these lines, important research has focused on the placement of household units in relation to wider social fields and institutions, from communities to states (see, for example, Cole and Wolf's 1974 discussion of inheritance strategies in two villages of the Tyrol, in relation to distinct political histories; Rebel's 1991 study of household ideologies in the Habsburg state; Donham 1990 on the wider relations of kinship and polity that envelop a "domestic mode of production").

In addition, a variety of scholars have explored the *emergence* of household economies in the context of modernization or capitalist development, upsetting the presumed primordial character of household organization (see Rebel 1982 on the Habsburg creation of peasant houses as bureaucratic units in early modern Austria; Fox-Genovese 1982 on the emergence of domestic economy in eighteenth-century France; Smith et al. 1984 on the formation of households in the world economy; Collins 1986 on household formation in the Andes; Roseberry 1991 on the emergence of a peasantry in the context of English enclosures; Gudmundson 1985 on the creation of a household-based smallholder class in nineteenth-century Costa Rica). These studies do not assert simply and mechanically that households are modern products or only appeared in the modern era. This would run counter to much anthropological knowledge and experience. This work does suggest, however, that some of the social, cultural, and economic characteristics (or activities) *attributed* to households *are* relatively modern and are imputations from the present upon the past. The most important of these is the apparent boundedness of the household itself. That is, a number of recent authors have emphasized the fluidity of interhousehold relations and the permeability of household boundaries in a variety of non-Western settings. The anthropologist who would take the bounded household as a primordial social unit, or as a basic unit for comparative social analysis, should do so with caution.

A comparative analysis of households, then, needs to develop both the *relational* and *historical* dimensions alluded to above. In historical terms, it should move beyond a view of household economies as simple evolutionary building blocks or primordial units and explore the diverse ways in which they emerge within historically specifiable processes of state formation, empire building, and economic expansion and contraction. In relational terms, it should examine the processes of state, empire, and commercial or industrial expansion and contraction themselves in relation to household formation. Do merchants in the nineteenth-century Venezuelan Andes enter into credit relations with farmers that have the effect of tying farmers as families to the land, "creating" household economies (Roseberry 1983)? Do planters in nineteenth-century São Paolo insist on employing *families* of immigrant laborers, solidifying a different kind of household economy in a different field of power (Stolcke 1988)? Do absolutist rulers in sixteenth-century Upper Austria or eighteenth-century France tax small properties, making a newly formed household economy the fiscal basis for their regimes (Rebel 1982)?

Conclusion

In the specific examples of class and household analysis, this essay has argued for an approach to political economy that is not content with assigning epochal labels (capitalist, feudal) or structural categories (bourgeois, peasant, proletarian) to social phenomena. Instead, it takes these designations and categories as necessary starting points for a more detailed sociological examination that pays attention to questions of context and relations. Without this kind of specificity, without a political economic focus on the appropriation of social labor within specifiable social fields, our social categories and evolutionary progressions remain empty. We would do well to heed Marx's warning that

> even the most abstract categories, despite their validity—precisely because of their abstractness—for all epochs, are nevertheless, in the specific character of this abstraction, themselves likewise a product of historic relations, and possess their full validity only for and within these relations. (1973, 105)

Recognizing this does not force us into a new nihilism. It simply means that there is much careful anthropological and historical work yet to be done.

REFERENCES

Chayanov, A. V. 1966. *Theory of Peasant Economy.* Homewood, IL: Richard Irwin Publishers.

Cole, J., and E. R. Wolf. 1974. *The Hidden Frontier.* New York: Academic Press.

Collins, J. 1986. The Household and Relations of Production in Southern Peru. *CSSH* 28:651–71.

Collins, J., ed. 1990. *Waged and Unwaged Labor.* Albany: State University of New York.

Donham, D. 1990. *History, Power, Ideology.* New York: Cambridge University Press.

Fox-Genovese, E. 1982. In *Fruits of Merchant Capital,* ed. E. Genovese and E. Fox-Genovese. New York: Oxford University Press.

Gailey, C. 1987. *From Kinship to Kingship.* Austin: University of Texas Press.

Gudmundson, L. 1985. *Costa Rica Before Coffee.* Baton Rouge: Louisiana State University Press.

Guyer, J. 1981. Household and Community in African Studies. *African Studies Review* 24:87–137.

Harris, O. 1981. Households as Natural Units. In *Of Marriage and the Market,* ed. K. Young, C. Wolkowitz, and R. McCullagh. London: CSE Books.

Leacock, E. 1972. Introduction. In *Origin of the Family, Private Property, and the State,* ed. F. Engels. New York: International.

Leacock, E. 1978. Women's Status in Egalitarian Society: Implications for Social Evolution. *Current Anthropology* 19:247–75.

Lofgren, O. 1984. Family and Household: Images and Realities: Cultural Change in Swedish Society. In *Households: Comparative and Historical Studies of the Domestic Group,* ed. R. Netting, R. Wilk, and E. Arnould, 446–69. Berkeley: University of California Press.

Marx, K. 1967. *Capital,* vol. 3. New York: International.

Marx, K. 1973. Introduction. In *Grundrisse.* New York: Penguin.

Medick, H. 1981. The Proto-Industrial Family Economy. In *Industrialization before Industrialization,* ed. P. Kriedte, H. Medick, and J. Schlumbohm, 36–73. Cambridge: Cambridge University Press.

Mintz, S., ed. 1985. *History, Evolution, and the Concept of Culture: Selected Papers by Alexander Lesser.* New York: Cambridge University Press.

Netting, R., R. Wilk, and E. Arnould, eds. 1984. *Households: Comparative and Historical Studies of the Domestic Group.* Berkeley: University of California Press.

O'Brien, J., and W. Roseberry. 1991. *Golden Ages, Dark Ages: Imagining the Past in Anthropology and History.* Berkeley: University of California Press.

Rapp, R. 1978. Family and Class in Contemporary America: Notes Toward an Understanding of Ideology. *Science and Society* (summer): 278–300.

Rebel, H. 1982. *Peasant Classes*. Princeton: Princeton University Press.

Rebel, H. 1991. Reimagining the Oikos: Austrian Cameralism in its Social Formation. In *Golden Ages, Dark Ages*, ed. J. O'Brien and W. Roseberry, 48–80. Berkeley: University of California Press.

Roseberry, W. 1983. *Coffee and Capitalism in the Venezuelan Andes*. Austin: University of Texas Press.

Roseberry, W. 1991. Potatoes, Sacks and Enclosures in Early Modern England. In *Golden Ages, Dark Ages*, ed. J. O'Brien and W. Roseberry, 19–47. Berkeley: University of California Press.

Sacks, K. 1974. Engels Revisited: Women, The Organization of Production, and Private Property. In *Woman, Culture, and Society*, ed. M. Rosaldo and L. Lamphere, 207–22. Stanford: Stanford University Press.

Sacks, K. 1982. *Sisters and Wives: The Past and Future of Sexual Equality*. Urbana: University of Illinois Press.

Sahlins, M. 1972. *Stone Age Economics*. Chicago: Aldine.

Silverblatt, I. 1991. Interpreting Women in States: New Feminist Ethnohistories. In *Gender at the Crossroads of Knowledge: Feminist Anthropology in the Postmodern Era*, ed. M. di Leonardo, 140–71. Berkeley: University of California Press.

Smith, J., I. Wallerstein, and H.D. Evers, eds. 1984. *Households and the World Economy*. Beverly Hills, CA: Sage.

Stolcke, V. 1988. *Coffee Planters, Workers, and Wives*. New York: St. Martin's Press.

Wilk, R., and R. Netting. 1984. Households: Changing Forms and Functions. In *Households: Comparative and Historical Studies of the Domestic Group*, ed. R. Netting, R. Wilk, and E. Arnould, 1–28. Berkeley: University of California Press.

Wolf, E. 1981. The Mills of Inequality. In *Social Inequality: Comparative and Developmental Perspectives*, ed. G. Berreman, 41–58. New York: Academic Press.

Wolf, E. 1982. *Europe and the People Without History*. Berkeley: University of California Press.

Yanagisako, S. 1979. Family and Household: The Analysis of Domestic Groups. *Annual Review of Anthropology* 8:161–205.

Chapter 4

The Development of Critical Medical Anthropology: Implications for Biological Anthropology

Merrill Singer

In 1966, when Alexander Alland proposed that "medical anthropology may serve as a major link between physical and cultural anthropology" (1966, 41), the fragmentation of anthropology at the borderlands of its major subdisciplines (biological, cultural, linguistics, and archaeology) already was becoming apparent. Uncertainty had emerged concerning the ability of anthropology to hold together both its seemingly disparate components as well as its global biocultural conception of humankind. Into the breach was thrust the relatively new subdiscipline of medical anthropology. With its targeted focus on health issues (including morbidity and mortality), medical anthropology was inherently biologically oriented. At the same time, in its recognition that the human conception of health was a cultural construction and that health status was extensively shaped by sociocultural practices (including both behaviors that cause illness and those that help remedy it), medical anthropology was simultaneously cultural in its focus. Thus, medical anthropology appeared to offer a useful bridge connecting symbols to selection, acculturation to adaptation, and ethnography to evolution, thereby allowing for the retention of a unified anthropology.

There is considerable room for debate over how well medical anthropology has fulfilled its promise as a disciplinary adhesive. Over time, biological and cultural anthropology have become, each in its own way, more highly specialized and aligned more closely with other disciplines, rather than with each other. Thus, many biological anthropologists have adopted microscopic levels of biological and biobehavioral analysis and have focused their attention on nonprimate and even nonmammalian species of only tangential concern to cultural analysis. At the same time, with the rise to prominence of postmodernism, some cultural anthropologists have come to define their work as a literary endeavor more concerned with text, text production, and text producer than with an external subject or scientific research. Consequently, many have questioned whether anthropology eventually will bifurcate along a science/antiscience divide that will leave the work of cultural and biological anthropologists forever disarticulated. As Peacock indicates,

> Physical anthropology and archaeology are often identified with a quasi-positivist perspective, cultural and linguistic anthropology of a certain persuasion with the interpretivist, even postmodernist line . . . Divisions—organizational, spatial, economic, political, personal— often polarize in this way. Some academic departments, for example, [already] have split along such fault lines. (1995, 1)

Despite these rifts and tensions, it is clear that medical anthropology has become an important meeting place between cultural and biological anthropology. Certainly, it is an arena in which debate and theory construction around biocultural issues have intensified dramatically in recent years (e.g., Johnson and Sargent 1990, Singer 1992). As a result, it has been suggested that medical anthropology now is moving "closer to achieving the type of biocultural synthesis that has long been among the major goals of anthropology as a field" (Johnson and Sargent 1990, 8).

In this light, contemporary debates within medical anthropology that bear on the topic of bioculturalism likely have important implications for the development of a political-economic biological anthropology and for the wider project of developing a critical biocultural synthesis. Of particular concern in this regard is the effort to create a critical, political-economically informed medical anthropology. Examining these issues in historic context is the aim of this chapter. This examination begins with a review of the demise and re-emergence of political economy as a field of study and of the subsequent creation of the political economy of health tradition in the social sciences (Baer, Singer, and Susser 1997). This is followed by an account of the development of critical medical anthropology as a synthesis of insights and understandings from medical anthropology and the political economy of health. The chapter concludes with an exploration of the emergent effort within critical medical anthropology to forge a critical bioculturalism, including a discussion of the key conceptual developments at the heart of this effort.

The Fall and Rise of Political Economy and the Political Economy of Health

As a distinct perspective within the social sciences, political economy is both old and new. The term is of fresh vintage in the sense that it constitutes an emergent approach that is looked to as a needed corrective to the reductionism of the recent past, especially within anthropology (Roseberry 1989; Wolf 1982). However, contemporary political-economic research rests on a deep tradition that stretches back in time to a period well before the rise of the modern social sciences. Because of this dual history, it is not always certain that the precise meaning of political economy is clear. In part, this confusion appears to stem from the fact that what is labeled by the term has undergone a very definitive change over the last hundred years.

Eric Wolf, who has examined this sociolinguistic transition and its underlying causes, points out that political economy as a field of study was parent to all of the contemporary social sciences, including sociology, anthropology, economics, and political science (1982, 7–8). All of these now seemingly distinct disciplines "owe their existence to a common rebellion against political economy" (19). As Wolf indicates, from the outset the goal of political-economic research has been to "lay bare the laws or regularities surrounding the production of wealth. It entailed a concern with how wealth was generated in production, with the role of classes in the genesis of wealth, and with the role of the state in relation to the different classes" (19).

However, the rise to prominence and the transforming effects of the capitalist mode of production fragmented the field, and "inquiry into the nature and varieties of humankind split into separate (and unequal) specialties and disciplines" (Wolf 1982, 7). This development disrupted not only the unity of social inquiry but the very sense of cohesiveness in society as well, leading to an intense concern in the dominant social class with maintaining social order and the economic and political privileges inherent in the existing configuration of society. Throughout the mid–nineteenth century, however, the specter of revolution hung in the air as the working class actively and sometimes militantly challenged the oppressive structures of inequality at the heart of capitalist society. Eventually this resistance found expression in a series of armed clashes that appeared to many as the harbinger of open class warfare throughout Europe.

In the midst of this mounting turmoil, questions about the underlying nature of social solidarity and social order were raised as burning issues of scholarly concern. The field of sociology splintered from political economy with the expressed mission of delving into the structure of social relations and social institutions. It defined its core problem as understanding the interpersonal bonds and associated cohesion-generating beliefs and customs that link individuals together to form families, small groups, institutions, and societies. Early sociologists came to view ties among individuals and the development of community as causal engines driving the functioning and unity of society. Auguste Comte, who coined the term *sociology* and helped to steer the discipline's early course, asserted that an understanding of these social dynamics would allow them to be both predicted and controlled. Meanwhile, the issues of concern to political economy, including how relations among individuals are shaped by the inequality among social classes in the production of national and international wealth, were dropped. In retrospect, it is evident that the guiding ideas of early sociology reflected the values, beliefs, and concerns of the dominant social class. As Marx noted at the time (1970, 64), "the ideas of the ruling class are in every epoch the ruling ideas, i.e. the class which is the ruling material force of society, is at the same time its ruling intellectual force."

While sociology focused its attention on the industrial societies brought into existence by the rise of capitalism, anthropology, its somewhat subordinate sister discipline, developed as the study of the small-scale, non-Western societies situated in the interstitial spaces between and within industrial centers. Cultural anthropology began as the study of evolutionarily conceived cultural forms, but during the twentieth century, through an emphasis on participant observation research on human beliefs and behaviors in natural contexts, it was transformed into the study of the subtle details and unique configurations of individual cultural cases. Each of these cases, or societies as they were called, was treated more or less as a social isolate, propelled by its own internal social dynamics, cultural logic, or adaptation to local conditions. Ignored in this close-to-the-ground empiricism were the sweeping processes and broader social relations that transcended micropopulations, historically uniting them with each other via broader developments in capitalist production. The problem, as Ollman (1971, 226) argues, is that "misinterpretation results from focusing too narrowly on facts which are directly observable and from abstracting these appearances from the surrounding conditions . . . which alone give them their correct meaning, a meaning that often runs counter to the obvious one." Moreover, as Giddens (1987, 20) keenly observes, "it is one of the ironies of the modern era that the systematic study of the diversity of human cultures—'field-work anthropology'—came into being at the very time when the voracious expansion of industrial capitalism and Western military power was accelerating their destruction."

Biological anthropology, in turn, began as the study of the biological differences among human groups and the discontinuities and evolutionary relationships between humans and other animals (living and extinct). Throughout much of its history, biological anthropology has treated human biology and contemporary human diversity as if they evolved in the context of natural conditions only and were not a product as well of thousands of years of "unnatural" (i.e., social) selection under socially produced environmental conditions. So too biological anthropology's handling of human adaptability (e.g., Armelagos et al. 1991).

A parallel narrowing of focus and jettisoning of the macroperspective of political economy gave birth to the fields of economics and political science. These disciplines were formed by defining economics and politics as separate, bounded domains of social action and value expression. Economics became the gradualist study of the role of demand in the creation of markets, independent of the actual social contexts in which production occurs, markets arise, or demand is generated, while political science became a study of government decision making, policy formation, and political culture, with little consideration of either the exercise of power for self-interested objectives or the interrelationship of politics and economics. In political science, concern with understanding class conflict gave way to a pluralistic view of society characterized by a "multiplicity of cross-cutting conflicts and alliances" in which antagonisms "are well contained within the fabric of the institutional order" (Giddens 1987, 32). In both cases, rapid, sweeping social change was discounted as a possible course or as a solution to any social problem no matter how pressing. The watchword became the (questionable yet venerated) Latin aphorism *Natura non facit saltum* (Nature does not proceed by leaps).

Although the social sciences, including anthropology and its several subfields, commonly are portrayed as natural outgrowths of normal intellectual interest in distinct arenas of human life, as the preceding account suggests, viewed in historic context the academic social science disciplines are best understood as the "reified products of sociopolitical processes" (Morsy 1990, 28), that is to say, as products of a particular political economy. With disciplinary fragmentation, the traditional topics of concern to the field of political economy were marginalized as issues of little merit in any of the emergent academic disciplines. For example, in reviewing the approaches taken by the health social sciences in analyzing the determinants of illness beliefs within a community, Elling (1980, 1–2) notes that:

> Much of the work on this question . . . has reflected the cultural concerns of anthropologists—the cross-cultural study of health and illness conceptions and behaviors. Recently, those who worked from this perspective have begun to realize that social structural forces—the very establishment of modern facilities, or the support by the government of one traditional medical group or another—bring about changes in health orientations and behaviors. But these changing perspectives often remain at a microcosmic level—the structural changes going on in the immediate area of a village one is studying and the concomitant changes in health and illness beliefs, values, attitudes, and behaviors. Or [as in much medical sociology], if a broader perspective is adopted, including national political forces, these may be treated as relatively free-standing or capricious aspects of some leader or party, without clear recognition of the intertwining of political and economic forces often extending into and stemming from an extranational world capitalist political economy.

Within the Weberian tradition, research has tended to be shaped by an interactionist perspective that focuses attention "on the immediate social relationships between individuals and groups in the medical context" while paying "relatively little attention to the political and economic structure of the medical care systems, or to its relationship with the wider society" (Doyal 1979, 15).

Despite the general turn from unified macroanalysis represented by the birth of the various social sciences, the desire to forge a global understanding of the impact on health of the intertwinement of the production of wealth and the exercise of power in a world of antagonistic social classes never completely disappeared. Indisputably, the key figure in sustaining a general commitment to addressing these issues was Karl Marx, and it is for this reason that today political economy is seen as a progressive perspective while during the nineteenth century its adherents ranged across the political spectrum (and Marx, himself, was quite critical of the mainstream political economy of his day). No doubt Marx's attention to social classes and their conflicted interests in specific historic context, indeed his elevation of class conflict as the key concept of social analysis and as the driving force in historical process, contributed in no small way to the urgency with which the nascent social sciences abandoned the concerns of political economy and developed their own socially acceptable arenas of narrow specialization, including confined approaches to questions of health and biology. Beyond Marx, modern political economy has been significantly influenced by the work of a variety of other theorists, including Antonio Gramsci on the nature of hegemony, E. P. Thompson on culture as a material product, Immanuel Wallerstein on the evolution and structure of the capitalist world system, and Andre Gunner Frank on dependency relations in underdeveloped countries. All of these workers were themselves deeply influenced by Marx and sought to extend ideas inherent in his analyses.

Specific concern with the development of a political-economic approach to health issues, a topic that was not a main concern for political economy, can be traced, on the one hand, to Marx's closest colleague, Friedrich Engels, and his study of the deplorable state of the working class of Manchester and, on the other, to Rudolf Virchow's examination (which was influenced by Engels's work) of structural factors in a typhus epidemic in East Prussia. Engels's seminal study examined the etiology of illness and early death in the working class in terms of an oppressive structure of class relations produced by industrial capitalism and its accompanying social and physical environments. Virchow, while a clinical pathologist at Charité Hospital, became interested in the underlying social causes of epidemics. When a typhus outbreak swept through the Upper Silesia region, a deeply impoverished section of East Prussia with a primarily Polish-speaking minority population, Virchow initiated a field study and in his subsequent writings emphasized political-economic factors in accounting for the epidemic, including unemployment, the failure of the government to provide food during a famine, the poor state of housing, and the intense overcrowding in the region. He wrote, "It is rather certain that hunger and typhus are not produced apart from each other but that the latter has spread so extensively only through hunger" (quoted in Waitzkin 1981, 84).

Through the work of Engels and Virchow, the foundation was set for the development of a political economy of health. This approach, however, did not receive a positive response from the managers of the emergent health care system of the nineteenth century. Instead the dominant approach to health, an orientation that was supported by the wealthiest social classes, came to view social conditions

> as natural phenomena, governed by natural, biological, and harmonious laws. Disease was explained as caused by an agent—the bacteria—always present in the diseased body. Within that theoretical construct, causality was defined as an association of the observable phenomena, with the subject for investigation being the micro-agent under the microscope. In focusing on the micro level, the macro social conditions were conveniently put aside. (Navarro 1985, 527)

This approach not only came to dominate biomedicine, but through the influence of biomedicine, had a profound effect on the various social sciences of health as they emerged from their respective disciplines over time.

The ideas of Engels and Virchow, however, were kept alive by a number of individuals who recognized the limitations of the biomedical model. A particularly important figure in this regard was Henry Sigerist, whose work had an important influence on the development of social medicine and public health. A critic of what Stark (1982, 432) aptly has called biomedicine's "undersocialized . . . views of disease," Sigerist migrated to the United States from Europe and brought with him the ideas of Marx, Engels, and Virchow. These found a receptive audience among health workers who daily saw the health consequences of social inequality as well as the immediate effects of a highly stratified health-care system.

As Baer (1982, 2) suggests, the political economy of health "is a subject which has been dropped and rediscovered several times since the mid-19th century." The period after the 1930s began one of the several lapses in attention to which Baer refers. This was an era during which biomedicine had fully "turned away from a broader social understanding of health and disease" (Singer and Baer 1995, 13) as part of a conservative response to the exploration of the social origins of disease initiated by Engels and Virchow. Notes Brown:

> It became clear to increasing numbers of physicians that the complete professionalization of medicine could come only when they developed an ideology and a practice that was consistent with the ideas and interests of social and politically dominant groups in society. . . . The med-

ical profession discovered an ideology that was compatible with the world view of, and politically and economically useful to, the capitalist class and the emerging managerial and professional stratum. (1979, 71)

The social sciences followed suit and did not return to a significant focus on the political economy of health for several decades.

Then in the early 1970s, Sander Kelman (1971) published a political-economic analysis of U.S. medicine from its origin as a cottage industry of independent practitioners to its development as a complex corporate and state system. Kelman's study helped to open the door to what has become a growing number of analyses of health-related issues from the political-economic perspective. Especially at first, these new studies were conducted by medical sociologists but, as discussed later, by the 1980s a critical medical anthropology had emerged as well (Baer 1986; Singer and Baer 1995; Singer 1997a).

Given the dominant perspectives within the social sciences, individuals who have attempted to promote political economy often have been marginalized within their respective disciplines. As Navarro argues, even the terms of political economic discourse have been tainted.

Concepts and terms such as class struggle, capitalism, and imperialism are frequently considered to be rhetorical and dismissed by the dominant functionalist and positivist schools. They are usually written between quotation marks, as if to alert the reader that they are subject to suspicion. Marxists contributing to social science journals are very frequently encouraged to rewrite their articles using more "understandable" and "less value-laden terms" more attuned to prevalent sociological thought. (1982, 7–8)

Despite discrimination, a strong tradition of political economy of health has survived, and the literature associated with this perspective has grown considerably during the 1980s and 1990s. The *International Journal of Health Services,* edited by Navarro, is one of its primary literary sources. Adherents see the political economy of health as offering a much needed "corrective for the disciplinary fragmentation of social science that obscures the relationship among economic systems, political power, and ideologies" (Morsy 1990, 27).

Reflections on the Emergence of Medical Anthropology
and Critical Medical Anthropology

As noted above, with the development of ethnographic research early in
this century and its elevation as the hallmark of anthropological inquiry,
cultural anthropology became the detailed examination of "living cultures." Whole vistas opened to anthropological insight as a result of this
important transition. Anthropologists became engrossed in comprehend-
ing the configuration of behaviors and beliefs that constitute ethnograph-
ically studiable social segments. In short order, however, the realization
that the "societies" that have been subject to anthropological inquiry are
but pieces of a larger whole, local components of a world system, was
backgrounded. In a telling example of methodological determinism,
ethnography "was turned into a theoretical construct by assertion, a priori. The outcome was a series of analyses of wholly separate cases" (Wolf
1982, 14), a pattern later duplicated for diverse medical systems with the
emergence of medical anthropology.

     Studies that would today be labeled medical anthropology have been
carried out by anthropologists since early in the discipline's history.
Indeed, some of the first field expeditions conducted under the banner of
anthropology collected information on folk healing beliefs and practices
as well as data on physical characteristics. Over the years, anthropologists
recorded and wrote about these topics, often with the intention of showing
how health-related ideas and behaviors are part and parcel of a wider cultural configuration. Exemplary is Evans-Pritchard's study of witchcraft
and magic among the Azande, which attempted to demonstrate the "intellectual consistency" of Zande beliefs about the causation and healing of
disease (and broader misfortune). At the time of his research, a period during which the British "colonial administration was undermining [the]
authority structure" of the Azande (Gillies 1976, xxiii), Evans-Pritchard
was employed by the colonial government of the Anglo-Egyptian Sudan.
Although Evans-Pritchard later asserted that during the fifteen years that
he worked in the Sudan he was "never once asked [his] advice on any question at all" by the colonial government (quoted in Kuper 1983, 104), his
studies, with their homeostatic functionalist bent, helped to form and
reflect the broader colonial era comprehension of colonized peoples and of
the world generally. Wolf (1982, 257) characterizes the anthropology of
this period as "'political economy' turned inside out, all ideology and

morality, and neither power nor economy." The problem, as he indicates, lay in anthropology's failure to come to grips with the phenomenon of power, including an inability to recognize the role of science in the maintenance of reigning structures of power.

It was not until the early 1960s that the term *medical anthropology* began to be used with any regularity. Recognition that a distinct field of study was unfolding was given added momentum when, in 1963, Norman Scotch selected "Medical Anthropology" as the title for his review of the literature on the social dimensions of health and illness published in the *Biennial Review of Anthropology*. In this paper, Scotch commented that "there are probably enough anthropologists now working either as researchers or teachers in medical settings so that it might be worth while to consider setting up a section of the American Anthropological Association analogous to the Medical Sociology section of the American Sociological Association" (59). This happened in due course. Through a series of sessions held during the annual meetings of the American Anthropological Association from 1967 through 1970, those with a concern with health issues moved from being an informal network of interested persons to a Group for Medical Anthropology, and ultimately to a Society for Medical Anthropology. By the late 1970s, Landy (1977, 8) was cautiously prepared to declare that "medical anthropology has begun to come of age." The subfield had become firmly established and well recognized within the discipline, courses and graduate programs in medical anthropology were being offered in many universities, journals dedicated to medical anthropology were being established, and medical anthropology texts were being published. Today, the Society for Medical Anthropology is one of the largest sections within the American Anthropological Association, while health-related issues have become a major area of study among anthropologists in the United Kingdom, various countries on the European continent, Latin America, and elsewhere.

Throughout its prehistory and during the early years after consolidation as a distinct subfield, medical anthropology always has been a critical project that challenged, at least to some degree, the adequacy of the disease model of biomedicine. However, as is plain in its very title, medical anthropology is marked by its long relationship with biomedicine. This relationship stretches back to the earliest studies of health-related topics, many of which were carried out by physician-anthropologists. For much of its history, medical anthropology's critique of biomedicine has been quite constrained. As Young (1982, 260) observes, "epistemological scrutiny is suspended for Western social science and Western medicine." Similarly, Landy has written:

> I perceive a contradiction in medical anthropological writing in regard to the treatment of American society. . . . Our society, our culture is one among many. But very frequently in the pages of medical anthropological writings we find that the medical system of that society, or of a broader conception that we imprecisely label as "Western" or "Euroamerican" society, is accepted as an established baseline against which to measure the disease concepts, classifications, and systemic processes (diagnosis, prognosis, treatment, cure, etc.) of other peoples. (1993, 304–5)

Critical medical anthropology (CMA) emerged in direct response to perceived shortcomings and limitations of this kind in conventional medical anthropology. The development of CMA reflects both a turn toward political-economic approaches in anthropology generally, as well as an effort to engage and extend the political economy of health approach by uniting it with the cultural sensitivity and in-depth local study of anthropology. Pivotal to the worldview of CMA is recognition of class and related race and gender antagonisms as the defining characteristics of capitalist society and the reigning world system. Classes have inherently conflicted social interests, in that, at its heart, capitalism is a system designed to promote the ability of one class to control and expropriate the labor of other classes. To maintain its dominance, the ruling class must keep conflict "on a terrain in which its legitimacy is not dangerously questioned" (Genovese 1974, 26). According to Genovese, "The success of a ruling class in establishing its hegemony depends entirely on its ability to convince the lower classes that its interests are those of society at large— that it defends the common sensibility and stands for a natural and proper social order" (quoted in Krause 1977, 259). As summarized by Abercrombie, Hill, and Turner (1980), ideology, the tool used to assert the appropriateness of inequality or to minimize its visibility, is consequential because of its capacity to set the terms of discussion.

> In all societies based on class divisions there is a dominant class which enjoys control of both the means of material production and the means of mental production. Through its control of ideological pro-

duction, the dominant class is able to supervise the construction of a set of coherent beliefs. These dominant beliefs of the dominant class are more powerful, dense, and coherent than those of subordinate classes. The dominant ideology penetrates and infects the consciousness of the working class, because the working class comes to see and to experience reality through the conceptual categories of the dominant class. (1980, 2) *like pharmaceutical co's heralding product to cure healthier, longer*

In this, biomedicine, as a core institution of capitalist society and as a system that reinforces dominance at the microsocial level, plays a vital function. *Foucault's biopower*

In response to the biomedical role in ruling class hegemony, CMA seeks to retrieve the lost threads of Virchow's and Engels's work in health-related anthropology. In so doing, its outlook is guided by questions like

(1) Who has power over the agencies of biomedicine? (2) How and in what form is this power *delegated*? (3) How is power expressed in the social relations within the health care system? (4) What are the economic, socio-political and ideological ends and consequences of the power relations that characterize biomedicine? and (5) What are the principal contradictions of biomedicine and arenas of struggle in the medical system? (Baer, Singer, and Johnsen 1986, 95–96)

In other words, this perspective is committed to the "making social" and the "making political" of health and medicine. In Morsy's (1990, 31) apt phrase, CMA strives to shift "anthropological obsession with what is inside peoples' heads to a scrutiny of what is on their backs." Further, high on the agenda of this approach is the exploration of the implications of all of these issues at the micro level of individual experience and behavior; with the ways in which social conflict and oppressive experience are somatized or embodied in illness; and with how illness serves as an arena for both resistance and political conscientization.

The problems addressed by CMA are several. First, critical medical anthropologists have argued that "disease cannot be perceived apart from a cultural context" (Pfifferling 1981, 198). For example, Emily Martin (1987) in her discussion of "Science as a Cultural System" shows how dominant cultural metaphors of an economic origin (e.g., "production," "control") shape discussions of the human body in biomedical textbooks. Similarly, she has argued that tropes of war and combat construct understandings of the immune system in biomedical education (Martin 1994). She speculates that one effect of such imagery "is to make violent destruction seem ordinary and part of the necessity of daily life" (1990, 417). Similarly, militarization characterizes biomedicine's approach to cancer, as seen the declaration of a "war on cancer" in the National Cancer Act of 1971. As Erwin (1987) observes, one consequence of medical militarization of this sort is that it encourages people to fight disease rather than to make the changes necessary to prevent it.

Second, critical medical anthropologists point out that there has been a significant level of biomedicalization within medical anthropology. Biomedicalization creates a tendency to transform the social into the biological. Alarming to many critical medical anthropologists, for example, is the level of medicalization of anthropological training. Over the last twenty years, several distinct graduate programs in medical anthropology have appeared that treat the discipline not as a social science, but as a technically oriented health science. Thus, Colby (1988, 691) has claimed that

> students are required to take so many graduate courses in traditional anthropology that there is little time to go outside their departments to learn about immunology and other matters vital to medical anthropology. Social theory is important, but it doesn't have to be taught; it can be picked up through reading at any time. In contrast, biological understanding requires laboratory experience, and quantitative sophistication requires courses in math and statistics.

Critical medical anthropologists oppose the biomedicalization of medical anthropology on the grounds that a "main but latent function of . . . medicalization is the resolution of social conflict" (de Swaan 1989, 1169) to the political and economic advantage of the dominant class. From the critical perspective, in adopting a subservient position vis-à-vis biomedicine, medical anthropology gains credibility, but at a painful cost. In Kapferer's assessment, medical anthropology, "largely directed and funded from within Western medical contexts" is "instrumental in a medical imperialism" (1988, 429).

Third, conventional medical anthropologists have made much of the distinction between 'disease,' the clinical indication of biological abnormality, and 'illness,' the sufferer's subjective experience and understanding of his/her condition. However, in the view of critical medical anthropology, this distinction is nothing other than a replication of the biomedical separation of 'signs' and 'symptoms,' an act that defines "the physician as active knower and the patient as passively known" (Kirmayer 1988, 59). Further, this distinction serves to reify the allegedly scientific and objective (and thus allegedly culture-free, politically neutral) nature of medical categories, understandings, and treatments. A cogent example is provided by Figlio in his discussion of the notion of "constitution" in nineteenth-century medicine.

> The history of the term shows the increasing emphasis upon the individual as industrialization took hold. Traditionally, it referred to the character of a locality at a certain time, including the people. . . . But during the nineteenth century the emphasis shifted away from depicting a total situation onto characterizing the general state of the individual. Constitutional weakness, stressed by an exciting cause, brought about disease . . . Disease was evidence that a predisposition existed . . . Thus, constitution as the central presupposition in medical thinking carried the implicit personal responsibility for illness into the hard core of medical theory. The ideological structure of medicine, which concealed the working conditions organized by capitalism, combined with the individualistic ideology of personal responsibility to promote individualism, not only in the marketplace, but also in the sickbed. (1983, 231–32)

While the terms have changed, the notion of constitution remains in late-twentieth-century biomedicine. For example, medical textbooks, "which, as in any profession, express and preserve orthodoxies" (Roberts 1985, 43), regularly conflate biological and politically conditioned social realities. Roberts cites as an example Craddock's *A Short Textbook of General Practice,* which informs medical students that "The vast majority of women have a basic need to have a home and children of their own" (Craddock 1976, 116). In their review of twenty-seven gynecological textbooks published since 1943, Scully and Bart (1973, 1014) found "a persistent bias towards greater concern with the patient's husband than with the patient herself. Women are consistently described as anatomically destined to reproduce, nurture and keep their husbands happy."

Fourth, following Engels and Virchow, CMA has been concerned with examining the social origins of disease—all disease. In the view of CMA, to the degree that it is a physical entity, disease generally is much more than "the straightforward outcome of an infectious agent or pathophysiological disturbance. Instead, a variety of problems—including mal-nutrition, economic insecurity, occupational risks, bad housing and lack of political power—create an underlying predisposition to disease and death" (Waitzkin 1981, 98). This insight suggests the importance of study-ing disease, including its manufacture and marketing, in terms of social structures. For example,

> an insulin reaction in a diabetic postal worker might be ascribed (in a reductionist mode) to an excessive dose of insulin causing an outpour-ing of adrenaline, a failure of the pancreas to respond with appropri-ate glucagon secretion etc. Alternatively, the cause might be sought in his having skipped breakfast because he was late for work; unaccus-tomed physical exertion demanded by a foreman; inability to break for a snack; or, at a deeper level, the constellation of class forces in U.S. society which assures capitalist domination of production and the moment to moment working lives of the proletariat. (Woolhandler and Himmelstein 1989, 1208)

As Woolhandler and Himmelstein suggest, unraveling the connection between social context and disease entails a careful, class-, ethic-, and gender-conscious analysis of the day-to-day living and working conditions of sufferers. Importantly, this synthetic analysis cannot begin with the immediate conditions at the time of diagnosis or even at the time of symp-tom onset, but must trace life pathways that may have created special vul-nerability in the sufferer. Significantly in this regard, there is an emergent body of research beginning to show the effects in adult life of adverse fetal and early childhood health conditions. For example, ischemic heart dis-ease, an ailment commonly associated historically with improved social conditions and prosperity, has been found to be disproportionate among the poor in wealthy, developed countries. Research by Barker and Osmond (1986) in England and Wales demonstrates a close association between geographic areas (i.e., country boroughs and urban districts) characterized by higher rates of current mortality from adult ischemic heart disease and past neonatal and postneonatal infant mortality. Child mortality rates were tied to poverty, including high rates of unemployment and overcrowding, which in turn were associated with poor maternal and early childhood nutrition. Barker and Osmond's study, in short, suggests that childhood poverty and the associated conditions of poor nutrition have lifelong health consequences. In a related study, Barker and coworkers (1990) found that poor maternal nutrition and fetal size are associated with hypertension in adulthood. Placental weight and birth weight, they found, predict the onset of hypertension by age 50. These researchers point to the childhood nutrition of the mother as a determinant of fetal size. In other words, they assert that "the nutrition of girls may . . . be linked to blood pressure in the next generation" (Barker et al. 1990, 262). Importantly, poor childhood nutrition continues to be a major health factor among impoverished social classes and oppressed ethic groups in developed countries despite an abundance of food in society generally.

Recent research among inner city Hispanic preschool children in Hartford, Connecticut (Pérez-Escamilla, Himmelgreen, and Ferris 1996)—the state with the highest per capita income in the United States—found that: (1) 90 percent of parents were anxious about the possibility of running out of food for their children each month; (2) 22 percent of parents reported that their children had been exposed to hunger because of a lack of household food supplies; (3) 10 percent of the children were found to be underweight; and (4) 21 percent of the children were born preterm and 22 percent had low birth weight. Early childhood conditions such as these set a course of health inequality throughout life and even across generations. But inadequate childhood nutrition and its sequalae presents just one of many intertwined biocultural predictors of poor adult health.

Another example is found in research by Koegel, Melamid, and Burnam (1995) from the Course of Homelessness project. This study showed that homeless adults in the United States came from families with disproportionately high rates of poverty, insufficient resources to pay for food, family breakup, and childhood homelessness. In other words, homelessness (and the wider conditions of poverty) in childhood begets homelessness in adulthood. The health effects of homelessness in both childhood and adulthood have been noted in a number of studies. Homeless children have more respiratory diseases, ear infections, skin infections, chronic physical disorders, and emotional and developmental problems than other poor children. Homeless adults also suffer higher rates of both common and more acute health problems, including significant rates of HIV disease and tuberculosis. Tuberculosis, in turn, is associated with poor housing conditions and poor nutrition, and is a cofactor for the spread of HIV (Baer, Singer, and Susser 1997). Life stress, such as that associated with poverty and discrimination, appears to be associated with improper immune system function and the onset and course of immune-based diseases like AIDS and cancer (Evens et al. 1997). Malnutrition also may be

a factor in lethality of HIV and other viral diseases because of the mutation patterns of viruses in nutrient-deprived hosts (AP 1996).

This discussion indicates that the nature of the interconnections
between social structure, early childhood health (and mother's health),
and adult health are complex, multifaceted, and require a critical biocultural analysis. Narrow focus on a limited set of variables—including both
biological analysis that ignores sociocultural conditions and sociocultural
analysis that ignores biology—risks misunderstanding the very nature of
health.

Finally, based on its critique of conventional medical anthropology,
CMA incorporates what Elling (1980, 236) termed the *progressive-holistic
perspective:* "Work from [this] perspective understands societies as involving class conflict and sees the state apparatus and medical-health systems
as mediating this conflict in favor of the ruling class in capitalist societies.
The historical developments and political-economic conditions are viewed
as primary, with value orientations and beliefs flowing from these fundamental conditions."

In other words, central to the critical paradigm is a concern with the
embeddedness of "webs of meaning" in "webs of power" (Singer 1997b).
Critical medical anthropology calls attention to the need for an alternative
approach in which symbols and meanings are neither obscured nor unduly
empowered and in which the analysis of the enactment of power is foregrounded and made pivotal to the project of medical anthropology and
beyond.

Nature, Adaptation, Unnatural Selection, and
the Environment

The understandings of health issues developed in CMA over the last
fifteen years have implications for biological anthropology around at least
three core issues: (1) the nature of nature; (2) the utility of the adaptationist perspective; and (3) the causes of ecological destruction. Each of these
will be examined in turn.

Efforts to expand conventional anthropological understanding of
nature have been central to the CMA engagement with issues of
human/environment relationship. Raymond Williams (1980, 6), in his
telling observation that "the idea of nature contains, though often unnoticed, an extraordinary amount of human history," captures a fundamental component of the CMA perspective. Further, in the CMA view, it is

not only the *idea* of nature (the way in which it is conceived) but, in addition, the actual physical reality of nature that has been profoundly influenced by the changing political economy of human society. This approach differs notably from the generally dominant Western worldview in which nature is seen as constituting an autonomous reality that operates in terms of its own principles separate from human society, an understanding that has its roots in the efforts of Enlightenment thinkers to disengage from the spiritual ideology of the eighteenth century.

> Where once nature was seen as sacred, the reflection of a divine plan or the embodiment of Ideas . . . , the Enlightenment task was to 'disenchant' nature and see 'God's world' as a mechanism, composed of physical matter obeying natural mechanistic laws rather than spiritual ones. . . . In the naturalist view, the universe consists of discrete material essences . . . which are fixed and stable in their identity. (Gordon 1988, 24)

Moreover, processes 'in nature' commonly are defined as having an existence that is separate from the workings of society. Nature, in fact, is understood as being "not only independent from culture but prior to it" (Gordon 1988, 27). In everyday speech, the term *nature* commonly is used to refer to areas that allegedly are untarnished by human presence (while the term *human nature* refers to built-in, biologically determined aspects of our behavior that are untainted by societal influence). In this way, it is possible to divide the world into two discrete and contrasting realms, the natural world and the human order. *dictionary – culture/nature*

CMA, by contrast, in attempting to apprehend "the relation of people to their environment in all its complexity" (Turshen 1977, 48) seeks to treat political economy and political ecology as inseparable (O'Connor 1989). As Parson (1977, xii) emphasizes, "economy is a matter of ecology; it has to do with the production and distribution of goods and services in the context of human society and nature." Crosby (1986), who uses the term *ecological imperialism* to label the biological expansion of European life forms into all corners of the globe, has contributed an important concept for the exploration of the impact of capitalist political economy on "nature." What has this impact consisted of? Notes Crosby (1986, 291–92), it involves "a condition of continual disruption: of plowed fields, razed forests, overgrazed pastures, and burned prairies, of deserted villages and expanding cities, of humans, animals, plants, and microlife that have evolved separately suddenly coming into intimate contact." For example:

> In primeval Australia, the weeds called dandelions might have lan-guished in small numbers or even died out, as the weeds the Norse brought to Vinland must have done. We shall never know, because that Australia has not existed for two hundred years. When dande-lions spread, they did so, in a manner of speaking, in another land, one containing and transformed by European humans and their plants, bacteria, sheep, goats, pigs, and horses. In that Australia, dan-delions have a more secure future than kangaroos. (Crosby 1986, 292)

Future theory development in CMA in this regard will benefit from current discussions in the political economy of ecology. This discourse seeks to transcend the productivist ethic and inattention to the contradic-tory aspects of societal-nature interaction that have characterized much political-economic analysis since Marx and Engels. Critical to this avenue of exploration is a reconsideration of human biology in light of political economy. In Duden's (1991) apt phrase, to fully appreciate human biology it is necessary to recognize that there is an entire "history beneath the skin." An important segment of this history has unfolded since the rise of social classes and inegalitarian social relationships, but the impact of this important development on human biology has been largely neglected.

Another critical issue involves the concept of adaptation and its use within the reigning adaptationist perspective (Singer 1989a). Darwinian adaptationism, as Levins and Lewontin (1985) note, is an example of Cartesianism and its tendency to see the world as comprised of atomic units with intrinsic properties, as independent things-in-themselves, as smaller wholenesses merely lumped together as aggregates the way a group of individual potatoes when packaged together constitutes a sack, to use a famous example from Marx. From the adaptationist perspective, there are two primary parts, preformed ecological niches and the organ-isms fitted to them, with adaptation being the process by which organisms adjust biologically and behaviorally to external conditions. However, Levins and Lewontin cogently argue,

> To maintain that organisms adapt to the environment is to maintain that such ecological niches exist in the absence of organisms and that evolution consists in filling these empty and preexistent niches. . . . But

the external world can be divided up in an uncountable infinity of ways, so there is an uncountable infinity of ecological niches. Unless there is a preferred or correct way in which to partition the world, the idea of an ecological niche without an organism filling it loses all meaning. . . . Adaptation cannot be a process of gradual fitting of an organism to the environment if the specific environmental configuration, the ecological niche, does not already exist. If organisms define their own niches, then all species are already adapted, and evolution cannot be seen as the process of *becoming* adapted. (1985, 68)

The whole notion of niches overlooks the shaping effects of "organisms" on the "environment." When these effects are considered, it is clear that "the environment is a product of the organism, just as the organism is a product of the environment" (Levins and Lewontin 1985, 69). Neither of these so-called parts has a privileged existence; both are changing and changing each other in the process. This understanding is grasped quickly in a consideration of the relationship between predator and prey species, where a drop or rise in the size of either group has immediate effects on the size of the other, raising questions about which is to be treated as "organism" and which as "environment." Yet the interrelationship is greater still. For example, "it is often forgotten that the seedling is the 'environment' of the soil, in that the soil undergoes great and lasting evolutionary changes as a direct consequence of the activity of the plants growing in it, and these changes in turn feed back on the organism's conditions of existence" (Levins and Lewontin 1985, 134). Indeed, the very oxygenation process that sustains life on Earth is a product of living organisms, reflecting the "co-evolution of the biosphere and its inhabitants" (Levins and Lewontin 1985, 47).

From the CMA perspective, it is evident that a holistic approach is needed, one that includes political economy as a primary force underlying complex dialectical relationships. Interestingly, advances in this orientation are proceeding most rapidly among Andeanist anthropologists, a group of scholars who until recently tended to construct their area of study as if it were an insulated, discrete, and natural category.

More than the "Oriental," the "Andean," derived from a geological formation, has a concrete ring to it. Perhaps this aura of naturalness helps to explain the historical lack of reflexivity amongst Andeanists about the use of the label. . . . Central to many . . . projections is the imagery of the highlands as a region of "remote," "isolated" mountain villages bracketed out of modernity. The same discourse that removes the peasants to a distant space also typically confines them to a primordial time of "traditional," "premodern," or "ancient" folkways. (Starn 1994, 19)

The adaptationist perspective led Andeanists to focus on physical adaptation to high altitude conditions, the topic still most likely to gain entry of Andean peoples in the texts of biological and biocultural anthropology. While Andeanists recognized the existence of poverty, their "stress on ecological adaptations and sophisticated symbolism had as a consequence a tendency to minimize the full extent of economic suffering across the countryside. Ethnographers usually did little more than mention the terrible infant mortality, minuscule incomes, low life expectancy, inadequate diets, and abysmal health care that remained so routine" (Starn 1994, 168).

In response to the unexpected level of peasant involvement in insurgent movements like Shining Path, as well as engagement with the literature of CMA and the political economy of health, adaptationist thinking among Andeanist anthropologists has given way to broader understandings. Carey (1990), for example, attempts a synthesis of medical ecology and CMA as a corrective to shortcomings in Andeanist research. His analysis of health among children in three communities of the Nuñoa District of Peru found an inverse relationship between altitude and morbidity, which is "directly opposite to what one would expect if physical stressors associated with altitude were the primary factors leading to poor health in the Nuñoa District population" (1990, 285). More significant in the health of the communities under study were social stressors. "Far from being the 'natural' order of things, these social stressors are created by social relations at the local level, which are shaped in turn by larger scale political-economic and sociocultural forces generated by the rest of Peru and beyond" (Carey 1990, 272). To the degree that they have an impact on who lives and who dies, such stressors are an example of unnatural (social) selection, one expression of the potential impact of political-economic factors on human biology (Grim and Wilson 1993; Singer 1996). While Darwin's theory of natural selection has since the 1930s been the dominant scientific understanding of the driving force of biological evolution, a narrow cultural conception of "nature" packed into this theory has diverted attention away from the effects of unnatural selection, that is, the process of differential survival and reproduction under precarious conditions created to serve the interests or as a result of the actions of dominant social groups. In many contexts, unnatural selection may be the primary arbiter of genetic inheritance.

In examining the ameliorative effects of interhousehold social support networks on household well-being, Carey returns to the concept of adaptation. Use of this notion in medical anthropology, however, commonly fails to address the question of "adaptive for whom?" (Singer 1989a). Human groups, even smaller scale communities, are rarely completely homogeneous, and hence "adaptation" tends to favor some strata over others (Leatherman, Carey, and Thomas 1995). In light of the foregoing discussion, CMA asserts that various practices that bioculturalist anthropologists have traditionally called "adaptations" might better be analyzed as social adjustments to the consequences of oppressive sociopolitical relationships. Unable to immediately overcome oppression, human groups commonly adopt a dual pattern: (a) they find ways to "get by" as best they can, while attempting to ameliorate the most painful aspects of the oppression; (b) they find ways to ignore, mock, or resist the oppression, overtly or covertly. Portraying psychosocial strategies of this sort as adaptation/adaptability distorts the actual social processes involved, processes that may, in time, lead, as they did in the Andes, to more open rebellion.

Finally, CMA has addressed the implications of ecological homogenization and outright environmental destruction. As Bodley reminds us, human societies have precipitated ecological crisis throughout their long history.

> Tribal hunters have contributed to the creation of grasslands; pastoral nomads have overgrazed their lands; peasant farmers have caused deforestation and erosion. From archeological evidence, it is clear that tribal cultures and early civilization at times faced their own local environmental crisis as imbalances occurred, and were forced to abandon certain regions or drastically alter their cultures. (1985, 27)

The dawn of agrarian states produced a far-reaching transformation in society/environment relations. The dangers of ecological self-destruction that plagued archaic and feudal state societies, however, pale by comparison with those of industrial capitalism. As contrasted with the relatively limited environmental modification wrought by pre-state and ancient state societies, the capitalist world system, with its culture of consumption, "introduces completely new environmental pollutants that disrupt natural biochemical processes" (Bodley 1985, 49). Capitalism, pushed by its inherent drive to reap greater profits, increase production, and capture new markets, historically has assumed that natural "resources" (i.e., those elements of the natural world valued by society at any point in time), not only minerals but water, fertile soil, trees, and much more, exist in unlimited supply in nature's bountiful storehouse. While the emergence of a capitalist world system contributed to the production of a plentiful (if not equitably distributed) food supply (including large quantities of nutritionally questionable foodstuffs), modern sanitation, and the powerful cures of biomedicine, these material benefits were obtained at the expense of the masses of people in the Third World and oppressed classes in the First World. Moreover, they were obtained often at the expense of perilous environmental damage. This destruction has significant implications for the health of many if not all human populations, including the potential well-being of future generations.

As Barnet and Cavanagh stress, capitalist production threatens the environment at four distinct points: (1) at the point of production significant quantities of toxic substances are poured into the environment and "are being spread around the world to countries willing to exchange breathable air for jobs" (1994, 289); (2) packaging of products for market appeal consumes large quantities of natural resources; (3) the products themselves increasingly are high consumers of fuel; and (4) planned obsolescence and reduced durability of products drives new wasteful production. Significantly, countries at the core of the capitalist world system have attempted to export pollutants to countries in the periphery, as exemplified by the case of the Khian Sea which set sail for Haiti in October 1987 with 13,000 tons of toxic incinerator ash from Philadelphia. The ash was dumped on a Haitian beach, only to be shoveled back aboard ship (minus 2,000 tons left behind on shore) when Haitian officials discovered it was not the fertilizer that had been promised. The Khian Sea spent the next fourteen months cruising the globe seeking a third world country from Senegal to Sri Lanka willing to accept its toxic cargo. World attention frightened off would-be takers, and the ash was eventually dumped into the Indian Ocean.

Within the capitalist world system, even postrevolutionary socialist-oriented countries have had a wretched environmental record. The former Soviet Union exhibited some of the worst historic occurrences of radioactive contamination, while the former Czechoslovakia and Poland had the highest levels of industrial pollution in Europe if not the world. Separation of these countries from their place in the world system, a common strategy of those whose primary agenda is disparaging socialism, leads to a mystification of the origins of widespread pollution in socialist-oriented countries. As Yih (1990, 22) notes, understanding the environmental record of these countries in part can be

> explained by the conditions under which socialist governments came into being—relative underdevelopment, external aggression, and, especially for the small dependent economies of the Third World, a disadvantaged position in the international market. The corresponding pressures to satisfy the material needs of the populations, ensure adequate defense, and continue producing and exporting cash crops and raw materials for foreign exchange, have led to an emphasis by socialist policy-makers on accumulation by the state, the uncritical adoption of many features of capitalist development, and a largely abysmal record vis-à-vis the environment (although there are exceptions, of course).

Full reincorporation of former socialist-oriented economies into the capitalist fold appears likely to exacerbate environmental problems rather than resolve them.

Conclusion

What are the implications of the emergence of a critical medical anthropology for future directions in biological anthropology? Before answering this question directly, it is important to address several issues that might lead some biological anthropologists to conclude that critical medical anthropology is not relevant to biological anthropology. Contrary to what has sometimes been asserted, as the foregoing discussion suggests, CMA does not advocate a rejection of biology as a critical area of anthropological study nor does it devalue the importance of the environment in shaping culture; that is to say, it does not heed the idealist or postmodern calls for a shift away from a materialist perspective in science. These points are important because there is a knee-jerk tendency to lump together all of one's critics and assume they embrace a common program. While CMA maintains a critical stance toward science, predicated on the recognition that science and its concepts are historically situated, culturally created, and socially influenced, and, as a result, cannot help but incorporate and promote tenets of the dominant ideology, CMA's ultimate objective is better science rather than a literary turn away from scientific ways of knowing (Singer 1993). Ignoring the sociocultural (and hence political-economic) nature of science does not seem a useful approach for avoiding unscientific influences on the research process (Blakey 1987).

Still these comments raise an unavoidable question. As posed by Radnitzky (1968, 35), "If all anthropological knowledge is relative [to time, place, and social structure], how do we meaningfully choose between alternatives?" On what basis can such choices be made? Growing from the long-standing anthropological identification with the experience and striving of the oppressed, CMA asserts that its mission is consciously emancipatory and partisan: it aims not simply to understand but to change culturally inappropriate, oppressive, and exploitive patterns in the health arena and beyond (Singer 1995). This stance does not express a disregard for sound empirical research nor does it indicate an acceptance of the conscious shaping of research findings to meet preconceived political expectations. Rather, it calls attention to the folly of so-called value-free science. As Bellah (1977, xi–xii) points out:

> Many of us, frightened by Weber's contempt for those who use the lecture platform for political or religious prophecy, have forgotten that value neutrality had for Weber a very specific and a very confined meaning, namely the obligation not to let our value predilections dictate the results of our research, and that it was itself a moral norm, a tenet of scholarship. What is dangerous is not the presence of value judgments—they can be found in almost every line that Weber wrote—but only those judgments that remain beyond the reach of critical reflection and are not subject to revision in the light of experience.

Gould (1992, 17) adds that "fair and scrupulous procedures do not demand neutrality, but only strict adherence to the rules of the craft." The rules of the craft in this instance, of course, include a set of scientific procedures to control bias in research. CMA embraces these standards because its goal is to produce the most accurate data possible so that praxis emanating from its research can be useful in changing oppressive conditions or relieving suffering. More broadly, the intent of CMA is to achieve a thoroughgoing synthesis of theory and the emergence of an integrated medical anthropology that is equally sensitive to bioenvironmental factors in health, the experience of suffering among those who are ill, and the primacy of political economy in shaping the impact of bioenvironmental factors on disease, sufferer experience, and the character of the health care system deployed in response to disease and illness.

The possibilities for a similar synthesis are under review now in biological anthropology. In part, concern with exploring this terrain grows from a recognition by some that the field has become overly specialized, exceedingly narrow, and atheoretical in its focus. No longer can whole trees, let alone the forest of which each individual tree is but an interacting part, be glimpsed by the microscopic lens adopted in much research in biological anthropology. Indeed, questions have been raised as to whether it is reasonable to call some of the work now done in the name of biological anthropology by that label. Certainly, many have complained about the inattention to living populations in the field's leading journal. At the same time, there is uneasiness that biological and cultural anthropology are drifting apart and will soon lose a common language and set of concepts by which to communicate about overlapping interests. Finally, there is a growing recognition that human evolution and, especially, human adaptability, unfold in a world in which unequal and oppressive social relations are ultimately determinant. In short, it would appear that biological anthropology, no less than medical anthropology, is, to use the poignant terminology of Eldredge and Gould, in an evolutionary punctuation, a period of potentially rapid change to a new order of being.

As it grapples with alternative frames of reference, seeking to take a broader, more encompassing, more politically aware view of its subject matter, biological anthropology will likely confront many of the issues now under discussion in medical anthropology, including the role of theory in the forging of research questions, the social responsibility of the scientist in an oppressive social world, the feasibility of value-free research, the influence of dominant ideology on scientific understandings, the shortcomings inherent in the notion of adaptation, the nature of nature in light of human history, the role of unnatural (social) selection in human evolution, the historic causes of disciplinary formation, and the importance of transcending the productivist ethic. What shape will the new biological anthropology take? Gould (1992, 21) offers a hopeful answer: "modern punctuationalism—especially in its application to the vagaries of human history—emphasizes the concept of contingency: the unpredictability of the nature of future stability, and the power of contemporary events and personalities to shape and direct the actual path taken among myriad possibilities. . . . Perhaps we will punctuate to a better place."

REFERENCES

Abercrombie, N., S. Hill, and B. Turner. 1980. *The Dominant Ideology.* London: George Allen and Unwin Ltd.

Alland, A. 1966. Medical Anthropology and the Study of Biological and Cultural Adaptation. *American Anthropologist* 68:40–51.

Armelagos, G., T. Leatherman, M. Ryan, and L. Sibley. 1991. Biocultural Synthesis in Medical Anthropology. *Medical Anthropology* 14 (1): 35–52.

Associated Press. 1996. Malnutrition May Heighten Danger of Virus Mutation. *Hartford Courant,* April 17, p. 6.

Baer, H. 1981. The Organizational Rejuvenation of Osteopathy: A Reflection of the Decline of Professional Dominance in Medicine. *Social Science and Medicine* 15A:701–11.

Baer, H. 1982. On the Political Economy of Health. *Medical Anthropology Newsletter* 14 (1): 1–3, 13–17.

Baer, H. 1986. Sociological Contributions to the Political Economy of Health: Lessons for Medical Anthropologists. *Medical Anthropology Quarterly,* o.s., 17:129–31.

Baer, H., M. Singer, and J. Johnsen. 1986. Toward a Critical Medical Anthropology. *Social Science and Medicine* 23:95–98.

Baer, H., M. Singer, and I. Susser. 1997. *Medical Anthropology and the World System.* Westport, CT: Bergin and Garvey.

Barker, D., and C. Osmond. 1986. Infant Mortality, Childhood Nutrition, and Ischaemic Heart Disease in England and Wales. *The Lancet* May 10: 1077–81.

Barker, D., A. Bull, C. Osmond, and S. Simmonds. 1990. Fetal and Placental Size and Risk of Hypertension in Adult Life. *British Medical Journal* 30:259–62.

Barnet, R., and J. Cavanagh. 1994. *Global Dream: Imperial Corporations and the New World Order.* New York: Simon and Schuster.

Bellah, R. 1977. Foreword. In *Reflections on Fieldwork in Morocco,* ed. P. Rabinow. Berkeley: University of California Press.

Blakey, M. 1987. Skull Doctors: Intrinsic Social and Political Bias in the History of American Physical Anthropology with Special Reference to the Work of Aleš Hrdlička. *Critique of Anthropology* 7 (2): 7–35.

Bodley, J. 1985. *Anthropology and Contemporary Human Problems.* Palo Alto, CA: Mayfield.

Brown, E. R. 1979. *Rockefeller Medicine Men.* Berkeley: University of California Press.

Carey, J. 1990. Social System Effects on Local Level Morbidity and Adaptation in the Peruvian Andes. *Medical Anthropology Quarterly* 4:266–95.

Colby, B. 1988. Comment on a Metology for Cross-cultural Ethnomedical Research. *Current Anthropology* 29 (5): 691.

Craddock, D. 1976. *A Short Textbook of General Practice.* London: H. K. Lewis and Co. Ltd.

Crosby, A. 1986. *Ecological Imperialism: The Biological Expansion of Europe, 900–1900.* Cambridge: Cambridge University Press.

de Swaan, A. 1989. The Reluctant Imperialism of the Medical Profession. *Social Science and Medicine* 28:1165–70.

Doyal, L. 1979. *The Political Economy of Health.* Boston: Southend Press.

Duden, B. 1991. *The Women Beneath the Skin.* Cambridge, MA: Harvard University Press.

Elling, R. 1980. *Cross-National Study of Health Systems.* New York: Transaction Books.

Erwin, D. 1987 The Militarization of Cancer Treatment in American Society. In *Encounters with Biomedicine,* ed. H. Baer, 201–27. New York: Gordon and Breach.

Evens, D., J. Leserman, D. Perkins, R. Stern, C. Murphy, B. Zheng, D. Gettes, J. Longmate, S. Silva, C. van der Horst, C. Hall, J. Folds, R. Golden, and J. Petitto. 1997. Severe Life Stress as a Predictor of Early Disease Progression in HIV infection. *American Journal of Psychiatry* 154:630–34.

Figlio, K. 1983. Chlorosis and Chronic Disease in Nineteenth-Century Britain: The Social Constitution of Somatic Illness in a Capitalist Society. In *Women and Health: The Politics of Sex in Medicine,* ed. E. Fee, 213–41. Farmingdale, NY: Baywood Publishing Company.

Genovese, E. 1974. *Roll, Jordan, Roll.* New York: Vintage Books.

Giddens, A. 1987. *Sociology: A Brief But Critical Introduction.* San Diego: Harcourt Brace Jovanovich.

Gillies, G. 1976. Introduction. In *Witchcraft Oracles and Magic among the Azande,* ed. E. E. Evans-Pritchard. London: Oxford University Press.

Gordon, D. 1988. Clinical Science and Clinical Expertise: Changing Boundaries Between Art and Science in Medicine. In *Biomedicine Examined,* ed. M. Lock and D. Gordon, 257–95. Dordrecht: Kluwer Academic Publishers.

Gould, S. J. 1992. Life in a Punctuation. *Natural History* 101 (10): 10–21.

Grim, C., and T. Wilson. 1993. Salt, Slavery, and Survival: Physiological Principles of the Evolutionary Hypothesis on Hypertension among Western Hemisphere Blacks. In *Pathophysiology of Hypertension in Blacks,* ed. J. Fray and J. Douglas, 123–35. Oxford: Oxford University Press.

Johnson, T., and C. Sargent. 1990. *Medical Anthropology: Contemporary Theory and Method.* New York: Praeger.

Kapferer, B. 1988. Gramsci's Body and a Critical Medical Anthropology. *Medical Anthropology Quarterly* 3:426–32.

Kelman, S. 1971. Toward the Political Economy of Medical Care. *Inquiry* 8:30–38.

Kirmayer, L. 1988. Mind and Body as Metaphors: Hidden Values in Biomedicine. In *Biomedicine Examined,* ed. M. Lock and D. Gordon, 57–94. Dordrecht: Kluwer Academic Publishers.

Koegel, P., E. Melamid, and A. Burnam. 1995. Childhood Risk Factors for Homelessness among Homeless Adults. *American Journal of Public Health* 85: 1642–49.

Krause, E. 1977. *Power and Illness: The Political Sociology of Health and Medical Care.* New York: Elsevier North-Holland.

Kuper, A. 1983. *Anthropology and Anthropologists: The Modern British School.* London: Routledge and Kegan Paul.

Landy, D. 1977. Introduction: Learning and Teaching Medical Anthropology. In *Culture, Disease, and Healing,* ed. D. Landy, 1–9. New York: Macmillan.

Landy, D. 1993. Medical Anthropology: A Critical Appraisal. In *Advances in Medical Social Science,* ed. J. Ruffini, 185–314. New York: Gordon and Breach Science Publishers.

Leatherman, T., J. Carey, and R. B. Thomas. 1995. Socioeconomic Changes and Patterns of Growth in the Andes. *American Journal of Physical Anthropology* 97:307–21.

Levins, R., and R. Lewontin. 1985. *The Dialectical Biologist.* Cambridge, MA: Harvard University Press.

Martin, E. 1987. *The Woman in the Body: A Cultural Analysis of Reproduction.* Boston: Beacon.

Martin, E. 1990. Toward an Anthropology of Immunology: The Body as Nation State. *Medical Anthropology Quarterly* 4 (4): 410–26.

Martin, E. 1994. *Flexible Bodies.* Boston: Beacon Press.

Marx, K. [1859] 1970. *A Contribution to the Critique of Political Economy.* New York: International.

Morsy, S. 1990. Political Economy in Medical Anthropology. In *Medical Anthropology: Contemporary Theory and Method,* ed. T. Johnson and C. Sargent, 26–36. New York: Praeger.

Navarro, V. 1982. The Labor Process and Health: A Historical Materialist Interpretation. *International Journal of Health Services* 12 (1): 5–29.

Navarro, V. 1985. U.S. Marxist Scholarship in the Analysis of Health and Medicine. *International Journal of Health Services* 15:525–45.

O'Connor, J. 1989. The Political Economy of Ecology of Socialism and Capitalism. *Capitalism, Nature, Socialism* 3:93–127.

Ollman, B. 1971. *Alienation: Marx's Conception of Man in Capitalist Society.* Cambridge: Cambridge University Press.

Parson, H. 1977. *Marx and Engels on Ecology.* Westport, CT: Greenwood.

Peacock, J. 1995. Claiming Common Ground. *Anthropology Newsletter* 4 (36):1, 3.

Pérez-Escamilla, R., D. Himmelgreen, and A. Ferris. 1996. *The Food and Nutrition Situation of Inner-city Latino Preschoolers in Hartford: A Preliminary Needs Assessment.* Hartford: University of Connecticut and Hispanic Health Council.

Pfifferling, J.-H. 1981. A Cultural Prescription for Medicocentrism. In *The Relevance of Social Science for Medicine,* ed. L. Eisenberg and A. Kleinman, 197–222. Dordrecht: D. Reidel Publishing Co.

Radnitzky, G. 1968. *Continental Schools of Meta-Science.* Göteborg: Akademiforlaget.

Roberts, H. 1985. *The Patient Patients: Women and Their Doctors.* London: Pandora Press.

Roseberry, W. 1989. *Anthropologies and Histories.* New Brunswick, NJ: Rutgers University Press.

Scotch, N. 1963. Medical Anthropology. In *Biennial Review of Anthropology,* ed. B. Siegel, 30–68. Stanford: Stanford University Press.

Scully, D., and P. Bart. 1973. A Funny Thing Happened to Me on the Way to the Orifice: Women in Gynaecological Textbooks. *American Journal of Sociology* 78 (4): 1045–49.

Singer, M. 1989a. The Limitations of Medical Ecology: The Concept of Adaptation in the Context of Social Stratification and Social Transformation. *Medical Anthropology* 10 (4): 218–29.

Singer, M. 1989b. The Coming of Age of Critical Medical Anthropology. *Social Science and Medicine* 28:1193–1204.

Singer, M. 1992. The Application of Theory in Medical Anthropology. *Medical Anthropology,* special issue, 14 (1).

Singer, M. 1993. A Rejoinder to Wiley's Critique of Critical Medical Anthropology. *Medical Anthropology Quarterly* 7 (2): 185–91.

Singer, M. 1995. Beyond the Ivory Tower: Critical Praxis in Medical Anthropology. *Medical Anthropology Quarterly* 9 (1): 80–106.

Singer, M. 1996. Farewell to Adaptationalism: Unnatural Selection and the Politics of Biology. *Medical Anthropology Quarterly* 10:496–515.

Singer, M. 1997a. *The Political Economy of AIDS.* Amityville, NY: Baywood.

Singer, M. 1997b. Articulating Personal Experience and Political Economy in the AIDS Epidemic: The Case of Carlos Torres. In *The Political Economy of AIDS,* M. Singer, ed. 1–74. Amityville, NY: Baywood.

Singer, M., and H. Baer. 1995. *Critical Medical Anthropology.* Amityville, NY: Baywood.

Stark, E. 1982. Doctors in Spite of Themselves: The Limits of Radical Health Criticism. *International Journal of Health Services* 12:419–57.

Starn, O. 1992. Missing the Revolution: Anthropologists and the War in Peru. In *Rereading Cultural Anthropology,* ed. G. Marcus, 152–80. Durham, NC: Duke University.

Starn, O. 1994. Rethinking the Politics of Anthropology: The Case of the Andes. *Current Anthropology* 35 (1): 13–38.

Turshen, M. 1977. *The Politics of Public Health.* New Brunswick, NJ: Rutgers University.

Waitzkin, H. 1981. The Social Origins of Illness: A Neglected History. *International Journal of Health Services* 11:77–103.

Williams, R. 1980. *Problems in Materialism and Culture.* London: Verso.

Wolf, E. 1982. *Europe and the People Without History.* Berkeley: University of California Press.

Woolhandler, S., and D. Himmelstein. 1989. Ideology in Medical Science: Class in the Clinic. *Social Science and Medicine* 28:1205–09.

Yih, K. 1990. The Red and the Green. *Monthly Review* 42 (5): 16–27.

Young, A. 1982. The Anthropologies of Illness and Sickness. *Annual Review of Anthropology* 11:257–85.

PART 2

Case Studies and Examples: Past Populations

Chapter 5

Linking Political Economy and Human Biology: Lessons from North American Archaeology

Dean J. Saitta

Archaeologists, with a unique view of relationships between environment, society, and human biology over large units of space and time, like to emphasize the importance of their discipline for understanding the human condition. Archaeology thus can provide a long-term, historical perspective on human survival problems and the relative costs and benefits of different strategies (e.g., technoeconomic, organizational) for coping with those problems.

The study of health in prehistory has amply demonstrated its relevance to archaeology's goal of understanding the biocultural consequences of different survival strategies. The study of human remains is perhaps the best means available for identifying patterns of resource deprivation and differential activity within and between human groups, and hence relative social inequality. Because many important stressors leave indelible marks on human bone, bioarchaeology can potentially circumvent some of the difficult problems with inferring social inequality from other lines of archaeological evidence such as house size variation, interhousehold wealth differentials, settlement hierarchies, and so on (e.g., see White 1985; Reid and Whittlesey 1990).

As with any set of archaeological observations, however, the social *meaning* of documented variation (or lack thereof) in biological well-being for any given case is not transparent. Biological markers could be the product of many different processes, and we cannot always read straightforwardly from observable patterns in bioarchaeological data to political-economic reality. A variety of historically specific "contextual" factors—ecological, biological, political, economic, and cultural—affect human health and thereby complicate bioarchaeological interpretation. Bioar-chaeologists have long been aware of this multiplicity of causes and have recently engaged in stimulating debate about it (e.g., Wood et al. 1992; Goodman 1993).

From the perspective of this chapter, the recognition of complexity is as exciting as it is sobering. It is exciting because it is in the complications of real-world archaeological and bioarchaeological data—especially the incongruities between expected and observed patterns, or what Binford (1987) and Leone (1988) term *ambiguity*—that clues to novel organiza-tional arrangements and alternative causal dynamics are to be found. The challenge in dealing with ambiguity so as to recognize novelty of process and cause, as bioarchaeologists have also pointed out, is to develop theory sensitive to the myriad contextual forces that shape human social life and biology, and to use multiple lines of evidence to evaluate that theory (see especially Goodman 1993).

This paper takes up the theoretical challenge from a Marxist, class-analytical perspective. This perspective takes human labor as the entry point to analysis of the social lives and biological well-being of humans. More pointedly, it sees the production and distribution of social labor as a useful entry point for integrating political economy and human biology.

The first part of the paper outlines the basic structure and organizing assumptions of a class-analytical Marxist theory. It specifies the kinds of social differences created by labor flows, the relationships between labor flows and other social processes, and the implications for understanding human health and nutritional patterns.

The second part examines case material from North American archae-ology as a way to further develop theory and open new research directions. Material from the Mississippian Southeast and the Anasazi Southwest—two areas abundant in empirical ambiguity and interpretive uncertainty—is especially useful in this regard.

The conclusion summarizes the theoretical and methodological chal-lenges facing bioarchaeological research in North America and beyond.

Human Labor and Biology in Marxist Theory

The distinctiveness of Marxist theory lies in its focus on the varied forms and conditions under which surplus labor is appropriated and distributed in society. By surplus labor, I mean the time and energy expended beyond the amount required (termed *necessary labor*) to meet the subsistence needs of individuals. That all societies produce surplus labor was one of Marx's key insights, and this basic idea has been developed in anthropology by, among others, Harris (1959), Wolf (1966), and Cook (1977). Surplus labor or its fruit (surplus product) is required to replace tools and other items used up in the production process; provide insurance against productive shortfalls; care for the sick, infirm, and other nonproducers; fund administrative positions; and satisfy common social and cultural needs (Cook 1977, 372).

Arrangements for mobilizing social labor vary widely in form. A vast literature examines these variations (e.g., Marx 1964; Hindess and Hirst 1975; Wessman 1981; Wolf 1982; contributors to Seddon 1978 and Kahn and Llobera 1981). Among the forms of the labor process that have been defined are the communal, tributary, and capitalist. Each form of surplus production is broadly governed by different social relationships: by kinship relations in the communal form; by political-jural relations in the tributary form; and by the marketing of human labor power in the capitalist form. In Marxist theory, any single organizational entity (e.g., a society, a community, a household) can contain one or more ways of producing surplus labor.

Because the organization of social labor governs activity patterns and the allocation of goods and services in society, it directly affects biological well-being. Extrapolating from Huss-Ashmore and Johnston (1985, 497–98), labor relations

1. determine the division between necessary and surplus labor or, in other words, between the "caloric minimum" required for the reproduction of individuals and the labor required for reproducing aggregates of individuals;
2. influence decisions about production strategies (including choice of strategy and the intensity of work) for meeting caloric minima and the variety of social demands for surplus. This in turn can place differential mechanical stresses on individuals;
3. govern consumption patterns within social units such as households; i.e., how resources are distributed, in what amounts, and to whom. This can disproportionately benefit some individuals and discriminate against others, often along lines of gender and age.

Understanding the social dynamic inherent in different forms of labor appropriation and its biological consequences requires theory that addresses difference at the level of individual human agents. Marx recognized that the process of producing and distributing surplus labor inevitably created such differences. Specifically, it sorted people into producers, appropriators, distributors, and recipients of surplus labor. For Marx, these differences defined positions in a set of *class* processes (1967). That is, Marx defined class as an individual's position in a *relationship* of surplus labor flow. This is in contrast to non-Marxist definitions of class as the differential possession of wealth, property, power, or some combination thereof (Resnick and Wolff 1986).[1]

The Marxist economists Resnick and Wolff (1987, 109–63) further clarify the nature of these labor relationships by breaking down the class process into two different, but closely connected kinds of surplus flow. One kind of flow is the initial production and appropriation of surplus labor. This can be termed the *fundamental* class process. Using conventional Marxist categories, we can distinguish communal, tributary, and capitalist forms of the fundamental class process. Producers and appropriators of surplus within each form are thus the fundamental classes in society—they occupy fundamental class positions.[2]

The second kind of surplus flow is the *subsumed* class process. This refers to the distribution of surplus labor *by* the appropriators *to* specific individuals who provide the political, economic, and cultural conditions that allow a particular fundamental class process—or multiple fundamental class processes—to exist. Such individuals may include people who make decisions about the allocation of labor to productive tasks; who regulate the distribution of necessary factors of production (e.g., tools and land); who distribute the surplus product to nonproducers; and who help create forms of consciousness among producers that are compatible with particular productive relationships. Distributors and recipients of surplus labor are thus the subsumed classes in society and occupy subsumed class positions. A number of different subsumed classes can exist in society, which in turn place a variety of drains on appropriated surplus.[3]

In Marxist theory, fundamental and subsumed class processes provide the conditions of each other's existence. Other conditions of existence are provided by a host of *nonclass* social processes. These nonclass processes do not involve flows of surplus labor, but rather other kinds of interactions that affect the production and distribution of surplus. For example, various kinds of power/authority relations can affect who is placed in what class position(s) and how they perform their roles. The nature and status of social exchange relationships (e.g., the existence of various forms of debt and obligation) can influence decisions about the conduct and intensity of household labor appropriation. Traffic in cultural meanings—meanings that shape the self and social consciousness of producers—can affect the willingness of people to participate in particular class (and other nonclass) processes. Nonclass processes are thus as important as class processes for understanding social production and reproduction. People confront each other not only in these nonclass relationships, but also in the rules that govern access to, and control over, nonclass social positions and practices. Some of these rules and practices are, as mentioned, provided and reinforced by the activities of subsumed classes.

Recognizing the potential for variable linkages between class and nonclass social processes is as important as recognizing individual human agency. This is especially crucial for understanding ambiguity in archaeological contexts, as I suspect that much ambiguity is created by novel combinations of class and nonclass processes. Marxist theory recognizes that any given fundamental class process can be sustained by a variety of nonclass processes. Some of these combinations may be counterintuitive. Communal forms of surplus appropriation, for example, do not require full *equality* of access to resources (Patterson 1991; Keene 1991; Lee 1992). What matters is the maintenance of some measure of *guaranteed* access to socially determined portions of necessary and surplus labor, or what Rosenberg (1990, cited in Lee 1992, 40) terms *entitlements*. Neither does communalism require the absence of formal, even institutionalized social hierarchy; what matters is the specific relationship between hierarchy and surplus appropriation (Resnick and Wolff 1988, 27–28). In short, communalism can be compatible with a variety of socially regulated forms of economic and political inequality as might be archaeologically indicated by house size variation, specialized craft production, prestige goods exchange, and settlement hierarchies, provided that most surplus labor is communally appropriated and access to social entitlements is guaranteed.

This Marxist analytical framework thus expects complexity in the social relations that organize labor flows at *all* ranges of societal scale, from kin-communal formations to industrial capitalist formations. Individuals are expected to participate in a variety of class and nonclass processes in both domestic and wider public spheres. In addition, they are expected to participate in a variety of class and nonclass struggles over labor flow and its various conditions of existence. Fundamental classes can struggle over the amounts of necessary and surplus labor produced in society, and over the form surplus labor takes (i.e., whether in goods, services, or some combination of the two). Subsumed classes can struggle with fundamental producers and also among themselves over the size and allocation of shares of appropriated surplus. Finally, people differentially positioned in nonclass processes can struggle over power relations, various economic conditions (e.g., how labor is divided and exchange regulated), and the cultural meanings that sustain fundamental and subsumed class processes. The precise character of these struggles and their outcome depends on the form of surplus appropriation and other local circumstances—making prediction difficult but not impossible.

Marxist theory thus eschews "classless" models of society that homogenize social labor processes and positions, as well as simple "two-class" models that oppose exploitative elites to subordinate commoners. Instead, individuals can have varied social positions, roles, and sources of support. Individuals can be producers of surplus labor at some institutional "sites" in society (e.g., field or workplace) but extractors at others (e.g., within households). Similarly, "elites" may be extractors of surplus (as in tributary formations), subsumed recipients of surplus who lack direct control over labor (as in communal formations), or both. The variable and problematic positions of individuals within class and nonclass processes create a mosaic of tensions, strategies and impulses to change which in turn can affect individual physiologies.

Finally, Marxist theory does not expect any particular form of surplus production to have necessary biological correlates or consequences, given the potential for variation in labor's nonclass conditions of existence and other historical factors. Class divisions may not lead to health and nutritional differences among people, if other complicating factors intervene. By the same token, health and nutritional differences may not necessarily reflect class divisions. I can imagine a scenario for communal formations in which economic goods and ritual items (i.e., prestige goods) have broadly equivalent cultural values and are reciprocally exchanged for each other, resulting in health differences between the exchanging parties without exploitation of one by the other. Such "unequal" exchanges could even become institutionalized as a way to create a complementarity of groups in a wider, integrated regional network. In this scenario, cultural factors intervene to create differing health profiles in the context of basically communal relations of production.

On the assumption that different political economies are not necessarily associated with specific patterns of biological advantage and deprivation, research must be contextual, with biological patterns viewed in the context of local cultures and histories. In the next section I examine case material from prehistoric North America as way to further develop a Marxist theory for understanding biocultural relationships in prehistory.

Class and Health in Prehistory: North American Cases

North American prehistory is a good place to explore organizational variation, including the complex relationships between social labor and human biology. Empirical research on prehistoric cultural and biological patterns attests to the diverse experiences of indigenous populations. These patterns challenge traditional interpretive models and suggest alternative political economies and causal dynamics.

Two geographical areas, the Mississippian Southeast and the Anasazi Southwest, are particularly interesting because of their potential to inform on alternative organizational possibilities. In this section I consider bioarchaeological patterns in each area and their broader social meaning, as understood through Marxist theory. Although it is difficult to provide conclusive interpretations given limitations of theory and data, some preliminary ideas can be sketched that raise new research questions and point the way to more exact interpretive models.

Mississippian Southeast

The traditional view of the Mississippian as a monolithic, homogeneous archaeological culture is currently yielding to one emphasizing a "mosaic" of regional variants and a diversity of developmental trajectories (Smith 1991, 168; see also Milner 1990, 21–23). Scholars have documented variation among Mississippians in the rate at which maize agriculture was adopted, in the uses to which early cultigens were put (whether economic or symbolic), and in the overall degree of agricultural dependence (Smith 1986; Rose, Marks, and Tieszen 1991). Variation has also been documented in rules of political succession, including combinations of ascription and achievement (Blakely 1977; Scarry 1992). Finally, differences have been mapped in the size, geographical scale, and developmental histories of political entities (Steponaitis 1991, 216).

The biological well-being of Mississippian peoples also appears to have varied considerably across time, space, and social context. At some major centers where social hierarchy appears well-established on architectural and mortuary evidence, biological differences between "elites" and "commoners" are not significant. Powell (1991, 1992), for example, shows that general health at Moundville was not compromised by political hierarchization. The Moundville chiefs were neither significantly better nourished nor less disease-ridden than the working populace. Powell also shows that biological patterns at other Mississippian centers present a similarly mixed picture (1992, 48–49). The finding that elites appear not to have benefited much from their "empowered" status violates an expectation of the traditional two-class model for ranked societies and opens the door to alternative interpretive possibilities (Smith 1991, 169).

Interestingly, general health at some other Mississippian centers appears to have been *inferior* to that at peripheral settlements. Humpf (1992) shows that the protohistoric mound center of Little Egypt (northwest Georgia) had poorer health as measured by enamel hypoplasias, dental caries, stature, and longevity than the outlying and presumably subordinate nonmound towns of Etowah and King. Possible explanations for this include Little Egypt's greater population density, political inability to sustain tribute collection from outliers, and earlier contact with disease-carrying Europeans. However, the lessons of other pre- and protohistoric Mississippian centers (including Moundville, which was similarly aggregated yet whose denizens nonetheless enjoyed good health) suggests that a single factor is not responsible for Little Egypt's generally poor health profile. Rather, causation must have been more complex.

In other parts of the Mississippian world, peripheral populations were clearly hurting, in the sense of having greater disease loads (pathologies, lesions, anemias) and reduced longevity. These areas include Dickson Mounds in Illinois (Goodman et al. 1984; Goodman and Armelagos 1985; Goodman, this vol., chap. 6) and Averbuch in Tennessee (Eisenberg 1991). Data from these areas directly raise the issue of exploitation in the Mississippian world. Goodman and Armelagos suggest that populations living in the vicinity of Dickson were suffering from unequal long-distance exchange relationships with, if not tributary exploitation by, the greatest of Mississippian political centers, Cahokia. Eisenberg (1991, 86) hints that tributary relations directly enmeshed Averbuch. Milner (1990, 26–27), however, challenges the inference of large-scale tributary relations emanating from Cahokia. He suggests that Cahokian exploitation of the Dickson area would have been logistically difficult and thus impractical given the distances involved, and he also questions the notion on empirical grounds (see also Emerson 1991). If Milner is correct, then some other factor or factors must be responsible for the biological deprivation evident at Dickson and, conceivably, at Averbuch as well.[4]

In short, the Mississippian record potentially reveals interesting discrepancies between health patterns and other demographic, settlement, and architectural patterns. Biological and material variation within and between Mississippian polities precludes simple unicausal or universal explanations (Humpf 1992, 130; Smith 1991, 168). It is unclear what social organizations are indicated by the combined biological and cultural patterns, or what the factors creating nutritional deprivation were. However the patterns do, I think, undermine any simple, two-class model of chiefly elites and subordinate commoners (see also Milner 1991, 53–54, for a similar view). In my opinion they invite more nuanced models of how labor and resources flowed through Mississippian political economies.

One alternative model would view Mississippian polities as variants of complex communal formations, where surpluses are collectively produced and distributed in the context of nonclass political, economic, and cultural relations of variable (and still dimly perceived) form and complexity. In these models "elites" are subsumed recipients of communal surplus labor, rather than fundamental classes of tribute-takers. In other words, elites receive subsumed class shares of communal surplus labor in either service (e.g., agricultural field work—see Scarry 1992), goods (e.g., animal protein—see Welch 1991), or both, as compensation for brokering trade in prestige goods (which can be viewed as communal *ritual* entitlements necessary for legitimating initiations, marriages, and other important life transition events), redistributing people over the landscape, administering communal undertakings such as moundbuilding, and so on.

Ethnography provides a warrant for expecting these kinds of relationships. Harrison (1987) describes a regional system among tribal polities in Melanesia in which a variety of material values (e.g., yams, fish, shell) are exchanged for various ritual values (e.g., totems, spirits, myths, spells, initiatory sacra). Piot (1992) documents a similar movement of economic values against ritual values within a single society (the Kabre) in West Africa. Harrison shows how the Melanesian exchanges can benefit the purveyors of symbolic goods and lead to incipient social ranking, while Piot shows how the African exchanges create social differences that are in fact *necessary* for the maintenance of complementarity and interdependency (and hence a broad equality) among different communities in an integrated regional system. The general point here is that each ethnographic example substantiates a complex relationship between tribal politics, economics, and ideology that conceivably can create health differences in the absence of fundamental class divisions.

Such complexity may also have characterized Mississippian social relationships, given the biological patterns discussed above and equivocal support for tributary models at even the most impressive Mississippian mound centers (e.g., see Welch's 1991 consideration of alternative models for Moundville). Populations in some areas (such as at Moundville) fared well under complex relationships of communality, while others (such as in the Dickson Mounds area), suffered. The key point is that the nutritional deprivation that existed in the Mississippian world may not have resulted from economic exploitation within the context of tributary relationships, but rather from historically specific sets of fundamentally communal class relations and their attending ideologies.

On this model of communal relations of production, tributary surpluses and class divisions are realized among Mississippians rarely if at all, and then only for the briefest periods of time. A look at even the most complex case of Mississippian development—Cahokia—suggests the plausibility of this model or some variant of it (Saitta 1994). Cahokia is generally interpreted as a tributary chiefdom (Dincauze and Hasenstab 1989; Peregrine 1991) although some suggest that it was a state (O'Brien 1992). Milner (1990) and Pauketat (1992), however, suggest that the Cahokia polity was more dynamic, unstable, and decentralized than usually supposed. Still, denying tribute and class divisions at Cahokia is difficult, especially during the Stirling Phase (A.D. 1050–1150). Tributary relations are perhaps most dramatically signaled by the famous Mound 72 retainer sacrifices (O'Brien 1992) and the stockading of the central elite precinct of the site (Pauketat 1992).

Nonetheless, these tributary relations were apparently short-lived and eventually truncated by popular resistance. It is interesting (and paradoxical for tribute models) that during the Stirling Phase "complexity" at Cahokia *increased* (i.e., political hierarchy deepened) as exchange in prestige goods *declined* (Pauketat 1992). If prestige goods had the status of communal ritual entitlements that moved against various economic values and labor, then their declining availability may have compromised the communal subsumed class incomes that sustained the Cahokian elites responsible for organizing long distance exchange. As a response, these communal subsumed classes may have begun to use their social position to foster exploitative (i.e., tributary) relations of production. Such relations may have been sustained and legitimized by Ramey incised ceramics (Pauketat and Emerson 1991), the construction and use of Woodhenge as an "authoritative resource" (Smith 1992), and elite annexation and fortification of other previously communal spaces. That this effort was effectively resisted by primary producers during the Stirling Phase is perhaps indicated by demographic flight to northern areas (Emerson 1991); a shift from extramural to intramural storage at outlying farmsteads (Pauketat 1992), perhaps as a way to conceal household surpluses from tribute-takers; and the eventual reclamation of annexed elite spaces for a return to residential use (Pauketat 1992). If we add to this the observation that health at Cahokia was comparable to Moundville—meaning generally good (Milner 1991, 67)—then we strengthen the warrant for investigating Cahokia with alternative models of political economy.

Anasazi Southwest

Health patterns in the Anasazi Southwest offer a similar warrant for exploring novelty in prehistoric political economies and biocultural relationships. At present there is little agreement about the complexity of Anasazi societies or the processes by which they were organized. For some scholars, these polities were always basically egalitarian, while others recognize a spectrum of organizational forms ranging from egalitarian to politically centralized and class-divided (Lightfoot and Upham 1989). Available evidence for resolving the issue is ambiguous if not contradictory, and opposed models can often find equivalent measures of support.

Patterns of variation in health and nutrition are as equivocal as the cultural patterns. Nelson et al. (1994), however, provide a useful synthesis that imposes some order on the existing data. Their information crosscuts environments, time periods, and various "organizational states" of Anasazi populations (e.g., dispersed, aggregated, and centralized). Although the data are limited, Nelson et al. suggest that biological disruption is dependent neither on environmental marginality nor on time. There is better support for biological disruption being dependent on organizational state, with the politically autonomous "dispersed" populations faring better than what the authors view to be politically centralized, class-divided cases.

Interestingly, however, the latter do not belong to a distinct pattern. Health at politically centralized and presumably class-divided Chaco Canyon, for example, was only slightly more disrupted than health among the dispersed settlements on Black Mesa. Nonetheless, the presumed tribute-taking elites at the great Chacoan towns (e.g., Pueblo Bonito) were healthier (in terms of fewer anemias and higher mean age at death) than nonelites living at the smaller Chacoan villages. The available data suggest to Nelson et al. that biological disruption in the Anasazi area resulted from a complex interaction of population density, environmental marginality, political economy, and unknown other factors.

I take the ambiguities noted by Nelson et al.—especially those characterizing their presumed politically centralized cases—as a warrant for exploring alternative models of Anasazi political economy. In keeping with the belief expressed for the Mississippian groups, I think that even the most "complex" of Anasazi polities can be modeled as variants of communal social formations. Substantiating communality is not a problem for the "dispersed" populations of Black Mesa and Arroyo Hondo, but it is a bit more difficult for areas like Chaco Canyon. However, there is still so much unknown about Chaco Canyon and especially the circumstances under which the Pueblo Bonito burial population was deposited (and archaeologically recovered) that perhaps we should not prematurely rule out the communal alternative.

For one thing, we cannot be certain that Pueblo Bonito was a distinct community with a full-time resident population of which the excavated burial population is a sample. That is, we cannot yet rule out the possibility that the Bonito burials were individuals drawn from a wider population that also included villagers. Chaco scholars have not eliminated the possibility that villagers were both the builders and the users of the great towns, and that they were also buried there. Several researchers have already built compelling cases in support of the Chacoan towns as seasonal aggregation sites rather than full-time residences (Windes 1984, 1987; Lekson et al. 1988).

Nor can we be sure that the Bonito burial population does not represent an accumulation of people from throughout the San Juan Basin who died just before or during periodic ceremonial aggregations (as envisioned by Judge 1989) and thus were accorded "status" treatment because of the timing and/or circumstances of their death rather than strictly because of their social position. If the Bonito burial population does sample individuals from a set of geographically dispersed and communally organized groups, this might explain why the Bonito burial population is not that different healthwise from the Black Mesa sample. One way to begin clarifying this issue might be to simulate what a burial population at a large aggregation site only periodically occupied under conditions like those found in the northern Southwest should look like. We might also consider whether such a scenario could account for certain problems with the Bonito burial sample, such as its relatively small number of infants.

Finally, the contrast to human biology provided by other kinds of material patterns at Chaco—for example, the striking architectural "modularity" of both Chacoan towns and villages (Johnson 1989) and the presence of strong egalitarian themes in architectural patterns on both local and inter-local scales (Fritz 1978)—further suggests that Chaco is marching to the beat of a different drummer, organizationally speaking. Whereas the proposed claim for communality is unsubstantiated, so too are claims for social complexity on a conventional two-class model.

Conclusion

I have argued that we need new theory for studying archaeological and bioarchaeological patterns so that complexity in prehistoric biocultural relationships can be better understood. Marxist theory strikes me as useful in this regard because, in contrast to conventional classless and two-class models of society, it problematizes labor flows and specifies the different ways that people can relate to these flows. At the same time, Marxist theory respects the relative autonomy of power relations and a variety of cultural processes in shaping class processes. This means that the form of class processes cannot be deduced from power relations (political hierarchy) or vice versa. It also means that biological patterns cannot be taken as a straightforward reflection of political economy (whether communal or noncommunal), because of intervening social and cultural (ideological) factors. The relative autonomy of social processes is what creates ambiguity in archaeological patterning, the stuff of which fresh insights about the past are made. By addressing the surplus labor process, its structural position in society, and the possibilities for variation in labor's conditions of existence, a class-analytical Marxism provides a basis for theorizing alternative organizational possibilities, impulses to change, and historical trajectories.

Bioarchaeological and other material patterns from prehistoric North America suggest complex relationships between political economy and human biology. As traditional two-class interpretive models do not always capture this complexity, I have suggested that models of communal society informed by class theory may prove useful for explaining patterns in the Mississippian Southeast and Anasazi Southwest. These models are, however, in need of greater theoretical development and empirical substantiation. The theoretical challenge is to more closely specify the precise relationship between flows of surplus, power, and meaning in each area; the extent to which communal and noncommunal class processes coexisted and how; and the potential for change under different historical and environmental circumstances. Development of such theory may help us better understand the complex interaction of population density, environmental marginality, political-economic processes, and other factors that affected human health in prehistory (Nelson et al. 1994).

The methodological challenge to future research is well put by Rathbun and Scurry: we need to rely on "empirical analyses of specific populations in their unique ecological and cultural settings" (1991, 164) rather than deductivist perspectives alone (see also Larsen and Ruff 1991, 111). The need for more fine-grained studies of intrapopulational health differences, especially as they relate to differential activity patterns among individuals (e.g., differences in degenerative joint disease), is also implicated by Marxist theory. Such variation is our best clue to the intensity and kinds of labors being performed by individuals. Studies of activity patterns and their relationship to health have a long history in bioarchaeology (e.g., see review of Bridges 1992). Much recent work usefully relates degenerative joint disease to different kinds of subsistence pursuits (e.g., Brock and Ruff 1988; Bridges 1991; Larsen and Ruff 1991). What is interesting in these studies is the amount of variability documented between sexes and across populations (Bridges 1992), variation that surely tips us off to different organizational arrangements.

Building from this work, it might also be fruitful to do more with the possible skeletal signatures of nonsubsistence related activities. I am thinking here of the interesting implication for the nature of status relationships that follows from the recognition of bony tumors in the ear cartilage of Middle Woodland central tomb males: namely, that status was tied to diving for pearl-bearing mussels (Streuver and Holton 1979). Long-distance running may have had a similar social function at certain times and places in the American Southwest, if recent findings about the nonutilitarian nature of Chacoan roads (i.e., their use as ceremonial raceways) are credible (see Roney 1992). Such an idea would certainly be testable with skeletal data. The more general point here, however, is that we will need attention to the skeletal signatures of both subsistence and nonsubsistence activities in order to achieve a better understanding of prehistoric class and nonclass relationships and their respective impacts on human biology.

Health data are critical for gaining insight into organizational variation and the causes and consequences of organizational change in prehistory. Unless we have a more complex theory of political economy for accommodating these data, their full implications might be missed. Problematizing labor—as the key link between political economy and human biology—is a start toward a more complex theory. In so doing we can hope to explain the empirical ambiguity that confounds traditional interpretive models and thereby gain new insights into relationships between human culture and biology. The results of bioarchaeological work might then prove even more useful in anticipating the biological consequences of social and economic change across space and time.

NOTES

1. Marx was not always consistent in his definition of class. In *Capital* and the *Grundrisse,* Marx waffles between property, power, and surplus labor definitions of class. Definitions of class as differential access to property and power, however, existed long before Marx came on the scene, and they continue to inform non-Marxist analyses of social life (Resnick and Wolff 1986). The surplus labor definition thus provides the most distinctively Marxist understanding of the term. It also makes the term applicable to kin-based societies. Although a distinction exists in Marxist anthropology between "preclass" and "class" societies (e.g., see Spriggs 1984), it is not clear that Marx ever meant to exclude kin-based societies from class analysis. A full defense of the surplus labor conception of class and its applicability to kin-based societies cannot be elaborated here. Suffice it to say that this conception meets the need expressed by Bloch (1985) and others who argue that the Marxist tradition should retrieve a concept of class in order to redress the ecodeterminism and teleology that have found their way into theories of change for "preclass" societies.

2. In capitalism the fundamental classes are capitalist buyers of labor power and the wage-earning sellers of labor power (Marx 1973, 108). In tributary social formations the fundamental classes can include what we term "chiefs" (depending on circumstances) and commoners, or "feudal" lords and peasants. In communal societies, primary producers are both performers *and* appropriators of surplus labor; that is, appropriation is collective in form and producers fill dual class positions (Amariglio, Resnick, and Wolff 1988). Communal formations are thus the only ones that lack a class *division* in which primary producers have no say over either the amounts or conditions of surplus production and hence are exploited (Wessman 1981). The absence of exploitation does not diminish the utility of the class concept for understanding communal societies, however, as there are still differences to be understood as concerns the distribution and receipt of surplus labor—the subsumed class process (see text following). For a broadly similar way of conceptualizing these social differences see Terray (1975).

3. Landlords, moneylenders, and merchants function as subsumed classes in

capitalism (Resnick and Wolff 1986, 1987); Big Men, "chiefs" (again, depending on circumstances), and various ritual specialists can function as subsumed classes in kin-based, communal social formations (Gailey and Patterson 1988). As Keesing (1991) points out, however, anthropologists have tended to take a narrow view of leadership in kin-based societies, in turn masking important variations and complexities in what can be termed subsumed class structures. A challenge for Marxist theory is to identify these subsumed classes, how they function to reproduce the conditions of labor appropriation, and how they draw support via allocated shares of surplus labor.

4. Contra Milner, Little (1987) establishes the plausibility of long-distance canoe travel—and hence exploitative core–periphery relationships—in the American midcontinent. However, archaeological substantiation of long-distance *exchange* relationships between areas via canoe would not in itself establish the existence of exploitative *class* relationships (see preceding text). One mechanism that prehistoric tribute-takers could have used for sustaining class divisions and economic exploitation over long distances was actual travel to peripheral areas with warrior entourages to collect tribute and reassert core supremacy (see Smith and Hally 1992). This mechanism remains to be established for the Mississippian cases at issue here, however. Thus, in the absence of secure *direct* evidence for long-distance tributary relationships in the Mississippian world, it would seem advisable to entertain a variety of interpretive models.

REFERENCES

Amariglio, J., S. Resnick, and R. Wolff. 1988. Class, Power, and Culture. In *Marxism and the Interpretation of Culture,* ed. C. Nelson and L. Grossberg, 487–501. Urbana: University of Illinois Press.

Binford, L. 1987. Researching Ambiguity: Frames of Reference and Site Structure. In *Method and Theory for Activity Area Research,* ed. S. Kent, 449–512. New York: Columbia University Press.

Blakely, R. 1977. Sociocultural Implications of Demographic Data from Etowah, Georgia. In *Biocultural Adaptation in Prehistoric America,* ed. R. Blakely, 45–66. Athens: University of Georgia Press.

Bloch, M. 1985. *Marxism and Anthropology.* Oxford: Oxford University Press.

Bridges, P. 1991. Degenerative Joint Disease in Hunter-Gatherers and Agriculturalists from the Southeastern United States. *American Journal of Physical Anthropology* 85:379–91.

Bridges, P. 1992. Prehistoric Arthritis in the Americas. *Annual Review of Anthropology* 21:67–91.

Brock, S., and C. Ruff. 1988. Diachronic Patterns of Change in Structural Properties of the Femur in the Prehistoric American Southwest. *American Journal of Physical Anthropology* 75:113–27.

Cook, S. 1977. Beyond the *Formen:* Towards a Revised Marxist Theory of Pre-Capitalist Formations and the Transition to Capitalism. *Journal of Peasant Studies* 4:360–89.

Dincauze, D., and R. Hasenstab. 1989. Explaining the Iroquois: Tribalization on a Prehistoric Periphery. In *Centre and Periphery,* ed. T. Champion, 67–87. London: Unwin Hyman.

Eisenberg, L. 1991. Mississippian Cultural Terminations in Middle Tennessee: What the Bioarchaeological Evidence Can Tell Us. In *What Mean These Bones?* ed. M. Powell, P. Bridges, and A. Mires, 70–87. Tuscaloosa: University of Alabama Press.

Emerson, T. 1991. Some Perspectives on Cahokia and the Northern Mississippian Expansion. In *Cahokia and the Hinterlands,* ed. T. Emerson and R. Lewis, 221–36. Urbana: University of Illinois Press.

Fritz, J. 1978. Paleopsychology Today: Ideational Systems and Human Adaptation in Prehistory. In *Social Archaeology: Beyond Subsistence and Dating,* ed. C. Redman et al., 37–59. New York: Academic Press.

Gailey, C., and T. Patterson. 1988. State Formation and Uneven Development. In *State and Society,* ed. J. Gledhill, B. Bender, and M. Larson, 77–90. London: Unwin Hyman.

Goodman, A. 1993. On the Interpretation of Health from Skeletal Remains. *Current Anthropology* 34:281–88.

Goodman, A., and G. Armelagos. 1985. Disease and Death at Dr. Dickson's Mounds. *Natural History* 94:12–18.

Goodman, A., J. Lallo, G. Armelagos, and J. Rose. 1984. Health Changes at Dickson Mounds, Illinois (AD 950–1300). In *Paleopathology at the Origins of Agriculture,* ed. M. Cohen and G. Armelagos, 271–305. Orlando: Academic Press.

Harris, M. 1959. The Economy Has No Surplus? *American Anthropologist* 61:189–99.

Harrison, S. 1987. Cultural Efflorescence and Political Evolution on the Sepik River. *American Ethnologist* 14:491–507.

Hindess, B., and P. Hirst. 1975. *Pre-Capitalist Modes of Production.* London: Routledge and Kegan Paul.

Humpf, D. 1992. Health and Demography in a Sixteenth Century Southeastern Chiefdom. In *Text-Aided Archaeology,* ed. B. Little, 123–32. Boca Raton: CRC Press.

Huss-Ashmore, R., and F. Johnston. 1985. Bioanthropological Research in Developing Countries. *Annual Review of Anthropology* 14:475–528.

Johnson, G. 1989. Dynamics of Southwest Prehistory: Far Outside, Looking In. In *Dynamics of Southwest Prehistory,* ed. L. Cordell and G. Gumerman, 371–89. Washington, DC: Smithsonian Institution Press.

Judge, W. J. 1989. Chaco Canyon-San Juan Basin. In *Dynamics of Southwest Prehistory,* ed. L. Cordell and G. Gumerman, 209–61. Washington, DC: Smithsonian Institution Press.

Kahn, J., and J. Llobera, eds. 1981. *The Anthropology of Pre-Capitalist Societies.* London: Macmillan.

Keene, A. 1991. Cohesion and Contradiction in the Communal Mode of Production: The Lessons of the Kibbutz. In *Between Bands and States,* ed. S. Gregg, 376–91. Center for Archaeological Investigations, Occasional Paper No. 9. Carbondale: Southern Illinois University Press.

Keesing, R. 1991. Killers, Big Men, and Priests on Malaita: Reflections on a Melanesian Troika System. In *Anthropological Approaches to Political Behavior,* ed. F. McGlynn and A. Tuden, 83–105. Pittsburgh: University of Pittsburgh Press.

Larsen, C., and C. Ruff 1991. Biomechanical Adaptation and Behavior on the Prehistoric Georgia Coast. In *What Mean These Bones?* ed. M. Powell, P. Bridges, and A. Mires, 102–13. Tuscaloosa: University of Alabama Press.

Lee, R. 1992. Art, Science, or Politics? The Crisis in Hunter-Gatherer Studies. *American Anthropologist* 94:31–54.

Lekson, S., T. Windes, J. Stein, and W. J. Judge. 1988. The Chaco Canyon Community. *Scientific American* 256:100–109.

Leone, M. 1988. The Relationship between Archaeological Data and the Documentary Record: Eighteenth Century Gardens in Annapolis, Maryland. *Historical Archaeology* 22:29–35.

Lightfoot, K., and S. Upham. 1989. Complex Societies in the Prehistoric American Southwest: A Consideration of the Controversy. In *The Sociopolitical Structure of Prehistoric Southwestern Societies,* ed. S. Upham, K. Lightfoot, and R. Jewett, 3–30. Boulder: Westview Press.

Little, E. 1987. Inland Waterways in the Northeast. *Midcontinental Journal of Archaeology* 12:55–75.

Marx, K. 1964. *Pre-Capitalist Economic Formations.* New York: International.

Marx, K. 1967. *Capital: A Critique of Political Economy,* vol. 3. New York: International.

Marx, K. 1973. *Grundrisse.* New York: Vintage Books.

Milner, G. 1990. The Late Prehistoric Cahokia Cultural System of the Mississippi River Valley: Foundations, Florescence, and Fragmentation. *Journal of World Prehistory* 4:1–43.

Milner, G. 1991. Health and Cultural Change in the Late Prehistoric American Bottom, Illinois. In *What Mean These Bones?* ed. M. Powell, P. Bridges, and A. Mires, 52–69. Tuscaloosa: University of Alabama Press.

Nelson, B., D. Martin, A. Swedlund, P. Fish, and G. Armelagos. 1994. Studies in Disruption: Demography and Health in the Prehistoric American Southwest. In *Understanding Complexity in the Prehistoric Southwest,* ed. G. Gumerman and M. Gell-Mann, 59–112. Reading, MA: Addison-Wesley.

O'Brien, P. 1992. Early State Economics: Cahokia, Capital of the Ramey State. In *Early State Economics,* ed. H. Claessen and P. van de Velde, 143–75. New Brunswick: Transaction Publishers.

Patterson, T. 1991. *The Inca Empire.* New York: Berg.

Pauketat, T. 1992. The Reign and Ruin of the Lords of Cahokia: A Dialectic of Dominance. In *Lords of the Southeast: Social Inequality and the Native Elites of Southeastern North America,* ed. A. Barker and T. Pauketat, 31–43. Washington: American Anthropological Association.

Pauketat, T., and T. Emerson. 1991. The Ideology of Authority and the Power of the Pot. *American Anthropologist* 93:919–41.

Peregrine, P. 1991. Prehistoric Chiefdoms on the American Midcontinent: A World-System Based on Prestige Goods. In *Core-Periphery Relations in the*

Pre-Capitalist World, ed. C. Chase-Dunn and T. Hall, 193–211. Boulder: Westview Press.

Piot, C. 1992. Wealth Production, Ritual Consumption, and Center/Periphery Relations in a West African Regional System. *American Ethnologist* 19:34–52.

Powell, M. 1991. Ranked Status and Health in the Mississippian Chiefdom at Moundville. In *What Mean These Bones?* ed. M. Powell, P. Bridges, and A. Mires, 22–51. Tuscaloosa: University of Alabama Press.

Powell, M. 1992. In the Best of Health? Disease and Trauma among the Mississippian Elite. In *Lords of the Southeast: Social Inequality and the Native Elites of Southeastern North America,* ed. A. Barker and T. Pauketat, 81–97. Washington, DC: American Anthropological Association.

Rathbun, T., and J. Scurry. 1991. Status and Health in Colonial South Carolina: Belleview Plantation, 1738–1756. In *What Mean These Bones?* ed. M. Powell, P. Bridges, and A. Mires, 148–64. Tuscaloosa: University of Alabama Press.

Reid, J., and S. Whittlesey. 1990. The Complicated and the Complex: Observations of the Archaeological Record of Large Pueblos. In *Perspectives on Southwestern Prehistory,* ed. P. Minnis and C. Redman, 185–95. Boulder: Westview Press.

Resnick, S., and R. Wolff. 1986. What Are Class Analyses? *Research in Political Economy* 9:1–32.

Resnick, S., and R. Wolff. 1987. *Knowledge and Class.* Chicago: University of Chicago Press.

Resnick, S., and R. Wolff. 1988. Communism: Between Class and Classless. *Rethinking Marxism* 1:14–42.

Roney, J. 1992. Prehistoric Roads and Regional Integration in the Chacoan System. In *Anasazi Regional Organization and the Chaco System,* ed. D. Doyel, 123–31. Albuquerque: Maxwell Museum of Anthropology.

Rose, J., M. Marks, and L. Tieszen. 1991. Bioarchaeology and Subsistence in the Central and Lower Portions of the Mississippi Valley. In *What Mean These Bones?,* ed. M. Powell, P. Bridges, and A. Mires, 7–21. Tuscaloosa: University of Alabama Press.

Rosenberg, H. 1990. Complaint Discourse, Aging, and Caregiving among the !Kung San of Botswana. In *The Cultural Context of Aging,* ed. J. Sokolovsky, 19–41. New York: Bergin and Garvey.

Saitta, D. 1994. Agency, Class and Archaeological Interpretation. *Journal of Anthropological Archaeology* 13:201–27.

Scarry, J. 1992. Political Offices and Political Structure: Ethnohistoric and Archaeological Perspectives on the Native Lords of Apalachee. In *Lords of the Southeast: Social Inequality and the Native Elites of Southeastern North America,* ed. A. Barker and T. Pauketat, 163–84. Washington, DC: American Anthropological Association.

Seddon, D., ed. 1978. *Relations of Production.* London: Frank Cass and Company.

Smith, B. 1986. The Archaeology of the Southeastern United States: From Dalton to De Soto, 10,500–500 B.P. In *Advances in World Archaeology,* ed. F. Wendorf and A. Close, 1–92. New York: Academic Press.

Smith, B. 1991. Bioarchaeology in a Broader Context. In *What Mean These Bones?*

ed. M. Powell, P. Bridges, and A. Mires, 165–71. Tuscaloosa: University of Alabama Press.

Smith, B. 1992. Mississippian Elites and Solar Alignments: A Reflection of Managerial Necessity, or Levers of Social Inequality? In *Lords of the Southeast: Social Inequality and the Native Elites of Southeastern North America,* ed. A. Barker and T. Pauketat, 11–30. Washington DC: American Anthropological Association.

Smith, M., and D. Hally. 1992. Chiefly Behavior: Evidence from Sixteenth Century Spanish Accounts. In *Lords of the Southeast: Social Inequality and the Native Elites of Southeastern North America,* ed. A. Barker and T. Pauketat, 99–110. Washington DC: American Anthropological Association.

Spriggs, M., ed. 1984. *Marxist Perspectives in Archaeology.* Cambridge: Cambridge University Press.

Steponaitis, V. 1991. Contrasting Patterns of Mississippian Development. In *Chiefdoms: Power, Economy, and Ideology,* ed. T. Earle, 193–228. Cambridge: Cambridge University Press.

Streuver, S., and F. Holton. 1979. *Koster: Americans in Search of Their Prehistoric Past.* Garden City: Anchor/Doubleday.

Terray, E. 1975. Classes and Class Consciousness in the Abron Kingdom of Gyaman. In *Marxist Analyses and Social Anthropology,* ed. M. Bloch, 85–125. London: ASA Monographs.

Welch, P. 1991. *Moundville's Economy.* Tuscaloosa: University of Alabama Press.

Wessman, J. 1981. *Anthropology and Marxism.* Cambridge, MA: Schenkman.

White, P. 1985. Digging Out Big Men? *Archaeology in Oceania* 20:57–60.

Windes, T. 1984. A New Look at Population in Chaco Canyon. In *Recent Research on Chaco Prehistory,* ed. W. J. Judge and J. Schelberg, 75–87. Albuquerque: National Park Service.

Windes, T. 1987. *Investigations at the Pueblo Alto Complex, Chaco Canyon,* vol. 1. Santa Fe: Department of the Interior.

Wolf, E. 1966. *Peasants.* Englewood Cliffs, NJ: Prentice-Hall.

Wolf, E. 1982. *Europe and the People Without History.* Berkeley: University of California Press.

Wood, J., G. Milner, H. Harpending, and K. Weiss. 1992. The Osteological Paradox. *Current Anthropology* 33:343–70.

Chapter 6

The Biological Consequences of Inequality in Antiquity

Alan H. Goodman

[handwritten annotation: - about social/political power affecting nutrition of local pop. - ↓ health indicies when food stuff traded for 'exotic' items - This example. Last week.]

Bioarchaeology, the study of human biological remains in archaeological contexts, is at a critical point of reconsidering methods and objectives. With the passing of the Native American Graves Protection and Repatriation Act (NAGPRA, US PL 101-601) and increased movement in many countries toward reburial of archaeologically recovered objects, not least of which are human remains, for the first time bioarchaeologists have begun to seriously consider the ethics of their work (Martin, this vol., chap. 7; Rose, Greene, and Greene 1996).

Somewhat paradoxically, this critical period comes after two decades of theoretical and methodological development during which bioarchaeology became more of an anthropological science, and more concerned with the lives of real peoples. Following from its parent fields of human adaptability and processual archaeology, in the 1980s bioarchaeology developed from a descriptive science (with primary goals of charting the geographic and temporal distribution of human types and infirmities) to an evolutionary and ecological science (focused on the processes by which past peoples became ill and other biocultural concerns). Descriptive bioarchaeology focuses simply on the question of presence/absence of a pathology, such as dental caries, in a specific time and place. In contrast, a more processual bioarchaeology calls for examining the *pattern* of caries in order to shed light on social and ecological variables such as diet, food preparation technologies, weaning practices, and oral hygiene. By testing among competing hypotheses to explain the distribution of disease, studies of disease in antiquity, paleopathology, became paleoepidemiology, a processual and populational science. By trying to understand the burden of disease in antiquity, bioarchaeologists became better equipped to understand how infirmities related to social formations and change.

Somewhat paradoxically, even with the development of a processual and epidemiological approach in bioarchaeology, the range of questions explored has not expanded to the point where bioarchaeology has much relevance to the lives of contemporary peoples. Part of this limitation may be traced to the material limits of what preserves well and to the questions amenable to study. However, bioarchaeology has also been limited by a still narrow theoretical focus and suppositions about the behavior of past individuals and groups. For example, a prevalent view of societies as integrated, functional wholes and a focus on evolutionary questions within a narrow ecological framework, adopted from processual archaeology and human adaptability, restricts analyses of the relationship between biological well-being and inequalities in access to and control of resources. Studies are infrequent of the distribution of disease and death within a group or in relationship to sociopolitical factors. As well, studies of health differences among groups have nearly invariably focused on differences in ecology and economics (food procurement strategies, settlement systems, etc.) to explain health patterns; few between-group studies of health consider differences in governance or access to ideology and political power. Of course "ideology" and "power" do not leave unambiguous archaeological signatures. However, these regional and class-based power differentials are the major determinants of health today (Navarro 1976; Waitzkin 1983), and I see no obligatory reason why they would not have been key to health in antiquity.

The focus of this chapter is on the problems and potentials for assessing inequality in antiquity and relating patterns of inequality to patterns of health. Presented first is a brief history of bioarchaeology. I highlight how the transition to an anthropological bioarchaeology has failed to consider health beyond a strictly defined ecological and evolutionary perspective. That is, relations of power have not been a focus. Next presented are examples of the study of health in the past, at Westerhus, Sweden, and at Dickson Mounds, Illinois, in relationship to variation in access to resource and power within geographically defined groups. Lastly, with examples from the Nile River Valley and Dickson Mounds again, I consider the case for inequalities based on geographic location.

A Brief History of Paleoepidemiology

Since before the time of Darwin, human skeletons have frequently been unearthed and studied by naturalists, medical professionals, and later on by physical anthropologists (Armelagos et al. 1971, 1982; Ubelaker 1982). For Westerners, at least, this activity appears to be driven by fascination with how long-deceased individuals looked, their maladies, and how they lived and died.[1]

Ubelaker (1982) divides the historical development of paleopathology, the study of health and disease in past peoples, into four periods, all beginning before the 1960s. The last of these periods extends from 1930 to the present and is defined by the development of "the paleoepidemiological approach, viewing disease with an ecological perspective" (1982, 337; also Armelagos et al. 1971). Ubelaker follows general convention in considering Earnest Hooton's (1930) study of the skeletal remains from Pecos Pueblo, New Mexico, to be the first example of a populational approach in paleoepidemiology. In this oft-cited pioneering study, Hooton, a professor at Harvard and the adviser to the majority of the next generation of physical anthropologists, estimated the prevalence of different morbid conditions in the Pecos human remains and tried to relate epidemiological patterns to culture and ecology.

Hooton's work notwithstanding, paleopathology before the 1960s was clearly not dominated by anthropologists, anthropological concerns, or ecological approaches. Until the last quarter of a century, most research on prehistoric maladies was neither very epidemiological nor ecological, had little concern for the role of culture, and seems to have been practiced more as an avocation of medical science than a field of anthropological inquiry. The focus of most studies was on understanding first occurrences and the geographic and historical limits of a condition, rather than its relationship to cultural processes and its significance within the lives of past individuals and groups (see Armelagos, Carlson, and Van Gerven 1982; Buikstra and Cook 1980). A tangible reminder of this period is found in skeletal collections of this period, which are biased toward the inclusion of crania and the best preserved individuals, a bias seen even in Hooton's Pecos Pueblo collection. Paleopathology existed as a field before the 1960s, but the field of paleoepidemiology, with a distinct ecological and anthropological flavor, was yet to be born.

Toward a More Ecological and Anthropological
Paleoepidemiology

By the end of the 1960s a transition took place toward a more ecological and anthropological approach to studies of health in the past. This perspective had clear leaders: Lawrence Angel, George Armelagos, and Jane Buikstra in the United States and Don Brothwell in the United Kingdom. Brothwell, for example, had already begun to explore a number of issues in the nutrition, demography, and diseases of past populations; in his work, one sees the clear formulation of the ecological perspective (Brothwell 1967). The field "arrived" with the publication of two edited volumes, Brothwell and Sandison's (1967) *Disease in Antiquity* and Jarcho's (1966) *Human Palaeopathology*, and a number of key articles such as Angel's (1966) "Porotic Hyperostosis, Anemias, Malarias, and Marshes in the Prehistoric Eastern Mediterranean," Kerley and Bass's (1967) "Paleopathology: Meeting Ground of Many Disciplines," and Armelagos's (1969) "Disease in Ancient Nubia," all significant for having been published in *Science,* the world's most widely circulated scientific periodical.

The literature of this period displays the ongoing tensions between focusing on diagnosis and history of conditions versus understanding maladies in cultural and ecological context. Jarcho's volume was dominated by a focus on first occurrences and diagnostic rigor. Whereas these remain as important issues for contemporary researchers, they do not reflect the excitement of a new (anthropological) paradigm. Similarly, in Kerley and Bass's (1967) *Science* article, they use the metaphor of paleopathology being a "meeting ground"; however, this meeting ground appears to be a place mainly envisioned for the gathering of biomedical scientists.

These tensions notwithstanding, by the end of the 1960s a clear and growing literature in anthropological paleopathology was evidenced. This new perspective on the field was soon to further develop in programs such as Buikstra's in North American bioarchaeology at Northwestern and similar programs at the Universities of Kansas, Massachusetts, and Tennessee, and the Smithsonian Institution, with offshoots at the Universities of California at Santa Barbara, Arkansas, Colorado, and Indiana, among others. A generation of paleoepidemiologists-bioarchaeologists emerged, mainly trained in North America and largely focused on North American skeletal remains.

As noted previously, the parents of paleoepidemiology were the "new archaeology" and human adaptability. The recently formulated new archaeology provided a set of scientific principles about the relationship between material remains and behavior and focused on ecological explanation (see Binford and Binford 1968). Human adaptability included a means of combining interests in evolutionary change with concern for the various adaptive problems faced by humans today, especially those living in limited and ecologically marginal environments (Baker 1962, 1966, 1969; Lasker 1969).

The ecological perspective—so evident in the new archaeology, human adaptability, and paleoepidemiology—did not come about by chance. The 1960s witnessed the development of ecological approaches throughout the social and biological sciences (Orlove 1980). Growing awareness of environmental destruction, the angst brought on by the Vietnam War, and concerns with the consequences of population growth were some of the popular issues that undoubtedly influenced the direction of the sciences. Within anthropology, this ecological perspective is marked by such key publications as Rappaport's (1967) *Pigs for the Ancestors* and Bennett's (1969) *Northern Plainsmen*. In his critical review of ecological anthropology, Orlove (1980) defines this stage of ecological anthropology by the development of neofunctionalism and neoevolutionism. Marvin Harris devotes the last chapter of his *Rise of Anthropological Theory* (1968) to "Cultural Materialism: Cultural Ecology" and unambiguously draws connections between archaeological and cultural anthropological research. Paleoepidemiology fit comfortably into the development of scientific and ecological approaches in anthropology.

*The Politics of Progress, Gathering-Hunting,
and the Development of Agriculture*

By the 1960s, gatherer-hunter studies also became a central ground for playing out new scientific and ecological perspectives in anthropology. The central publication was Lee and DeVore's *Man the Hunter* (1968; the result of a 1965 conference). What was so singularly significant about this volume was the view espoused in a variety of chapters that contemporary gatherer-hunters often failed to live a Hobbesian existence. The Zen economics of Sahlins (1968) promoted a view that contemporary gatherer-hunters were materially satisfied, if not well off. Lee's (1968) data on San time allocation presented clear evidence that this group was not teetering at the brink of survival. Arguing on ecological and epidemiological principles, Dunn (1968) suggested that gatherer-hunters would not be expected to suffer as much from infectious disease as agriculturalists. Rather than just surviving, gatherer-hunters may actually have lived a rather stress-free life; humans may be particularly adapted to this life-style.[2]

This new perspective on contemporary gatherer-hunters suggested the importance of studying the health of past gatherer-hunters, especially in relation to subsequent agriculturalists. It is into this world that paleoepidemiology was born. The dominant question of the subsequent two decades of paleoepidemiological research centered on comparing the health of hunter-gatherers with later horticulturalists (Cohen and Armelagos 1984). Unfortunately, the spotlight on group-level change over time obscured any focus on health differences within and among contemporaneous groups. It is this problem that I focus upon in the following.

Health Variation and Within-Group Inequalities

Social Class and Health at Westerhus, Sweden

A widely held assumption is that most societies studied by archaeologists, especially those before the advent of agriculture, were not highly stratified or differentiated (Rothschild 1979). Most everyone did the same things and shared the same interests. Surplus accumulation was minimal. Even so, differences might exist, most obviously by age and sex cohorts, that might affect access to resources.

A clear example of health differentiation in relationship to class-like control over resources is seen in the research of Swärdstedt (1966) on linear enamel hypoplasia prevalences at Westerhus, a medieval Swedish population. Linear enamel hypoplasias are lines or bands of decreased enamel thickness caused by a disturbance to enamel development (Goodman and Rose 1990; Kreshover 1960; Sarnat and Schour 1941). The ameloblasts that make enamel fail to secrete sufficient enamel, thus leaving behind a visible area of reduced enamel thickness. These defects are useful for reconstructing health during the time of tooth formation, around birth to six years for the commonly studied permanent anterior teeth and from the second trimester of pregnancy through one year of age for deciduous teeth. As these defects are indelible and not remodeled, the record of stress is fixed in the location of the defects on tooth crowns (Goodman and Rose 1990).

Swärdstedt (1966) showed clear differences in enamel defect frequencies among social groups buried at Westerhus (fig. 1). Individuals in social group 1 are landowners and individuals of high status, group 2 includes peasants who own their own land but are clearly below group 1 in status and wealth, and individuals in group 3 are "indentured slaves" who neither own their own land nor control their means of production. They are at the bottom of this caste-like society.

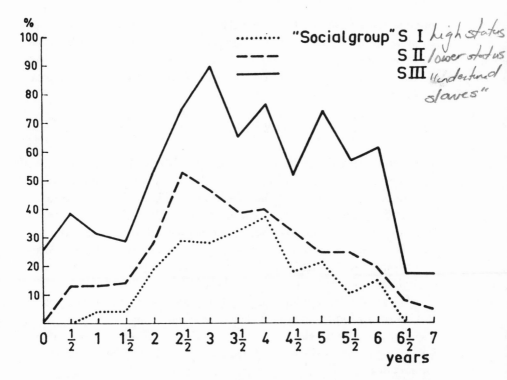

Fig. 1. The frequency of linear enamel hypoplasias (LEH) by half-year developmental periods for social groups from Westerhus, medieval Sweden. (Redrawn from Swärdstedt 1966.)

The age-specific pattern of enamel defects divided by half-year development periods is similar in all groups. The peak frequency or percent of defects is found between two and five years developmental age. What differs is the frequency of defects among groups. For all half-year developmental periods the highest percentage of enamel defects is found in the slave group (3), and conversely, the lowest, indicating less stress, in the landowners (1). The data fit the expected pattern extremely well—the landowners with greater wealth were less stressed.

This analysis succeeded in the sense that hypoplasias (stress markers) vary in predicted ways with social status. Enamel hypoplasia, a relatively reliable and easily identified measure, was used, and, perhaps even more critically, clearly demarcated differences among social groups were studied. Here, status differences are archaeologically unambiguous: there is historical documentation of social class, and these are reliably preserved by place of burial relative to the church. There is little guesswork in reconstructing meaningful social groupings in life. Unfortunately, this is not typical of most efforts to reconstruct status in life from archaeological remains.

Social Class and Health at Dickson Mounds, Illinois

Following Swärdstedt's lead, and Rothschild's (1979) analysis of grave goods as indicators of social status at Dickson, I looked for similar social class differences in health at Dickson Mounds, Illinois. Dickson Mounds is located near the confluence of the Spoon and Illinois Rivers, close to the town of Lewiston, Illinois. The skeletal sample studied spans from the Late Woodland, a hunting and gathering occupation (ca. A.D. 900–1000) and assumed to be highly egalitarian, to Middle Mississippian (ca. A.D. 1150–1300), assumed to be more highly stratified.

The most salient point emerging from the archaeological analysis of the Dickson Mounds area is evidence for rapid change in economy and social organization (Harn 1978, 1980). For heuristic purposes, Lallo (1973) divided individuals into three roughly sequential phases (also see Goodman et al. 1984a).

The first phase, called the Late Woodland (LW) occupation (ca. A.D. 950–1050), is characterized by a generalized hunting and gathering economy with seasonal campsites and a relatively small (75–125) group of people. Artifacts from this time period suggest a relatively autonomous group; there is little evidence of trade or other forms of contact with Mississippian peoples at Cahokia, about 100 miles to the south (near present day East Saint Louis, Illinois) and at other sites in the American Bottoms.

Toward the end of this time period, evidence accrued for contact and increased "Mississippianization" of the local population. This signals a new transitional horizon called Mississippian Acculturated Late Woodland (MALW; ca. A.D. 1050–1175). In addition to a mixed gathering-hunting and agricultural economy, during the MALW one begins to find permanent living sites and the beginning of a village-like settlement pattern. Evidence for long-distance trade is seen in the increasingly diverse, exotic, and changing nature of village refuse and mortuary offerings (Lallo 1973; Harn 1978).

Around A.D. 1175, the local population seems to have fully entered into the Mississippian sphere of influence. During this period, called Middle Mississippian (MM) (ca. A.D. 1175–1300), a more complex settlement pattern emerges with ceremonial centers, hamlets, and surrounding campsites. Population size, density, and sedentism continued to increase. Long-distance trade flourished. In broad outline it appears that utilitarian items were traded along an east–west axis, while items of symbolic value were obtained from the south, presumably traveling up the Mississippi River via Cahokia (Harn 1978).

In summary, the main changes in life-style at Dickson, through roughly 350 years of occupation, include

- intensification of and greater reliance on agriculture,
- increased population density and sedentism, and
- expanded and intensified trade.

Following Rothschild (1979) individuals were sorted into those: (1) without any grave offering, assumed to signify lowest status in life, (2) individuals buried with only utilitarian items, called class I offerings, assumed to be intermediate social status, and (3) individuals with exotica, called class II/III offerings, assumed to be individuals of highest social status. As in the Swärdstedt study, the measure of "stress" is linear enamel hypoplasia. Individuals were characterized as having no hypoplasias, one hypoplasia, or two or more hypoplasias between 3.5 and 7.0 years of developmental age.

There is not a statistically significant association between number of hypoplasias/stress and grave goods/social status, in part because the sample sizes for some subgroups are small. However, a trend is evident in which individuals with no grave goods are more likely to have two or more hypoplasias (17.6 percent) compared to those with utilitarian items (14.1 percent) and those with exotica (8.7 percent).

Why is the relationship between social status and health not stronger? One hypothesis is that status, while affecting health, does so in more subtle ways in this past population. Perhaps, as Rothschild (1979) suggests, the Middle Mississippian at Dickson is a more egalitarian society than assumed, thus differences are less dramatic because status differences are less striking. Alternatively, it could be that status is more complexly patterned, and that it cannot be sufficiently captured by any single measure such as grave offerings at time of death. In short, grave offerings provide an imperfect measure of status in life. I assume both hypotheses are partly true. But, if status is not well measured, or is "different" from our ethnographic notions of it, then how can it be better evaluated? This is a question we will return to later in the discussion.

Sociopolitical Power, Health, and Regional Systems

Nile River Kingdoms and Health at Sudanese Nubia

Differential access to resources also occurs among groups who occupy different geographic areas, and these patterns may change over time as political-economic patterns shift. These shifts may have consequences for health. This process is the focus of the next two examples: the first is from the Nile River Valley, and the last returns to Dickson Mounds.

The Nile River Valley is unique in that it is a very narrow strip of fertile land bordered by a very unproductive desert. Because the land outside of the valley is largely uninhabitable, those living along the valley have limited adaptive options. They must adjust to the ecology and presumably the sways of power. Through the ages different political groups have ascended to power, but most often the seat of power was to the north of the Wadi Halfa and Kulubnarti regions, where Van Gerven's and Armelagos's bioarchaeological programs have taken place (Armelagos 1969; Martin et al. 1984; Van Gerven et al. 1981, 1995). Van Gerven and colleagues (1981, 1995) find that health of local groups varies in direct relationship to the florescence of kingdoms. Health suffers when kingdoms are powerful, and when kingdoms lose power health gets better in these peripheral groups. Van Gerven et al. (1981, 1995) suggest that during economically expansive times kingdoms exert greater control and doubtlessly extract surplus labor and tribute from locals. However, during times of collapse, locals are left to govern themselves, and with greater local political control comes greater access to resources and improved health. Specifically, when either the kingdom of Meroe to the south or the Christian kingdom to the north expands during periods of great power, Nubians lose political autonomy and their health suffers. Conversely, when the kingdoms decline in power they are less able to control areas as far away as Kulubnarti, and health in the political periphery improves. Infants and children appear to be particularly affected by these regional processes (Martin et al. 1984). In summary, health in Nubia is highly related to one's position in relationship to sociopolitical systems. Here, being just over the border of a system of control allows for better health, something we also see in less accessible parts of the American Southwest, such as on the top of Black Mesa (Martin et al. 1991). Conversely, being on the periphery of a system (rather than outside of a system) can be extremely stressful as this is a place where control over power is minimal.

Mississippian Political Systems and Health Changes at Dickson Mounds

A millennium ago, and centuries before Columbus "discovered" the Americas, the eastern half of North America was densely occupied by Native Americans. Settlements typically were along waterways and varied in size from small seasonal campsites to cities such as Cahokia, near present day East St. Louis, Illinois, which was among the largest of its time. One of many thousands of sites of this time is the Dickson Mounds site.

The effects of changes on health status can be evaluated because of the availability of a large skeletal collection, including individuals who lived during the pre-agricultural, transitional, and agricultural phases. The following summary of the paleoepidemiology of Dickson Mounds focuses on seven measures of morbidity and mortality: (1) long bone growth, (2) enamel developmental defects, (3) porotic hyperostosis, (4) infectious lesions, (5) traumatic lesions, (6) degenerative lesions, and finally (7) mortality, the ultimate indicator of adaptive failure (Goodman et al. 1984a).

Stature and other anthropometric measures are commonly used as general indicators of nutritional status during infancy and childhood (Sutphen 1985). Rather subtle decreases in growth are meaningful because they are associated with increased morbidity and mortality, and decreases in functions such as work capacity (Allen 1984; Chavez and Martinez 1982; Martorell 1989). These anthropometric measures of living individuals provide a basis from which to derive inferences from studies of long bone growth in length and circumference in past populations.

Lallo (1973) calculated the average length and circumference of long bones at Dickson by developmental age (based on dental maturity) and cultural horizon. He found little difference in length and circumference until around two years of age. At this age there is a distinct decrease in growth velocity, especially in circumference, for children in the Middle Mississippian. For example, comparing the average length of tibia for the 5 to 10 year age groups, Lallo (1973) found that the mean Mississippian tibial length is significantly less than the LW or MALW tibial lengths ($p < .05$; 209.0 mm vs. 228.6 and 229.2 mm respectively; table 1). An even more pronounced difference is seen in comparing attained tibial circumferences.

The mean tibial circumference of 5 to 10 year old MM children is significantly less than that of their age-matched LW and MALW peers (p < .05; 25.2 mm vs 33.3 mm and 32.8 mm respectively; table 1). Once the greater attained growth of the LW and MALW samples is achieved, they remain relatively constant until maturity, and this tibial growth pattern is typical of the other long bones. Finally, the age at which this growth faltering occurred—around two years—suggests possible stresses associated with a weaning diet (Goodman et al. 1984a; Lallo 1973).

Data on the prevalence and chronological pattern of enamel hypoplasias provide an independent means of assessing growth disruption. Goodman and co-workers (1980) found an increased frequency of hypoplasia from 0.90 defects per individual during the Late Woodland to 1.61 per individual in the Middle Mississippian period. The prevalence of individuals with one or more hypoplasias increases from 45 percent during the LW to 80 percent during the MM (table 1).

The chronology of enamel hypoplasia on permanent teeth shows that the Dickson Mounds population experienced peak stress between the ages of two and four, which may correspond to the age at completion of weaning (Goodman et al. 1984b; fig. 2). The comparison of chronologies between the earlier groups and the Middle Mississippian at Dickson Mounds shows an earlier age of onset of hypoplasia in the MM, suggesting an earlier onset of stress. Although these data do not pinpoint a time

TABLE 1.   Summary of Select Skeletal Indicators of Health at Dickson

	Late Woodland	MALW[a]	Middle Mississippian
Mean tibial length[b] (mm)	228.6	229.2	209.0
Mean tibial circumference[b] (mm)	33.3	32.8	25.2
Percentage of enamel hypoplasias—Adults	45.0	60.0	80.0
Percentage of porotic Hyperostosis—Subadults	13.6	31.2	52.0
Percentage of tibial infectious lesions	26.0[c]		84.0
Percentage of traumatic lesions—Males	17.9	16.4	38.0
Percentage of traumatic lesions—Females	23.5	16.4	31.1
Percentage of degenerative lesions—Males	38.5	42.6	76.0
Percentage of degenerative lesions—Females	41.2	41.0	67.4
Life expectancy at birth (years)[d]	22–26[c]		20–22

[a]MALW = Mississippian Acculturated Late Woodland
[b]Based on 5–10 year age group
[c]Combined MALW and Late Woodland
[d]Calculations from Johansson and Horowitz (1986)

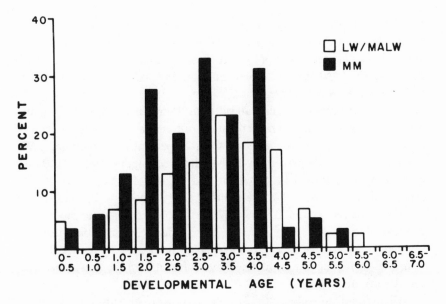

Fig. 2. Frequency distribution of enamel hypoplasias by half-year periods in two Dickson Mounds samples; MM = Middle Mississippian, LW/MALW = combined Late Woodland and Mississippian Acculturated Late Woodland samples (after Goodman et al. 1984b).

of weaning, they are consistent with a pattern of earlier weaning in agricultural versus gathering-hunting societies.

Porotic hyperostosis, the third measure, is a general term used to identify bony lesions found most often on the superior border of the orbits and the external surface of the crania. These porotic lesions, which are characterized by a thinning of the subperiosteal cortical bone and corresponding expansion of the diploe, develop as a result of an anemia. The frequent endemic and mild nature of these defects in North American skeletal materials suggests that the anemia was due to a nutrient inadequacy, most likely related to iron metabolism, rather than a hereditary anemia (Mensforth et al. 1978; Mensforth 1991).

Lallo, Armelagos, and Rose (1977) found that among subadults these lesions significantly increased from 13.6 percent in the LW to 31.2 percent in the MALW and 51.5 percent in the MM (table 1). Furthermore, during the Late Woodland porotic hyperostosis is limited to the superior border of the orbits, a condition specifically referred to as cribra orbitalia. However, in the MALW and MM, individuals tend increasingly to have porotic involvement at other sites, suggesting a more extensive and severe manifestation. Porotic hyperostosis both increases fourfold in frequency and increases in percentage of "severe" cases from none in the LW and 6.5 percent in the MALW to 17.8 percent in the MM (Goodman et al. 1984a; Lallo, Armelagos, and Rose 1977).

The fourth measure, generalized tibial bone infection, also dramatically increases over time. The percentage of tibiae with evidence for infection (periosteal reactions) increases from 26 percent in a combined LW-MALW sample to 84 percent in the Middle Mississippian (table 1). Based on extent of periosteal involvement and degree of tissue destructions, Lallo and co-workers (1978) determined that all but 7 (8 percent) of 90 cases of tibial infection in the LW-MALW were slight to moderate, whereas of the 163 cases of infection in the Middle Mississippian nearly a fourth (23 percent) were severe. Paralleling the porotic hyperostosis pattern, these data suggest an increase over time in *both* the prevalence and severity of infections.

Changing from subadult morbidity indicators, the fifth and six measures focus on traumatic lesions and degenerative lesions in adults. The most common bones with postcranial fractures (traumatic lesions) at Dickson are the humerus, clavicle, ulna, and radius (Goodman et al. 1984a; Lallo 1973). Since the distribution of traumas by bone is not significantly different among cultural horizons, all postcranial fractures were combined. Adults females from the Late Woodland and MALW have a lower frequency of fractures than those from Middle Mississippian (23.5 percent and 16.4 percent vs 31.1 percent), and this is even more dramatic for males (17.9 and 16.4 percent vs 38.0 percent; table 1; Lallo 1973; Goodman et al. 1984a). Based on the type and location of fractures, few of these lesions seem to have resulted from strife and violence. Rather, almost all of the fractures seem to have resulted from an increase in work and activity.

The possibility of an increase in activity and activity-induced pathology also is seen in the pattern of osteoarthritis, degeneration of joints, and osteophytosis, degeneration of vertebral bodies. For all adults, there is a significant increase in the frequency of degenerative pathologies (either osteoarthritis or osteophytosis) from 39.7 percent in the LW to 41.8 percent in the MALW and 65.8 percent in the MM. This trend is similar in both sexes (table 1; also Goodman et al. 1984a; Lallo 1973).

The last indicator of health is life expectancy. Assuming no migration or population growth, Lallo and co-workers (1980) computed mean life expectancies at birth of 19 years in the Middle Mississippian and 26 years in the combined LW-MALW earlier groups. In general, age-specific mortality and probability of dying consistently increase while survivorship and age-specific life expectancy consistently decrease through the cultural horizons. In all age classes there is a general trend toward an increased probability of dying during the Mississippian.

Johansson and Horowitz (1986) have challenged the assumption of zero population growth. They model a modest decrease in rate of growth during the LW and a growth rate of around 0.5 percent per year after agriculture. These changes have an effect of lessening the degree of difference in life expectancy among groups (table 1). However, a modest decrease in life expectancy from the Late Woodland to the Middle Mississippian remains. *why - because of ↑ agr ? ↑ sed. life ?*

All indications point toward a decline in health and nutritional status at Dickson (table 1). While morbidity and mortality levels before Middle Mississippian were already high, they increase dramatically. What caused this deterioration in health?

Most of the indications of deficient health are potentially explainable by local ecological factors, specifically a decline in dietary quality and perhaps quantity. This was the original hypothesis put forward by Lallo (1973) and the one that has guided most research in Dickson paleoepidemiology. In fact, Dickson is a powerful test case for a scientific approach to the study of health in past populations. A clear hypothesis can be designed and tested.

The results of this hypothesis-testing exercise were positive. The Middle Mississippian peoples, assumed to be more heavily agricultural, were found to suffer more growth disruption, increased mortality, and increased infection and anemia. All of these data made sense in light of the fact that maize is a poor source of the essential amino acids lysine and tryptophan and has lower bioavailability of essential trace elements such as zinc and iron, which are consequential for growth and immune system functioning. Lastly, the population increase associated with agricultural intensification, coupled with intensification of contact with outsiders, could create an increased opportunity for the spread of infectious diseases. On these grounds, the decline in health at Dickson appears to be well explained by economically driven changes in settlement pattern and diet.

agr. corn!

sedetory life

Paradoxes, however, are also apparent. The dietary shift, including the effect of demographic change, does not easily account for the increases in degenerative and traumatic pathologies. A society experiencing difficulties providing enough food for its people might overexploit local resources and degrade agricultural lands, but no evidence for this exists. The most paradoxical fact is that a balanced diet seems to have been available. Archaeological evidence strongly suggests that gathering-hunting was never completely abandoned in this species-rich area; many nearby Mississippian sites have yielded a great concentration of animal bones and projectile points used for hunting (Munson and Harn 1966). Yet, data on health and nutritional status (Goodman et al. 1984a), trace elements (Gilbert 1975), and stable carbon isotope ratios (Buikstra, Rose, and Milner 1989) suggest that the Mississippian diet was nutritionally poor and heavily reliant on maize. There is a disparity between the food that was produced and locally consumed.

I have previously suggested that the explanation to this paradox may come from consideration of regional and interregional processes, focusing specifically on the relationship between Dickson and Cahokia, a center of Mississippian culture (Goodman et al. 1984a; Goodman and Armelagos 1985). The builders of the Dickson Mounds received many of their symbolic items, such as copper-covered ear spools and marine shell necklaces, from or through the Cahokia region (Harn 1978); it is less clear what villagers at Larson, the largest Middle Mississippian village at Dickson, "traded" in exchange for these highly valued symbolic items.

Much of the health data could be explained if Dickson had been trading perishable foodstuffs for these luxury items. In particular, the diversion of meat or fish downriver to Cahokia could explain the discrepancy between food availability and intake. In order to generate a surplus of foods for trade Dicksonites may have had to intensify their agricultural production while continuing to hunt and gather. The increase in degenerative and traumatic conditions could have resulted from this increased work load. This system also could have put increased social strains on the community, leading to internal strife. In addition, the accumulation of luxury items may have required protection from outside groups, such as Oneonta to the north. This would also explain why the Larson site was pallisaded.

Was it possible that the peasants at Dickson were involved in a tributary/exploitative relationship with Cahokia? Some archaeologists maintain that there is too great a distance between Dickson and Cahokia for Cahokia to have exerted systemic control and that Cahokian political power was in decline while health was deteriorating at Dickson (Milner 1990). Conversely, Cahokian influence is evident as far away as northern

New York (Dincauze and Hasenstab 1989) and waterways were easily navigable, thus making such long-distance relationships more probable (Little 1987; also see Saitta, this vol., chap. 5).

More generally, recent research on trade and regional relationships in archaeology (Rowlands, Larsen, and Kristiansen 1987), along with studies on the concept of precapitalist social formations, and core and periphery areas by Wallerstein (1976, 1977) and others (Amin 1976; Arghiri 1972; Frank 1967; Polyani 1966; Williams 1966) suggests that intergroup relationships throughout most of human prehistory were more complex, intense, and pervasive than has been generally realized. Extrapolating from this research suggests the need to look at health in prehistory in relationship to regional systems and interpopulation contact.

How is it that increased involvement with larger economic systems might have a negative effect on the health of local populations? The process may be as simple as trading foods for items of symbolic value. While this might initially seem harmless, health can be compromised when the interaction continues to the point where needed foods are being traded away. Similar scenarios have often occurred in recent times: a group with little political or economic clout learns that it can trade something it has access to (sugar cane, alpacas, turtles) for something it greatly admires (radios, metal products, alcohol), but can only obtain through trade with a more powerful group. Because deterioration is slow and only begins to take a toll over time, group members do not perceive that the long-term consequences are unfavorable. Nor are all such "trading agreements" strictly voluntary, especially once entered into.

Although the causal web of factors leading to the decline in health may never be fully explicated, I contend that the health decline cannot be explained by local/ecological factors alone. In order to understand adaptation in the past, the struggle to get by, one needs to understand the proximate conditions, the "microenvironment," what one eats, the pathogens one is exposed to, and the biophysical conditions that reach the body. However, a deeper understanding of the "adaptive process" requires going beyond the proximate microenvironment to consider how it is shaped and structured by larger conditions. The web of causation needs to be broadened (Krieger 1994). The problem, then, is to better understand the nature of "border-crossing" social, economic, and political relations, how they influenced biologies, and how the connections to biology can be better understood.

Discussion and Conclusion

Just as one would obtain a very limiting picture of disease etiology in the present without considering the role of access to and control of resources, ideology, and power, so also must it be limiting for understanding infirmities in the past. Cohen (1989) has suggested that intragroup differences in health are noise relative to the signal of differences due to changing patterns of subsistence. Unfortunately, what Cohen characterizes as "noise" is for others an important signal. Furthermore, I contend that one can more clearly understand how health changes with agricultural intensification if one considers relative positions of power. Agriculture undoubtedly has differential benefits depending on location relative to seats of power, and hypothetically it benefits least individuals on the fringes of sociopolitical systems.

Second, we need to further conceptualize the working of power in past societies. It is surely problematic to think of power as operating on only one level and along a single dimension. Power tends to vary within regions, within communities, and within households. As well, power may not operate in a clear, linear way. Roseberry (this vol., chap. 3) has referred to the notion of fields of power, and this concept might provide a good way to think about how power is manifest in many past contexts. Following Roseberry, power may reside in multiple overlapping fields. These fields of power may move actions and beliefs in conflicting directions, and the contours of such fields may shift through one's lifetime and over historical time.

Nelson's (1995) recent work in breaking down the complexity of archaeological sites suggests other fruitful research directions. Nelson shows that sites such as Chaco Canyon, New Mexico, and La Quimada, Zacatecas, Mexico, are not equal in their complexity. Chaco Canyon may have involved a larger population over a larger area, with more buildings and public works, but La Quimada may have been more hierarchical (also see Saitta 1997). Such a deconstructing of the elements of complexity might lead to interesting inferences for health. Finally, Saitta's focus (this vol., chap. 5) on the relationship between labor flows and social processes might also be fruitfully extended to consequences for bone and teeth.

In summary, inequalities in the past are not transparent, but this does not mean that they are not there in "simple" and prehistoric societies. Given the great interest of archaeologists in these processes, we can look forward to more creative ways of measuring inequality and status differentials. While assuming that status is directly related to burial position, care in burial, grave offerings, and such should be problematized, the relationship between status and health is worth the research effort.

Following the Westerhus example (Swärdstedt 1966), a productive area of research may be studies of populations with some historical documentation of social position and status. An obvious example of this is work in the United States on African-American biohistory (Rose and Rathbun 1987; Blakey, this vol., chap. 16). Finally, it is hoped that more bioarchaeologists will undertake regional analyses that consider how health varies in relationship to both ecology and power. Central Mexico is one of the places where this work has started (Márquez Morfín, this vol., chap. 9).

What is most exciting is the potential for merging ecological perspectives with a more resolutely political-economic perspective. In this way we might be able to open up a political ecology of bioarchaeology in which health is conceptualized and studied in relationship to interaction between local, ecological determinants and more encompassing fields of power. Challenges remain to better operationalize this broadening of horizons.

NOTES

Parts of this chapter were initially presented as a paper at the Wenner-Gren Symposium No. 115 and at the 13th International Congress of Anthropological and Ethnological Sciences, Mexico City, July 31, 1993, and subsequently published in a different form in *Rivista di Antropologia.* Debra Martin, George Armelagos, and Thomas Leatherman provided useful comments. This paper is dedicated to Leslie L. Goodman and his sense of social justice.

1. Many of the scientific debates over fossil human finds in the nineteenth century centered on questions of normality and pathology (Armelagos, Carlson, and Van Gerven 1982). During the first quarter of this century Don Dickson, a chiropractor, became so interested in the bones found in the Mississippian mounds on his family's land that he quit his medical practice in order to devote time to exploring the mounds (Goodman and Armelagos 1985). In July 1996 a single skeleton, dubbed Kennewick Man, was found along the banks of the Columbia River and soon generated a wealth of fascination across the United States (Chatters 1997). Dated at circa 9200 years of age, and according to Chatters showing "Caucasoid" features, the skeleton raised a number of questions about early human colonization and habitation of the Americas, while also raising ethical questions about scientific study (Goodman 1997).

2. By the 1980s one popular book urged Westerners to adopt a Paleolithic diet and life-style (Eaton, Shostack, and Konner 1988), and this view of happy and healthy gatherer-hunters had become a staple of popular culture (Goodman 1990).

REFERENCES

Allen, Lindsay. 1984. Functional Indicators of Nutritional Status of the Whole Individual or the Community. *Clinical Nutrition* 35:169–75.

Amin, S. 1976. *Unequal Development.* New York: Monthly Review Press.

Angel, J. Lawrence. 1966. Porotic Hyperostosis, Anemias, Malarias and Marshes in the Prehistoric Eastern Mediterranean. *Science* 153:760–63.

Arghiri, E. 1972. *Unequal Exchange.* New York: Monthly Review Press.

Armelagos, George J. 1969. Disease in Ancient Nubia. *Science* 163:255–59.

Armelagos, George J., D. S. Carlson, and D. P. Van Gerven. 1982. The Theoretical Foundations and Development of Skeletal Biology. In *A History of American Physical Anthropology,* ed. F. Spencer, 305–28. New York: Academic Press.

Armelagos, George J., James Mielke, and J. Winter. 1971. Bibliography of Human Paleopathology. Res. Report No 8, University of Massachusetts Department of Anthropology.

Baker, Paul T. 1962. The Application of Ecological Theory in Anthropology. *American Anthropologist* 64:15–22.

Baker, Paul T. 1966. Human Biological Variation as an Adaptive Response to the Environment. *Eugenics Quarterly* 13:81–91.

Baker, Paul T. 1969. Human Adaptation to High Altitude. *Science* 163:1149–56.

Bennett, J. W. 1969. *Northern Plainsmen: Adaptive Strategies and Agrarian Life.* Chicago: Aldine.

Binford, S. R., and L. R. Binford, eds. 1968. *New Perspectives in Archaeology.* Aldine: Chicago.

Brothwell, Don. 1967. The Bio-Cultural Background to Disease. In *Disease in Antiquity,* ed. D. Brothwell and A. T. Sandison, 56–68. Springfield, IL: C. C. Thomas.

Brothwell, Don, and A. T. Sandison, eds. 1967. *Disease in Antiquity.* Springfield, IL: C. C. Thomas.

Buikstra, Jane E., and Della Cook. 1980. Paleopathology: An American Account. *Annual Review of Anthropology* 9:433–70.

Buikstra, Jane, Jerome C. Rose, and George Milner. 1989 Maize Consumption in the Prehistoric Central Mississippi Valley: Delta[13]C Values and Diet. Paper presented at the annual meetings of the Society for American Archaeology.

Chatters, James C. 1997. Encounter with an Ancestor. *Anthropology Newsletter* 38 (1): 9–10.

Chavez, Adolfo, and Celia Martinez. 1982. *Growing Up in a Developing Community.* Mexico City: Instituto Nacional de la Nutricion.

Cohen, Mark N. 1989. *Health and the Rise of Civilizations.* New Haven: Yale University Press.

Cohen, Mark N., and George J. Armelagos, eds. 1984. *Paleopathology at the Origins of Agriculture.* New York: Academic Press.

Dincauze, Dina F., and R. J. Hasenstab. 1989. Explaining the Iroquois: Tribalization on a Prehistoric Periphery. In *Centre and Periphery: Comparative Studies in Archaeology,* ed. T. C. Champion, 67–87. London: Unwin.

Dunn, F. L. 1968. Epidemiological Factors: Health and Disease in Hunter-Gatherers. In *Man the Hunter,* ed. R. Lee and I. DeVore, 221–28. Chicago: Aldine.

Eaton, Boyd, M. Shostack, and M. Konner. 1988. *The Paleolithic Prescription.* New York: Harper and Row.

Frank, Andre. 1967. *Capitalism and Underdevelopment in Latin America.* New York: Monthly Review Press.

Gilbert, Robert. 1975. Trace Element Analysis of Three Skeletal Amerindian Populations at Dickson Mounds. Ph.D. thesis, University of Massachusetts, Amherst.

Goodman, Alan H. 1990. The Paleolithic Prescription: A Guide to Modern Living? Paper presented at Sixth International Conference on Hunting and Gathering Societies (CHAGS 6), Fairbanks, AK, May 27–June 1.

Goodman, Alan H. 1997. Racializing Kennewick Man. *Anthropology Newsletter* (October): 3, 5.

Goodman, Alan H., and George J. Armelagos. 1985. Death and Disease at Dr. Dickson's Mounds. *Natural History* (Sept.): 12–18.

Goodman, Alan H., G. J. Armelagos, and J. C. Rose. 1980. Enamel Hypoplasias as Indicators of Stress in Three Prehistoric Populations from Illinois. *Human Biology* 52:515–28.

Goodman, Alan H., J. Lallo, G. J. Armelagos, and J. C. Rose. 1984a. Health Changes at Dickson Mounds, Illinois (AD 950–1300). In *Paleopathology at the Origins of Agriculture,* ed. M. N. Cohen and G. J. Armelagos, 271–306. New York: Academic Press.

Goodman, Alan H., George J. Armelagos, and Jerome C. Rose. 1984b. The Chronological Distribution of Enamel Hypoplasias from Prehistoric Dickson Mounds Populations. *Am. J. Phys. Anthrop.* 65:259–66.

Goodman, Alan H., and Jerome C. Rose. 1990. Assessment of Systemic Physiological Perturbations from Dental Enamel Hypoplasias and Associated Histological Structures. *Yearbook of Physical Anthropology* 33:59–110.

Harris, Marvin 1968. *The Rise of Anthropological Theory.* New York: Columbia.

Harn, Alan. 1978. Mississippian Settlement Patterns in the Central Illinois River Valley. In *Mississippian Settlement Patterns,* ed. B. Smith, 233–68. New York: Academic Press.

Harn, Alan. 1980. The Prehistory of Dickson Mounds: The Dickson Excavation, Report No. 36. Illinois Museum, Springfield.

Hooton, E. 1930. *The Indians of Pecos Pueblo: A Study of Their Skeletal Remains.* New Haven: Yale University Press.

Jarcho, Saul, ed. *Human Palaeopathology.* 1966. New Haven: Yale University Press.

Johansson, Sheila R., and Sheryl Horowitz. 1986. Estimating Mortality in Skeletal Populations: Influences of the Growth Rate on the Interpretation of Levels and Trends During the Transition to Agriculture. *Am. J. Phys. Anthrop.* 71:233–50.

Kerley, E. R., and W. Bass. 1967. Paleopathology: Meeting Ground for Many Disciplines. *Science* 157:638–44.

Kreshover, S. 1960. Metabolic Disturbances in Tooth Formation. *Annals of the New York Academy of Science* 85:161–67.

Krieger, Nancy. 1994. Epidemiology and the Web of Causation: Has Anyone Seen the Spider? *Social Science and Medicine* 39:887–903.

Lallo, John. 1973. The Skeletal Biology of Three Prehistoric American Indian Societies from Dickson Mounds. University of Massachusetts, Amherst.

Lallo, John, George J. Armelagos, and R. P. Mensforth. 1977. The Role of Diet, Diseases and Physiology in the Origin of Porotic Hyperostosis. *Human Biology* 49:471–83.

Lallo, John, G. J. Armelagos, and J. C. Rose. 1978. Paleoepidemiology of Infectious Disease in the Dickson Mounds Population. *Medical College of Virginia Quarterly* 14:17–23.

Lallo, John, J. C. Rose, and G. J. Armelagos. 1980. An Ecological Interpretation of Variation in Mortality within Three Prehistoric American Indian Populations from Dickson Mounds. In *Prehistoric North America*, ed. D. Bowman, 203–38. The Hague: Mouton.

Lasker, Gabriel. 1969. Human Biological Adaptability. *Science* 166:1480–86.

Lee, Richard. 1968. What Hunters Do for a Living or How to Make Out on Scarce Resources. In *Man the Hunter*, ed. R. Lee and I. DeVore, 30–48. Chicago: Aldine.

Lee, Richard, and DeVore, I., eds. 1968. *Man the Hunter*. Chicago: Aldine.

Little, Elizabeth. 1987. Inland Waterways of the Northeast. *Midcontinental Journal of Archaeology* 12:55–76.

Martin, Debra L., George J. Armelagos, Alan H. Goodman, and Dennis P. Van Gerven. 1984. The Effects of Socioeconomic Change in Prehistoric Africa: Sudanese Nubia as a Case Study. In *Paleopathology at the Origins of Agriculture*, ed. M. N. Cohen and G. J. Armelagos, 193–214. New York: Academic Press.

Martin, Debra L., A. H. Goodman, G. J. Armelagos, and A. L. Magennis. 1991. *Black Mesa Anasazi Health: Reconstructing Life from Patterns of Disease and Death*. Carbondale: Southern Illinois University Press.

Martorell, Reynaldo. 1989. Body Size, Adaptation, and Function. *Human Organization* 48:15–20.

Mensforth, Robert P. 1991. Paleoepidemiology of Porotic Hyperostosis in the Libben and BT-5 Skeletal Populations. *Kirtlandia* 46:1–47.

Mensforth, Robert P., C. O. Lovejoy, J. W. Lallo, and G. J. Armelagos. 1978. The Role of Constitutional Factors, Diet and Infectious Disease on the Etiology of Porotic Hyperostosis and Periosteal Reactions in Prehistoric Infants and Children. *Medical Anthropology* 2 (1): 1–59.

Milner, George R. 1990. The Late Prehistoric Cahokia Cultural System of the Mississippi River Valley: Foundations, Florescence and Fragmentation. *J. of World Archaeology* 4 (1): 1–43.

Munson, P., and A. Harn. 1966. Surface Collections from Three Sites in the Central Illinois River Valley. *Wisconsin Archaeologist* 47:150–68.

Navarro, V. 1976. *Medicine Under Capitalism*. New York: Prodist.

Nelson, Ben. 1995. Complexity, Hierarchy, and Scale: A Controlled Comparison between Chaco Canyon, New Mexico and La Quimada, Zacatecas. *American Antiquity* 60:597–618.

Orlove, B. 1980. Ecological Anthropology. *Annual Review of Anthropology* 9:235–73.

Polyani, K. 1966. *Dahomey and the Slave Trade.* Seattle: University of Washington Press.

Rappaport, R. A. 1967. *Pigs for the Ancestors.* New Haven:Yale University Press.

Rose, Jerome C., Thomas J. Greene, and Victoria D. Greene. 1996. NAGPRA Is Forever: Osteology and the Repatriation of Skeletons. *Annual Review of Anthropology* 25:81–103.

Rose, J. C., and T. A. Rathbun. 1987. African American Biohistory Symposium: Preface. *Am. J. Phys. Anthrop.* 74:177.

Rothschild, Nan A. 1979. Mortuary Behavior and Social Organization at Indian Knoll and Dickson Mounds. *American Antiquity* 44:658–75.

Rowlands, Michael, M. Larsen, and K. Kristiansen. 1987. *Core and Periphery in the Ancient World.* Oxford: Cambridge University Press.

Sahlins, M. 1968. In *Man the Hunter,* ed. R. Lee and I. DeVore. Chicago: Aldine.

Saitta, Dean. 1997. Power, Labor and the Dynamics of Change in Chacoan Political Economy. *American Archaeologist* 62:7–26.

Sarnat, B. G., and I. Schour. 1941. Enamel Hypoplasias (Chronic Enamel Aplasia) in Relationship to Systemic Diseases: A Chronological, Morphological and Etiological Classification. *Journal of the American Dental Association* 28:1989–2000.

Sutphen, J. 1985. Growth as a Measure of Nutritional Status. *Journal of Pediatrics, Gastroenteritis and Nutrition* 4:169–81.

Swärdstedt, T. 1966. *Odontological Aspect of a Medieval Population from Jamtland/Mid-Sweden.* Stockholm: Tiden Barnangen, AB.

Ubelaker, Douglas H. 1982. The Development of American Paleopathology. In *A History of American Physical Anthropology 1930–1980,* ed. F. Spencer, 337–56. New York: Academic Press.

Van Gerven, Dennis P., M. K. Sanford, and J. R. Hummert. 1981. Mortality and Culture Change in Nubia's Batn el Hajar. *Journal of Human Evolution* 10:395–408.

Van Gerven, Dennis P., Susan G. Sheridan, and William Y. Adams. 1995. The Health and Nutrition of a Medieval Nubian Population. *American Anthropologist* 97 (3):468–80.

Waitzkin, H. 1983. *The Second Sickness.* New York: Free Press.

Wallerstein, I. 1976. *The Modern World System: Capitalism, Agriculture and the Origin of the European World Economy in the Sixteenth Century.* New York: Academic Press.

Wallerstein, I. 1977. Rural Economy in Modern World-Society. *Studies in Comparative International Development* 12 (1): 29–40.

Williams, E. 1966. *Capitalism and Slavery.* New York: Capricorn Books.

Chapter 7

Owning the Sins of the Past: Historical Trends, Missed Opportunities, and New Directions in the Study of Human Remains

Debra L. Martin

*- looks at the socio/political aspects of
violence on skeletal remains → finds ? have
7 skeletal anomalies → gender descrimination*

This study suggests the ways in which a political-economic perspective in bioarchaeology can redirect current research into new and productive areas. Criticisms aimed at skeletal analyses are considered and shown to be related to the historical decoupling of the study of past populations from their living descendants, in this case, Native Americans. Examples are drawn from the American Southwest because it is here, at the turn of the century, that many biological anthropologists (as well as ethnologists and archaeologists) were trained. Their studies set in motion a way of imagining Native Americans (vis-à-vis the precontact past) that created a physical anthropology unconcerned with the struggles of contemporary native people. This in turn led to the denouncement by Native Americans and others of skeletal analyses as irrelevant, disrespectful, and oppressive to indigenous people, and to the enactment of legislation prohibiting the excavation and analysis of remains without the consent and collaboration of direct descendants.

In this paper, a brief account of the historical trends in the study of Southwest human remains is provided to clarify how early descriptive studies led to the use of reductionist models for explaining the past. A political-economic perspective enriches and expands studies utilizing archaeological remains and serves to link studies of the past with concerns of people in the present. An example is provided that looks at patterns of violence directed against women in the precontact Southwest. Here I try to position past health conditions within the context of social relations, constrained by differential access to resources and asymmetrical gender relationships. Studies such as these broaden the interpretations of past cultures and challenge oversimplified, and ultimately belittling, scenarios of how men, women, and children lived. In this way, some of the major criticisms regarding bioarchaeological studies are addressed.

The training and graduate school experience of myself and others parallels the ironies and problems inherent in the practice of physical anthropology. For those of us drawn into these subfields, isolated fieldwork and solitary lab research consumed our energies and served to disconnect us from native people, the descendants of those whose lives we were most interested in. For bioarchaeology students in particular (that is, biological anthropologists whose work was primarily with North American skeletal remains), the laboratory walls exploded open in the 1980s. Native Americans began an organized campaign that publicly decried the act of excavating, analyzing, and storing non-European human remains, and they demanded the repatriation of all such remains currently held in federal and state repositories.

As we labored in our labs during this time, we began to keep our work clandestine for fear that materials might be snatched out of our hands before completion of our dissertations. At first, we did not see ourselves (or our subdiscipline) as being responsible for the anger and rancor in the Native American community. We saw ourselves as conducting studies that contributed to scientific knowledge. Now, in retrospect, it is difficult to see how we could have been so naive; Native American distrust of anthropologists in general and physical anthropologists in particular comes as no great surprise. Historically the indigenous people of the United States have been decimated and subjugated by colonizers from Europe, and it is in precisely this arena of domination and resistance that bioarchaeological studies have been carried out (Spotted Elk 1989; Deloria 1986). Thus, the act of "doing science" on Native Americans and their ancestors is linked to larger patterns of domination (Deloria 1995). Human remains have been measured, X-rayed, analyzed, and reduced to analytical components, and biological anthropologists applied their trade with virtually no recognition or acknowledgment that there might be a social, political, religious, or ethical realm to what they did and how they did it. To some degree, this arrogance continues into the present.

Native American resistance included the long battle for and historic passage of legislation in 1990 (PL 101–601, "Native American Graves Protection and Repatriation Act"). This legislation ensures that American

Indians have final say about the nature of archaeological studies that rely on ancestral human remains and sacred objects found on federal or tribal lands. Biological anthropologists, specifically bioarchaeologists, can no longer assume access to either the remains or the information inferred from them (Masayesva 1991). The repatriation effort has already served to redefine the direction of studies that involve human remains (Jenkins 1991), and this important resistance to and action against the community of scholars who have built entire careers on studying human remains is in itself an interesting case study of the intersection of science, ideology, and power. *says more about researcher than those researched.* *Hager's book!*

The American Southwest as a Living Laboratory

The American Southwest has long been a key training ground and laboratory for many of anthropology's most distinguished scholars. The record of human habitation in the American Southwest is both long and continuous, and the arid conditions that contributed to the preservation of artifactual and biological remains is on a par with areas such as the Upper Nile Valley in Egypt. For anthropologists, an additional contingency of history was the fact that the Pueblo people are intact and in situ communities in spite of the genocidal policies and colonial pressures exerted during and after colonization.

The Pueblo Indians are the continuation of ancient peoples referred to as the Anasazi, Mogollon, and Hohokam in scientific literature, but contemporary Pueblo Indians rarely use those terms when speaking of their ancestors. Instead, words for "ancestor" in a number of languages (e.g., Zuni, Hopi, Tewa, and Keresan) are used. Criticism of the label "Anasazi" (a Navajo word) is justified since it has little relevance to contemporary Pueblo people (Ladd 1991). The term *Pueblo* was applied by the Spanish conquistadors to American Indians living in compact farming villages near the Rio Grande in the 1500s; today it is used by Pueblo groups to refer collectively to the large and heterogeneous Indian populations living in the Southwest.

There are a number of Pueblo communities in Arizona and New Mexico, and continuities of these communities with precontact groups are evident in material culture, subsistence patterns, religious and ideological behaviors, and biology. What is clear about the Pueblo people is the unbroken cultural continuity that exists into the present. The Puebloans, as descendants of New World explorers who settled in Mesoamerica and

North America thousands of years ago, have maintained a persistent hold on traditional values while adapting to novel and changing economic, ecological, political, and cultural conditions (Ortiz 1979).

For archaeologists, the Southwest has been a major training ground since the turn of the century (e.g., Fewkes 1904; Kidder 1927). There are literally tens of thousands of known archaeological sites in the Southwest, and this geographic region was among the first to be studied by ethnographers and archaeologists, from the late 1800s and into the present. An impressive wealth of data already exists for many aspects of Pueblo precontact history as reconstructed from the archaeological record (see syntheses in Cordell 1998; Crown and Judge 1991; Gumerman 1994). Since the 1930s, thousands of sites have been excavated, and the reconstruction of health, environment, climate, trade networks, population movement, settlement patterns, housing, subsistence activities, and other facets of prehistoric Pueblo existence continues with documention and study.

In a similar manner, the Southwest became the training ground for American ethnologists such as Elsie Clews Parsons and Ruth Benedict, and, as such, it continues to be the subject of intense focus and numerous ethnographic studies (see Basso 1979 for review). There is virtually no facet (at least within the context of ethnography and archaeology) of historic and contemporary Pueblo society and behavior, from language to religion to worldview, that has not been studied (Smithsonian's *Handbook of North American Indians,* vols. 9 and 10).

Human remains encountered at Southwest archaeological sites were usually sent to eastern museums and universities for analysis. Starting with the earliest analyses by Hrdlička from a variety of Southwest sites (1908) and Hooton from Pecos (1930) and continuing through the present, there is an enormous literature on precontact skeletal remains for this region (Martin 1995). Readers of this early literature are simultaneously impressed that these researchers write with such descriptive detail and frustrated by their inability to see these ancestral peoples in broader regional and historical contexts. The focus of many of the reports on health and disease was and continues to be a tabulation of measurements, medical anomalies, and pathologies for individual skeletons (e.g., Hrdlička 1935; Reed 1946, 1965; Bennett 1966, 1973, 1975; Miles 1966, 1975).

At the root of the problem was the persistent focus upon descriptive morphology and racial typology. The literature from the earliest studies was focused quite specifically on Native American craniometry. Hrdlička, one of the founding fathers of American physical anthropology, cut his teeth on the skeletal remains from a variety of Southwestern sites. Trained as a physician, he turned all of his energy toward analysis of comparative morphology. His monograph on "Physiological and Medical Observations among the Indians of the Southwestern United States and Mexico" (1908) was one of the first systematic examinations of skeletal remains. Although this study made note of diseases present, its major focus was on the detailed reporting of genetic anomalies and epigenetic traits, with a heavy dose of craniometrics. Hrdlička demonstrated a very close biological relationship (based on cranial metrics) between the earliest Pueblo people (ca. 200 B.C.) and the historic Zuni. This study and many that followed (Hrdlička 1935; Reed 1946, 1948; Bennett 1973, 1975; Corruccini 1974; Miller 1981; Birkby 1982) sought to demonstrate a physical and genetic relationship among precolonial Southwestern groups across time and space. Native American critics point out the irony of this body of findings, showing that every origin story of the Pueblo Indians speaks to the relatedness of all of the Pueblo people in spite of cultural and linguistic variability (Anyon et al. 1996). Anyon and colleagues further show how use of native knowledge and oral tradition was thwarted in the early 1900s by ethnographers such as Kroeber and Lowie who argued that Pueblo people are "ahistorical" and that they (anthropologists) could not "attach to oral traditions any historical value under any conditions whatsoever" (Anyon et al. 1996, 14). Nothing could be further from the truth (Fine-Dare 1997).

In a similar vein, hundreds of human remains from the Pecos Pueblo, New Mexico (A.D. 1200–1838) excavated by Kidder in the 1920s were sent directly to the Peabody Museum at Harvard. Hooton, also an important founding father of physical anthropology, provided one of the first major tomes on precolonial skeletal remains. In this work, Hooton (1930) provides information on age and sex, but the real focus of the volume was a presentation of metric data from the adult crania. In the concluding chapter (344–63), it is revealing that only one small paragraph is dedicated to a summary of pathology (348), and fourteen pages fall under the subtitle "Conclusions on the American Race Problem." In this section, supported by a lengthy appendix of over a hundred photographs of individual skulls in frontal and side views (reminiscent of police mug shots), Hooton uses detailed craniometric observations to conclude that the indigenous inhabitants of Pecos were not Europeans.

Hooton's focus on craniometry represents one of many, many missed opportunities for skeletal biologists to examine, firsthand, the effects of colonization. The Pecos remains were unique because the collection represented individuals from the precolonial and colonial period. Hooton's interest was centered on analysis of the crania, and he paid little attention to the historical processes of colonization that caused people to die and thus become part of the collection he was studying.

For most physical anthropologists conducting research on Native American biology since the days of Hooton and Hrdlička, the laboratory window shades were drawn to contemporary problems of racism, poverty, and disease affecting Native Americans. In the early 1900s, reports surfaced that demonstrated that American Indian rates of infant mortality and adult morbidity were alarmingly high and disproportionate to the rates for the general U.S. population (Moore, Silverberg, and Read 1972). Their rate of diabetes was three times higher than that of other Americans, and the rate of tuberculosis sevenfold higher (Adair, Deuschle, and Barnett 1988). In the 1980s, for example, life expectancy, 46 years at birth for Navajo and Hopi men, was 20 years less than the average "American" (Kunitz 1983). These data typically were not examined with an eye toward understanding the impact and effects of colonization and economic and racial oppression related to the placement on reservations.

Bioarchaeology studies add a dimension of history and context to the preceding studies and could serve to link past processes of poor health with present conditions. In reporting on the biology of precolonial populations living in the American Southwest, it was clear that many of the health problems facing people worldwide today were endemic and vexing difficulties for prehistoric groups. For example, iron deficiency anemia was ubiquitous among children and adults throughout the occupation of the Southwest (Walker 1985). Congenital defects such as vertebral fusion have been documented (Merbs and Euler 1985). Children experienced disruptions in their growth probably due to a combination of infectious disease and undernutrition (Martin et al. 1991). Helminthic parasites such as pinworm and hookworm are found in desiccated feces (Reinhard 1990). Tuberculosis likewise has been demonstrated to exist in a number of Southwestern skeletal series (Palkovich 1984).

The archaeological occurrence of these health problems is interesting, but they cannot be fully understood without some understanding of the social relations within the groups these people lived in and a more intricate understanding of the local and regional factors affecting the flow of resources. Nor does this laundry list of potentially life-threatening illnesses address the reverberations at the household or community level. As Leatherman and colleagues (1986) so convincingly demonstrate for families in the Andes, when one member of the household becomes ill it has implications for all members in domains of work load, productivity, and participation in social activities. Thus, the science of bioarchaeology was separated from the contemporary human condition, and the opportunity to contribute to understanding the biological effects of oppression and genocide was bypassed.

Health studies *can* be used as means for addressing larger social issues such as the specific relationship between colonization and disease, disability, and death. The lack of understanding of patterns of disability and disease as it relates to dominance and access to resources is not unique with respect to Native Americans, although it is highly ironic, since Native Americans were studied so doggedly over the years by biological anthropologists and medical personnel. It is easy to see why Native Americans thought it foolhardy that scientists could make important contributions to Indian lives today through studies of Indian bones. Not only is much of the data neither helpful nor relevant, but it has been used in ways that aid in the continued tyranny over native people today. Silko laments: "It is only natural that they insist on measuring us with the yardstick they use for themselves . . . the interpretation of our reality through patterns not our own serves only to make us ever more unknown, ever less free, ever more solitary" (1987, 83). Without the explicit collaboration and textured layering of the voices of those most closely related to the people studied, we are destined to create scenarios that, although grounded in theoretical modeling and scientific empirical observations, are wanting in relevance and significance.

It is incumbent upon the scientific community to use information that has been collected over the years from artifacts and human remains in a way that does not trivialize or diminish the lives of the living descendants of those being studied. One way to do this is to transform biological anthropology into a more dialogical process, similar to Wood and Powell's (1993) proposal for archaeology. This includes decision making and research as a collaborative and reflexive process among coparticipants (that is, Native Americans and biological anthropologists).

An example of both the importance of the past for the present and how this cooperative process can work is drawn from recent collaborative investigations into endemic health problems of the indigenous groups who refer to themselves as the Pima or the Tohono O'odham in southern Arizona. High rates of diabetes, hypertension, and obesity have plagued members of this group since the 1940s. Recent multidisciplinary efforts to understand the etiology of these patterns of ill health have combined Native American, anthropological, archaeological, and epidemiological information on diet and health to understand the progression of these health problems over time. Some researchers reduced these health problems to one of genetic susceptibility (Weiss, Ferrell, and Hanis 1984), a form of blaming the victim (Cowen 1990). Others took a multivoiced anthropological and epidemiological approach and suggested a more complex etiology (Brand et al. 1990; Smith, Schakel, and Nelson 1991). Research from a number of disciplines was combined including data on past health status (paleopathology), precolonial indigenous food sources (archaeology and oral tradition), historical use of traditional foods (ethnobotany and oral tradition), quality of contemporary diet (nutrition), and changing patterns of sedentism (exercise science). It was revealed that when these groups abandoned their traditional diets, the rates of obesity and diabetes dramatically increased. These studies point to historical dietary and behavioral variables as important causal factors in diabetes, hypertension, and obesity. Armed with this scientific information, Pima groups have voluntarily and enthusiastically begun to incorporate traditional foods such as lima beans, tepary beans, mesquite pods, and corn back into their diets with positive results (Cowen 1990). Such multidisciplinary research examines the larger interacting spheres of culture, environment, and biology, and these kinds of nonreductionist studies on "ancestral menus" and ancestral health may continue to provide crucial clues to solving health problems. The time depth afforded by these data are critical, but more importantly, the Pima Indians were coparticipants and collaborators in the design and implementation of the studies.

The linking of political processes and their biological effects is essential for understanding the relationship between historical changes and illness, and the relationship between social stratification, differential access to resources, and health (see Whiteley 1996 for a particularly focused account of these variables as they affect Hopi Indians). Such questions cross over numerous disciplinary boundaries and thus demand a multidimensional approach. For example, poverty is a multicomponent stressor that can cause, on the biological level, increased exposure to undernutrition, infectious pathogens, and biotic extremes, as well as a limited access to dwindling resources. The causes of poverty in the contemporary world are usually the end result of "sociopolitical and economic processes whose origins might be displaced in both time and space" (Goodman et al. 1988, 193). The challenge is to locate these processes, and to formulate responses that take both history and social relations in their full context into consideration.

Women, Violence, and Social Relations in the Precontact Southwest

Historically, the anthropological portrayal of Pueblo Indians as passive and docile in both literature and photographs did a great disservice to Native Americans (Deloria 1995). In moving away from this unrealistic picture of Pueblo life, more recent research has begun to (over)emphasize the "dark side" of the ancient Pueblo people with studies purporting to demonstrate cannibalism (White 1992), institutionalized violence (Turner 1993), and endemic warfare (Haas and Creamer 1993). These studies tend toward particularism and ahistorical essentialism because they fail to provide linkages of the data taken from archaeological remains to broader social and historical processes. In speaking with Pueblo Indians, I have found them to be most concerned with the reduction of Pueblo culture to one behavior, in this case, cannibalism, to the exclusion of all others. Thus, one of the major complaints regarding recent studies is the inability to capture the complexity and dynamic nature of Pueblo culture and social relations by outsider anthropologists.

What is useful about a political-economic perspective, to the extent that it can be realized utilizing fragmentary data sets from archaeological contexts, is that it provides a way to contextualize scientific data within broader social frameworks. It acknowledges that science cannot be separate from the people it studies and their conditions. It involves critical self-reflection, inclusion of social history and regional context, and exploration of social relations and fields of power. Two well-studied archaeological sites (La Plata and Black Mesa) are used to highlight how indicators of poor health can be linked to social dynamics and provide an example of how to situate bioarchaeological studies within a political-economic perspective. This study seeks to demonstrate the utility of employing a political-economic perspective in analysis of precontact human remains.

Located near the borders of New Mexico and Colorado, the La Plata River Valley was a permanently watered, productive agricultural area in which more than 900 sites have been reported (H. W. Toll 1994). The valley was continuously occupied from A.D. 200 until about A.D. 1300. Large communities were maintained throughout the occupation. This area was lush by local and regional standards, and density of available resources was high. Agricultural potential was likewise very good; there is also ample evidence of hunted and domesticated game in the diet (M. S. Toll 1994). This area is located in the middle of a large and interactive political sphere of influence with Mesa Verde to the north and Chaco Canyon to the south. Trade items and nonutilitarian goods are abundant. Based on site size and density, it was a major population center, with communities up and down the river valley in close proximity.

In contrast, Black Mesa (A.D. 800–1150) in northeastern Arizona is located within the desert plateau region and is a relatively isolated and marginal environment with an ephemeral water source. Although agriculture was practiced, maize was never abundant, and many other local resources such as rabbits and other rodents were exploited (Ford 1984; Semé 1984). Black Mesa never was a major population center, nor was it a "focal point for trade or Anasazi culture innovation" (Gumerman 1984, 6). There is virtually no evidence of exotic trade items nor is there an abundance of nonutilitarian goods (Powell 1983). It was populated largely by farmers living in dispersed small groups.

La Plata and Black Mesa represent two extremes on the Pueblo continuum in terms of availability of resources (abundant versus poor), organizational state (aggregated versus dispersed), position and location vis-à-vis other spheres of power (central versus marginal), health (low morbidity versus high morbidity), and quantity of trade items (abundant versus none). For the human remains from both Black Mesa and La Plata, extensive studies were conducted (see Martin et al. 1991; Martin et al. in press).

La Plata. Evidence for violence from the La Plata burial series includes healed fractures and trauma, that is, nonlethal injuries that were incurred sometime during adult life. Cranial wounds found on individuals from La Plata fit the description of depression fractures caused by blows to the head (Walker 1985). The frequencies of healed trauma for adults at La Plata reveal that females have a threefold increase in the frequency of cranial trauma over males (14.2 percent versus 42.8 percent), and a twofold increase in postcranial trauma (18.7 percent versus 35.7 percent). Adult frequencies greatly outnumber those for subadults who have an overall rate of 4.7 percent for cranial trauma and virtually no cases of postcranial trauma.

La Plata adults with cranial and/or postcranial trauma clearly demonstrate different patterns between males and females. For males, there are three cases of healed cranial trauma (out of eighteen males). Six females (out of fourteen) demonstrate healed cranial trauma (largely in the form of depression fractures), and the ages of these women range from approximately twenty-two to thirty-eight years. However, the inventory of healed nonlethal cranial wounds for the females is longer and more extensive, with three of the six cases involving multiple head wounds. For example, the youngest female (ca. age twenty) has a healed broken nose. Another young female (ca. age twenty-two) demonstrates two depression fractures, one on the forehead and one on the back of the head. A mid-twenties female has multiple depression fractures about the front and side of her head. A young thirties female has a large non-reunited but healed series of fractures at the top of her head. Of the two females approaching age forty, one has a healed fracture above her right eye, and one has a depression fracture at the back of the head.

Five females demonstrate postcranial trauma. However, two features of lower body trauma are distinctly different from the male pattern: (1) In four out of six cases, the cranial and postcranial fractures co-occur, and (2) the postcranial fractures in the females occur in younger age categories, ranging from twenty to thirty-eight. For example, the youngest female (age twenty) has fractures in the atlas and axis of the neck vertebrae (she also had a broken nose). A twenty-five-year-old has several fractures (right shoulder, left upper arm, neck) along with multiple depression fractures about the head. This female also had a severe case of osteomyelitis that affected numerous bones. There appear also to be localized, trauma-induced osteophytes (painful bone growths) on the third through fifth cervical vertebrae. It is possible that this woman was struck with an object hard enough to cause not only cranial fracturing, but also lacerated wounds on the shoulders and chest area.

In reviewing other factors associated with health for adult males and females at La Plata, females have more cases of infection (30.7 percent) than males (6.2 percent) and some of these may be related to sequelae from the injuries that produced the fractures. Females demonstrated higher frequencies of enamel hypoplasias indicating more childhood growth disruption. A final observation regarding women with cranial trauma is that several exhibit more left/right asymmetry in long bone widths and more pronounced cases of postcranial ossified ligaments, osteophytes at joint surfaces, and localized periosteal reactions (enthesopathies). Whether these observations are the result of occupational stress (Kennedy 1989) or the sequelae of injuries that caused biomechanical problems is not clear. Regardless of the etiology, these markers suggest increased physiological trauma.

An association emerged when the mortuary contexts of the individuals with cranial trauma were examined. The majority of the burials from La Plata are flexed or semiflexed, and placed within abandoned structures or in storage pits. Often burials contain associated objects, usually ceramic vessels or ground stone. Every female at La Plata with cranial trauma had a mortuary context that did not follow this pattern. All were found in positions that were loosely flexed, prostrate, or sprawled. The mortuary context of females with cranial trauma reveals that, unlike their age-matched counterparts without signs of trauma, they were generally haphazardly placed in abandoned structures with no grave goods.

Black Mesa.   The overall frequencies of trauma on the remains from Black Mesa are negligible. Two males (out of 39; 5.1 percent) had unambiguous trauma: one male over the age of forty had a healed broken rib, and one male, a very robust twenty-year-old, showed a healing traumatic injury to the left side of the mouth and cheek. The body was in a flexed position with several accompanying grave goods.

For Black Mesa females, only one young sixteen-year-old (out of 52; 1.9 percent) demonstrated cranial lesions. However, this young female was placed in a tightly flexed position with at least nine bowls, ladles, and pots. No subgroup could be identified as being particularly at-risk for intentional violence or biomechanical stress. Other indicators of health at Black Mesa suggest the presence of nutritional and infectious disease stress. A picture emerges of endemic, mild-to-moderate nutritional stress that had an impact on almost all age and sex groups. The generally mild nature of the iron deficiency, the pervasiveness of childhood growth disruption, as well as the clustering of pathologies around infancy and weaning, all point to a difficult existence in an unforgiving environment, but there is no evidence of violence, differential treatment, or subgroups at risk.

Political-Economic Perspective on Gender, Trauma, and Violence.   Violence and fear of injury may have played a significant role in repressing some members of the La Plata community. Trauma is absent in children and generally benign in adult males (particularly the postcranial trauma which was all minor and occurred in elderly males). Females carry the unequal burden of traumatic injuries in this group. The location and size of the cranial injuries showed that by overall dimensions and size in area, female injuries covered a larger area, involved more bony elements, often

> how are these "traumatic injuries" occuring?

occurred in multiples, and caused internal (endocranial) damage in some cases. Furthermore, the comorbidity factors of cranial and postcranial trauma, infections, and decreased life expectancy (there were very few females represented in the older age categories) suggest unduly hard times for some adult females. Females with these health problems are in mortuary contexts suggesting rapid disposal with no grave offerings. As a group, they were younger when they died than females who had traditionally prepared graves.

An examination of other attributes suggests that women with evidence of trauma at La Plata were part of the larger Pueblo culture to the extent that most of these women have occipital or lambdoidal flattening consistent with the use of cradleboarding during infancy (Morris 1939). The one physical characteristic that distinguishes at least several of the women with trauma is a pattern of nonpathological lesions and abnormalities associated with occupational stress or habitual use of select muscle groups. Particularly, the upper arm bones are most affected and this may be attributed to an increase in activities such as corn grinding (Trinkaus, Churchill, and Ruff 1994).

Although the small sample sizes limit a detailed quantitative analysis of occupational stress markers, one hypothesis suggests division of labor by sex and possibly by "class" as well. Spencer and Jennings (1965), Titiev (1972), and Dozier (1970) summarize sexual division of labor for Pueblo people suggesting that, traditionally, women ground corn, prepared food, gathered wood, built and mended houses, made pottery and clothing, gathered wild foods, and made baskets. Men were responsible for farming, occasional hunting, and religious and ceremonial activities. The difficult task of grinding a season's crop of corn into meal to be stored for the year belonged to the women, who might spend as many as eight to nine hours a day at the grindstone. In traditional subsistence societies, with agricultural intensification there is often a concomitant pressure on women to increase their productivity simultaneous with a decrease in birth spacing (Harris and Ross 1987, 49). This places an enormous burden on women to partition their time, energy, and activities between very different and competing tasks: economic labor, and bearing and rearing children.

As the La Plata Valley population increased (through a combination of immigration and increased fertility), several conditions could have arisen. There would be a need to increase food production to feed the increasing numbers of people, and therefore a need for an increased labor pool. As more people moved into the La Plata Valley, it is possible that the more local or "native" populations maintained access and control of the resources. That is, natal groups would have had preferred access to food and other resources over nonrelated newcomers. This could effectively establish an underclass of people who were exploited in any number of ways. Reproductive-aged females would be the most advantageous group to exploit because they could aid in laborious domestic tasks and food production, as well as in child rearing. La Plata communities may have felt it necessary to construct rigid rules about resource allocation, and this would dictate strategies that targeted a subgroup within the population such as reproductive-aged women who migrated either voluntarily or involuntarily into the area. These women could have become indentured servants to others. How they came to be servant/laborers is less clear; it could have been through raiding and abduction of women from other villages.

Black Mesa, with few resources, chose a local and regional strategy that employed a more egalitarian distribution of resources, dependance on strong reciprocal trade networks among extended families and communities, and reliance on a diverse and flexible subsistence strategy through shared storage and redistribution of food (Plog and Powell 1984; Gumerman 1988). Ironically, archaeologists have written that La Plata was a "bread basket" and a favored place to live (H. W. Toll 1994), while Black Mesa has been referred to as a "backwater" region with the inhabitants as "poor cousins" to their more prosperous neighbors (Gumerman 1988). Resource availability and ecological richness, however, did not ensure equality for La Plata women; women may have been subject to increased violence either as captured or enslaved laborers, or as recipients of physical exploitation caught in the struggle for control over labor, production, and resources.

The environment, while playing a crucial role in constraining the productivity and use of the landscape, is not a good predictor of social dynamics and emergence of groups at risk. Population growth is not, in and of itself, the major factor underlying illness and decline. It is likely that the pattern of violence is related in this case to the interaction of environment and population with social rules about gender and labor. Thus, the study of violence in archaeological contexts must necessarily go beyond the proximate causes of individual cases but to do so requires the use of a theoretical framework that is responsive to historical and contextual factors.

A Political-Economic Perspective Applied to Bioarchaeological Research

In working with Pueblo men and women during a series of NAGPRA consultations, it became clear to me that what Pueblo people most want is an opportunity to be part of the ongoing interpretations of their past. My interest in violence against women was received with some interest, and Pueblo women in general were eager to know why it was present in the past and why it continues to persist in the present. As an example, in the Laguna Pueblo of Paguate today, women are negotiating for equality and access to formal political power (Linthicum 1996). Laguna women have never held elected offices nor had an equal voice in political decision making at the level of the tribal council or government office. Although women have played supportive roles through matrilineal practices that dictate marriage patterns, land use, and some ritual practices, decisions on a wide range of political, economic, health, and resource issues have been made largely by Laguna men.

Does this differential access to power have biological consequences for women in terms of health, productivity, and longevity? For Pueblo women in general, statistics demonstrate increasing cases of teen pregnancies, single-mother households, domestic violence, and chronic diseases (State of New Mexico Public Health Services Division 1993). These problems adversely affect both women and children. A more active role for women in decision making is strongly recommended around issues such as these that bear directly on the quality (and quantity) of their individual and collective lives. It is revealing, and no coincidence, that one of the Laguna women challenging the status quo is the former director of the local domestic violence shelter.

The La Plata/Black Mesa study begins to address the concerns of these Pueblo women, because it suggests the complex ways that violence is tied to gender, social relations, power and access to resources. The study also points to the contexts within which violence *is not* found, and why that may be the case. Although this study on violence in the past may not be met with unequivocal support by Native Americans, I have been encouraged by conversations with some that this kind of study is useful in showing the complexities and painting a picture of Pueblo people that is neither "all good" nor "all bad" (R. Martin, personal communication).

A critical look at the bioarchaeological work done prior to NAGPRA legislation demonstrates a body of data detached from the social realities of the time and unable to address real problems in health and health care. Examples drawn from the bioarchaeological literature reveal that a political-economic perspective can provide a lens for health problems and can generate a new set of questions regarding processes of inequality, asymmetrical gender relations, and resource distribution. Further, the linkage of these kinds of processes to health conditions illustrates the mechanisms used to establish and reinforce positions of dominance and how these ultimately affect rates of morbidity and mortality.

It is abundantly clear that anthropologists interested in the biological past need to reassess their motivations and methods regarding analyses utilizing indigenous archaeological resources. Invigorating the practice of biological anthropology with a new ethos involving scientific research that is nonreductionist and responsive to and inclusive of Native Americans necessitates a more reflexive and dialogical process. It is my hope that invigorating the practice of biological anthropology with a political-economic perspective and new methodologies will contribute to a more relevant and engaging enterprise, especially for those who previously were disenfranchised from the process.

NOTE

I thank the Wenner-Gren Foundation for providing the opportunity to imagine a new bioarchaeology. Hampshire College's Southwest Field Studies Program provided funding and support for data analysis. The Museum of New Mexico Office of Archaeological Studies provided funding and laboratory space for the La Plata research. Special thanks to Alan Goodman, Nina Payne, Wolky Toll, Brooke Thomas, and the "SAR All-Women Group" for critical insight and helpful comments.

REFERENCES

Adair, J., K. W. Deuschle, and C. R. Barnett. 1988. *The People's Health: Anthropology and Medicine in a Navajo Community.* Albuquerque: University of New Mexico Press.

Anyon, Roger, T. J. Ferguson, Loretta Jackson, and Lillie Lane. 1996. Native American Oral Traditions and Archaeology. *Society for American Archaeology Newsletter* (March/April): 14–16.

Basso, K. H. 1979. History of Ethnological Research. In *Southwest,* ed. A. Ortiz, 14–21. Handbook of North American Indians, vol. 9, W. C. Sturtevant, general editor. Washington, DC: Smithsonian Institution.

Bennett, K. A. 1966. Human Skeletal Remains. App. III. In *Archaeological Investigations in Lower Glen Canyon, Utah, 1959–1960,* ed. P. V. Long, 73–74. Bulletin No. 42. Phoenix: Museum of Arizona.

Bennett, K. A. 1973. *The Indians of Point of Pines, Arizona. A Comparative Study of Their Physical Characteristics.* Anthropology Papers No. 23. Tucson: University of Arizona Press.

Bennett, K. A. 1975. *Skeletal Remains from Mesa Verde National Park, Colorado.* Publications in Archaeology, 7F, Wetherill Mesa Study. Washington, DC: National Park Service.

Birkby, W. H. 1982. Biosocial Interpretations from Cranial Non-metric Traits of Grasshopper Pueblo Skeletal Remains. In *Multidisciplinary Research at Grasshopper Pueblo, Arizona,* ed. W. A. Longacre, S. J. Holbrook, and M. Graves, 36–41. Anthropological Papers No. 40. Tucson: University of Arizona Press.

Brand, Janette C., B. Janelle Snow, Gary P. Nabhan, and A. Stewart Truswell. 1990. Plasma Glucose and Insulin Responses to Traditional Pima Indian Meals. *American Journal of Clinical Nutrition* 51:416–20.

Cordell, Linda S. 1998. *Prehistory of the Southwest.* New York: Academic Press.

Corruccini, R. S. 1974. The Biological Relationships of Some Prehistoric and Historic Pueblo Populations. *American Journal of Physical Anthropology* 37:373–88.

Cowen, Ron. 1990. Seeds of Protection: Ancestral Menus May Hold a Message for Diabetes-Prone Descendants. *Science News* 137:350–51.

Crown, Patricia L., and W. J. Judge. 1991. *Chaco and Hohokam: Prehistoric Regional Systems in the American Southwest.* Santa Fe, NM: School of American Research Press.

Deloria, V. 1986. A Simple Question of Humanity: The Moral Dimensions of the Reburial Issue. *NARF Legal Review* 14:1–12.

Deloria, V. 1995. *Red Earth, White Lies: Native Americans and the Myth of Scientific Fact.* New York: Scribner.

Dozier, E. P. 1970. *The Pueblo Indians of North America.* New York: Holt.

Fewkes, J. W. 1904. *Two Summers' Work in Pueblo Ruins.* Bureau of American Ethnology. Washington, DC: Government Printing Office.

Fine-Dare, K. S. 1997. Disciplinary Renewal out of National Disgrace: Native American Graves Protection and Repatriation Act Compliance in the Academy. *Radical History Review* 68:25–53.

Ford, R. 1984. Ecological Consequences of Early Agriculture in the Southwest. In *Papers on the Archaeology of Black Mesa, Arizona,* vol. II, ed. S. Plog and S. Powell, 127–38. Carbondale: Southern Illinois University Press.

Goodman, A. H., R. B. Thomas, A. C. Swedlund, and G. J. Armelagos. 1988. Biocultural Perspectives on Stress in Prehistoric, Historical, and Contemporary Population Research. *Yearbook of Physical Anthropology* 31:169–202.

Gumerman, George J. 1984. *A View from Black Mesa: The Changing Face of Archaeology.* Tucson: University of Arizona Press.

Gumerman, George J. 1988. A Historical Perspective on Environment and Culture in Anasazi Country. In *Anasazi in a Changing Environment,* ed. George J. Gumerman, 1–24. Cambridge: Cambridge University Press.

Gumerman, George J. 1994. Patterns and Perturbations in Southwest Prehistory. In *Themes in Southwest Prehistory,* ed. G. J. Gumerman, 3–10. Santa Fe, NM: School of American Research.

Haas J., and W. Creamer. 1993. *Stress and Warfare Among the Kayenta Anasazi of the Thirteenth Century A.D.* Chicago: Field Museum of Natural History Press.

Harris, Marvin, and E. B. Ross. 1987. *Death, Sex, and Fertility: Population Regulation in Preindustrial and Developing Societies.* New York: Columbia University Press.

Hooton, E. A. 1930. *The Indians of Pecos Pueblo: A Study of Their Skeletal Remains.* Papers of the Southwestern Expedition 4. New Haven: Yale University Press.

Hrdlička, A. 1908. Physiological and Medical Observations Among the Indians of the Southwestern United States and Northern Mexico. *Bureau of American Ethnology Bulletin* 37:103–12.

Hrdlička, A. 1935. The Pueblos, With Comparative Data on the Bulk of the Tribes of the Southwest and Northern Mexico. *American Journal of Physical Anthropology* 20:235–460.

Jenkins, L. 1991. Tribal Initiatives in Research: A New Partnership between Science and Native Peoples. Paper presented at the 90th Annual Meeting of the American Anthropological Association, Chicago.

Kennedy, K. A. R. 1989. Skeletal Markers of Occupational Stress. In *Reconstruction of Life from the Skeleton,* ed. M.Y. Iscan and K. A. R. Kennedy, 129–60. New York: Alan R. Liss.

Kidder, A. V. 1927. Southwestern Archaeology. *Science* 66:489–91.

Kunitz, S. J. 1983. *Disease Change and the Role of Medicine: The Navajo Experience.* Berkeley: University of California Press.

Ladd, Edmund. 1991. Comments. In *The Anasazi: Where Did They Go?* ed. J. Judge, 25–28. Dolores, CO: Bureau of Land Management Series Press.

Leatherman, T. L., J. S. Luerssen, L. B. Markowitz, and R. B. Thomas. 1986. Illness and Political Economy: The Andean Dialectic. *Cultural Survival Quarterly* 10:19–21.

Linthicum, L. 1996. Laguna Vote May Open Politics to Women. *Albuquerque Journal* (Dec. 1): A1, A10.

Martin, D. L. 1995. Stress Profiles for the Prehistoric Southwest. In *Themes in Southwest Prehistory,* ed. G. J. Gumerman, 87–108. Santa Fe, NM: School of American Research Press.

Martin, D. L., N. J. Akins, A. H. Goodman, and A. C. Swedlund. In press. *Harmony and Discord: Bioarchaeology of the La Plata Valley.* Santa Fe: Museum of New Mexico Press.

Martin, D. L., A. H. Goodman, G. J. Armelagos, and A. L. Magennis. 1991. *Black Mesa Anasazi Health: Reconstructing Life from Patterns of Death and Disease.* Southern Illinois University at Carbondale, Center for Archaeological Investigations, Occasional Paper No. 14.

Masayesva, V. 1991. Research and Indian People: A Time to Examine the Real Human Issues. Paper presented at the 90th Annual Meeting of the American Anthropological Association, Chicago.

Merbs, C. F., and R. J. Euler. 1985. Atlanto-Occipital Fusion and Spondylolisthesis in an Anasazi Skeleton from Bright Angel Ruin, Grand Canyon National Park, Arizona. *American Journal of Physical Anthropology* 67:381–91.

Miles, J. S. 1966. Diseases Encountered at Mesa Verde, Colorado. Evidences of Disease. In *Human Palaeopathology,* ed. S. Jarcho, 91–97. New Haven: Yale University Press.

Miles, J. S. 1975. *Orthopedic Problems of the Wetherill Mesa Populations.* Publications in Archaeology 7G, Wetherill Mesa Studies. Washington, DC: National Park Service.

Miller, R. J. 1981. *Chavez Pass and Biological Relationships in Prehistoric Central Arizona.* Ph.D. diss., Department of Anthropology, Arizona State University, Tempe.

Moore, W. M., M. M. Silverberg, and M. S. Read. 1972. *Nutrition, Growth and Development of North American Indian Children.* DHEW Publication No. 72–26 (NIH). Washington, DC: U.S. Government Printing Office.

Morris, E. H. 1939. *Archaeological Studies in the La Plata District.* Washington, DC: Carnegie Institute.

Ortiz, A. 1979. Introduction. In *Southwest,* ed. A. Ortiz, 1–4. *Handbook of North American Indians,* vol. 9, W. C. Sturtevant, general editor. Washington, DC: Smithsonian Institution.

Palkovich, A. M. 1984. Agriculture, Marginal Environments, and Nutritional Stress in the Prehistoric Southwest. In *Paleopathology at the Origins of Agriculture,* ed. M. N. Cohen and G. J. Armelagos, 425–61. New York: Academic Press.

Plog, S., and S. Powell. 1984. Patterns of Culture Change: Alternative Interpretations. In *Papers on the Archaeology of Black Mesa, Arizona,* vol. II, ed. S. Plog and S. Powell, 209–16. Carbondale: Southern Illinois University Press.

Powell, S. 1983. *Mobility and Adaptation: The Anasazi of Black Mesa, Arizona.* Carbondale: Southern Illinois University Press.

Reed, E. K. 1946. The Distinctive Features and Distribution of the San Juan Anasazi Culture. *Southwestern Journal of Anthropology* 2:295–305.

Reed, E. K. 1948. The Western Pueblo Archaeological Complex. *El Palacio* 55:9–15.

Reed, E. K. 1965. Human Skeletal Material from Site 34, Mesa Verde National Park. *El Palacio* (autumn): 31–45.

Reinhard, K. J. 1990. Archaeoparasitology in North America. *American Journal of Physical Anthropology* 82:145–63.

Semé, M. 1984. The Effects of Agricultural Fields on Faunal Assemblage Variation. In *Papers on the Archaeology of Black Mesa, Arizona,* vol. II, ed. S. Plog and S. Powell, 139–57. Carbondale: Southern Illinois University Press.

Silko, Leslie Marmon. 1987. Landscape, History and the Pueblo Imagination. In *On Nature,* ed. D. Halpern, 83–94. Albuquerque: University of New Mexico Press.

Smith, Cynthia J., Sally F. Schakel, and Robert G. Nelson. 1991. Selected Traditional and Contemporary Foods Currently Used by the Pima Indians. *Journal of the American Dietetic Association* 91:338–41.

Spencer, R. F., and J. D. Jennings. 1965. *The Native Americans: Prehistory and Ethnology.* New York: Harper and Row.

Spotted Elk, C. 1989. Skeletons in the Attic. *New York Times,* March 8.

State of New Mexico Public Health Services Division. 1993. *The Health of Mothers and Infants in New Mexico.* Albuquerque, NM: Government Documents.

Titiev, M. 1972. *The Hopi Indians of Old Oraibi.* Ann Arbor: University of Michigan Press.

Toll, H. W. 1994. The Role of the Totah in Regions and Regional Definition. Paper presented at the 5th Occasional Anasazi Symposium, San Juan College, Farmington, NM.

Toll, M. S. 1994. The Archaeobotany of the La Plata Valley in Totah Perspective. Paper presented at the 5th Occasional Anasazi Symposium, San Juan College, Farmington, NM.

Trinkaus, E., S. E. Churchill, and C. B. Ruff. 1994. Postcranial Robusticity in Homo II: Humeral Bilateral Asymmetry and Bone Plasticity. *American Journal of Physical Anthropology* 93:1–34.

Turner, C. G., II. 1993. Cannibalism in Chaco Canyon. *American Journal of Physical Anthropology* 91:421–39.

Ubelaker, D. H. 1988. North American Indian Population Size, A.D. 1500–1985. *American Journal of Physical Anthropology* 77:289–94.

Walker, P. L. 1985. Anemia among Prehistoric Indians of the American Southwest. In *Health and Disease in the Prehistoric Southwest,* ed. C. F. Merbs and R. J. Miller, 139–63. Anthropological Research Papers No. 34. Tempe: University of Arizona.

Weiss, Kenneth M., Robert E. Ferrell, and Craig L. Hanis. 1984. A New World Syndrome of Metabolic Diseases with a Genetic and Evolutionary Basis. *Yearbook of Physical Anthropology* 27:153–78.

White, T. D. 1992. *Prehistoric Cannibalism at Mancos 5MTUMR-2346.* Princeton: Princeton University Press.

Whiteley, Peter. 1996. Paavahu and Paanaqawu: The Wellsprings of Life and the Slurry of Death. *Cultural Survival Quarterly* (winter): 40–45.

Wood, J. J., and S. Powell. 1993. An Ethos for Archaeological Practice. *Human Organization* 52:405–13.

Chapter 8

Nature, Nurture, and the Determinants of Infant Mortality: A Case Study from Massachusetts, 1830–1920

Alan C. Swedlund and Helen Ball

In the latter half of the nineteenth century, rates of infant mortality in American cities were a matter of grave concern. As many as 15 to 20 percent of newborns died within their first year, and in the worst neighborhoods or most afflicted cities, rates could go much higher (Phelps 1912; Woodbury 1926; Swedlund 1990; Meckel 1991). Since the mid–nineteenth century, countless studies of infant mortality have been undertaken. Those of the time were aimed primarily at the illumination of causes and the prevention of loss (e.g., Phelps 1912; Woodbury 1926). Recent twentieth-century studies have attempted to portray the historical events and factors involved and to reevaluate earlier data in terms of new methodologies and theoretical perspectives (e.g., Preston and Haines 1990; Meckel 1991). Several of these have addressed the political climate of the late Victorian (ca. 1870–1890) and Progressive (ca. 1890–1920) Eras and identified social, ideological, and economic dimensions of the problem (see especially Meckel 1991; Klaus 1993; Ladd-Taylor 1994).

In earlier work (Swedlund 1990; Ball and Swedlund 1996) we took a regional approach to the issues and focused our attention mostly on Massachusetts. The Commonwealth of Massachusetts experienced some of the country's highest rates of infant and childhood loss in the second part of the nineteenth century and became a center for the national debates that ensued. The health community was early and actively involved in studying and trying to prevent infant mortality (e.g., Knowlton 1845; Shattuck et al. 1850; Boston Board of Health 1875; Massachusetts Board of Health 1879). Moreover, a variety of sources of data were readily available to us for both rural and urban communities.

1830 - 1920

National and international comparisons have contributed significantly to an appreciation of the factors associated with this historical
period of epidemiological transition. Nevertheless, we contend that a
finer-grained approach in a specific regional context might uncover relationships that are masked at larger scales of analysis.[1] In this respect we
agree with Kunitz (1994), who has argued the importance of location and
historical contingency in explaining disease processes, but we are quick to
acknowledge that the issues we address were also part of a Western experience occurring in the United Kingdom and continental Europe as well.
Some aspects of urbanization, industrialization, and other effects of
modernity were shared by all regions of the West, were interconnected,
and cannot be understood without recourse to this larger system. In other
respects, each nation and region had its own distinctive aspects that
affected at least the course of debate, if not the nature of the transition (see
Wolf 1982 and Roseberry 1989 for discussions on this connectivity).

We argue that for New England and the northeastern United States,
the critical factors for infant mortality had to do with the significant
amount of foreign immigration and the history of women's labor participation consequent to early factory industrialization. These factors gave
rise to some regional distinctiveness, and they form the centerpiece of our
discussion. Debates on the excessively high infant mortality rates in the
late-nineteenth-century and turn-of-the century West often focused on
issues of class, gender, and ethnicity, but in the eastern United States race
and ethnicity reached a level of interest and attention that was not
matched in England or France (Meckel 1991; Klaus 1993). Understanding
how these three factors were treated—and often conflated—is a central
aim of this chapter.

Through the Massachusetts example we investigate a number of questions pertinent to critical and political-economic approaches in biological
anthropology. We also address the important issue of how to critique an
episode in the history of science and at the same time do "good science."
This involves fresh consideration of categories of analysis that are generally thought to be straightforward and unambiguous in their social science
and epidemiological etymologies but that may be legitimately contested
and problematized. It also involves deciding whether or not data that are
collected and defined in a historically contingent context, and that may
well carry certain subjectivities, may still be "recycled" and made useful
for inferences about their historical significance and epidemiological precision. That is, can they satisfy the modern standards of validity and relia-

bility requisite for meaningful hypothesis testing? To answer this question we present an exercise in using historical data to see whether we can track some arguments made in the past. We locate ourselves in this work as positivist and empiricist and as employing a biomedical perspective. We also employ an interpretive approach, however, and acknowledge its value in gaining a deeper understanding of our research problem.

We situate this work at the intersection of medical anthropology and physical anthropology. Infant mortality had definitely become medicalized by the late nineteenth century. And while our approach obviously deals with measurable states of health (morbidity-mortality), it also incorporates—as did the thinking of the time—notions about a "natural" state of being, about issues of race and ethnicity, about gender, and about order and change (evolution). One may question the place of physical anthropology in the history of infant mortality in the United States, but it is our aim to show that the discourse of physical anthropology was important as a site of opinion on the causes of death and debility in infants and children. Racialist and gendered explanations frequently invoked notions of "inherent," or instinctive, aspects of character, morality, and intelligence (or ignorance) on women and the foreign-born. Such explanations found their greatest manifestations in the eugenics movements of the first quarter of the twentieth century. We suggest that the roots of these explanations are entangled in the early history of physical anthropology.

We begin the main body of the paper with a consideration of some of the categories that require elaboration. Next, we proceed with a series of analyses that employ historical data and that sequentially address the questions posed by investigators of the period, but also questions that linger in the health literature today. These particular analyses reflect the questions as posed in the nineteenth century having to do with the relative effects of proportions of foreign-born and wage-earning women, along with the constellation of variables that were commonly associated in this debate. Since these questions tended to be most focused on urbanized places in the past, we have selected smaller cities and rural parts of Massachusetts to include in the analyses. Indeed, the assumption that the problem was localized in cities historically tended to deflect attention from the fact that less urbanized areas and members of the "native born" and middle classes were not immune from high rates of infant loss.

We conclude that while women's wage work and foreign nativity were certainly important risk factors for losing an infant or young child, they should best be thought of as structural and remote causes rather than as proximate or ultimate causes. Finally, taking up the theme of this volume, we suggest that considerations of cultural milieu and historical contingency are not merely addenda to the physical anthropology project, but are fundamental to the research problem. The study of infant mortality is so socially and historically embedded that any brief attempt to engage the basic data and render some conclusions simply will not suffice.

Background

Some of the earliest reports on health in the United States observed that the foreign-born population experienced much higher mortality than its native counterpart. In Massachusetts as early as the 1840s, mortality rates for the Irish were noted as being especially high (e.g., Shattuck et al. 1850). For 1871, the Boston Board of Health reported: "We see by [these] figures that, of the nine States compared, Massachusetts, with the highest death-rates by cholera infantum and diarrhoeal disease, also has the largest proportion of Irish population . . ." (1875, 151–52).

Ethnicity and country of origin were major categories of analysis and were singled out as "etiological factors" even though many theories of mortality were concerned with the sanitary condition—or environment— of the urban center under investigation. As Rosenberg (1979, 5–7) and others have pointed out, it was thought to be the differential vulnerability, or ability to "adjust" to these environmental conditions, that made groups more or less susceptible to illness and death. Observers of the times were not unaware that immigrant groups were forced by poverty to live in some of the most substandard housing in some of the most wretched neighborhoods, but even this observation was mediated in part by explanations that attributed poverty to ignorance and people's choice of residential location to a desire to be with "their own."

From the mid–nineteenth century onward, extraordinarily high levels of infant mortality were recorded in the industrializing centers of both Europe and the United States (Swedlund 1990; Meckel 1991). By the third quarter of the nineteenth century, as contagion theories of disease gave way to a more coherent germ theory, the proximate causes of death were becoming increasingly clear (see Massachusetts State Registrar 1918; Warner 1986). As infant death rates exceeded 150 per thousand births in many English and U.S. cities, the symptoms of afflicted children were recognized to be of similar origin in a vast majority of cases. Most common were infections of the sort we now recognize as the pneumonia-diarrhea complex. Complications of infant and weanling diarrheas were probably the single most significant cause. Because these conditions were known to be closely associated with the care and feeding of children, it was all too easy to place the responsibility for these children's failure to thrive upon their mothers and families. When the ailing child's mother worked outside the home, the culpability argument became more strident. If the parents were also foreign-born, it became that much more so.

In another paper (Ball and Swedlund 1996) we outlined the development of attitudes and perceptions toward working mothers during the nineteenth and early twentieth centuries. Experts' views shifted from emphasizng the role of negligence in infant mortality to gradually encompassing a fairly comprehensive epidemiological model. This period of blaming represents an important episode in the history of Western medicine because it demonstrates in concrete ways both the epidemiological and the social transitions that occurred during the late nineteenth century. An understanding of the role of women's work in infant mortality grew out of active, applied (empirical) work on the social and environmental conditions of working-class life. Some of the first questions asked were about the life-styles of working-class women. Thus, women's work, women's "ignorance," and ethnicity (the foreign-born) became the principal independent variables in the explanations of rates of infant mortality. Also, we suggest, a subtext was present in the debates on the perceived relationships among these variables that requires some further consideration of their meaning.

Infant Mortality

Infant and childhood mortality has been regarded as a significant marker of how well a population or community is doing socially (see Preston and Haines 1990; Swedlund 1990; Wise and Pursley 1992 for discussions). The argument maintains that communities value children and tend to be proactive on their behalf. This by no means is to suggest that societies do not permit a certain amount of prenatal or postnatal loss (e.g., Scrimshaw 1978, 1984; Johansson 1987; Ginsberg and Swedlund 1986; Scheper-Hughes 1992), but only that levels of infant and childhood mortality are a good index of a group's ability to manage its social and physical environment. Thus, when high rates of infant and childhood mortality occur, the stage is set for debates over the reasons. This was not always so. In the early part of the nineteenth century childhood mortality was often not distinguished from general mortality, nor was infant mortality distinguished from childhood mortality (see Meckel 1991). In addition, there was much debate about whether infants were "naturally" strong and resistant to external forces or fragile and weak and in need of exceptional care.

The rise of statistical and sanitary sciences during the 1800s gave interested observers both data and circumstantial evidence showing that infant mortality was indeed substantially higher than that of older children in the population and that this "at risk" group must be attended to in an effort to bring the rates down. Furthermore, health advocates recognized that there was greater political value in emphasizing the loss of infants and young children than in describing losses in terms of the general population. In these ways, infant mortality became identified, objectified, and designated a significant health problem in the Victorian and Progressive Eras (for useful discussions see Armstrong 1986; Meckel 1991, 11–39; Wright 1987).

The Foreign-born

The literature on immigration to the United States between about 1840 and 1920 is vast and cannot be summarized adequately here, but certain points are essential to the goals of this chapter. Key among them is that, for issues such as employment, health, and community representation, the percentage and composition of foreign-born in the population held considerable consequence for observers of the times. In the case of health, it has been pointed out that whereas in France and England it was largely possible to confine socioeconomic theories and analyses to issues of class, in the United States class was virtually always confounded with, if not substituted by, the analysis of race and ethnicity (Meckel 1991; Klaus 1993). Indeed, as Kraut (1994) amply illustrates, the United States historically has tended to identify the most recent immigrants as principal bearers of infectious diseases and inferior genes. The assignment of inferiority was also extended to other ethnic minorities resident in the United States (especially to African-American descendants of early African slave populations). Such a tendency has often led to studies in which the effects of income and class are difficult to separate from the effects of ethnicity, and in several cases to studies in which income and class are shown to be necessary but not sufficient to account for health or mortality differences (see Preston and Haines 1990). The latter finding, in turn, has often prompted assumptions of "inherent" biological or biocultural differences. These assumptions were seldom questioned: the supposed *natural inferiority* of African Americans went virtually unchallenged (by the health establishment) until well into the twentieth century. In other cases, assumptions were questioned: the assumed *natural inferiority* of the Irish did not go unchallenged in the nineteenth century.

We do not have to look far to see the contemporary remnants of such thinking. Explanations for differences in adult life expectancy, infant mortality, and susceptibility to AIDS have all been subjected to ethnic and racial hypotheses in recent years, much as high infant mortality, shorter life expectancies, and tuberculosis were attributed to the "inferior" genes of immigrants in the past (Kraut 1994). Recent calls for research along ethnic lines have a familiar ring, implying inherent differences between groups, whether in genes or life-style or both.[2] What is often missing is any analysis of differential access to health care and other resources. The search for enlightened explanations of diseases of complex etiology offers an opportunity for new insights through a biocultural approach, particularly one informed by a political-economic perspective.

It is important to recall this history of disease attribution among ethnic groups, and to remind ourselves that the mid- to late nineteenth century was the time of Virchow in Germany, Broca in France, Galton and Spencer in England, Lombroso in Italy, and Louis Agassiz and Samuel George Morton in the United States, to name a few (Stocking 1968; Gould 1981; Kevles 1985). These scientists were instrumental in defining the debates about group differences in health, and as we shall see, their ideas influenced research on infant mortality in Europe and the United States.

Women's Work and Women's Roles

We now focus our attention on women's work and child survival because it was women's work that concerned early researchers and reformers after some had dismissed the direct effects of nativity. By women's work we refer specifically to wage-earning labor outside the home, which many thought to be prima facie evidence of neglect of children. To understand the importance of women's status as an explanatory variable in infant mortality, we must again look at the historical conditions under which research on the problem transpired. That some mothers may have been forced circumstantially in certain times and places to neglect their children is not the issue, but the discourse on women's roles in the high levels of mortality that obtained in the late-nineteenth- and early-twentieth-century

United States was not about isolated instances, but about systematic and widespread neglect owing to either willful action or ignorance. Again, there is no way to do justice to the wide array of studies that have addressed this arena (much of it by recent feminist scholars), but an overview of the reification of this constellation of women's status variables is necessary.

Unlike the situation in England and continental Europe, where a large urban, working-class population was available, the labor force for early industrialization in the northeastern United States consisted primarily of the rural unemployed, including large numbers of young single women who came to work in the textile industry and other manufactures. The decentralized locations of many early mill communities in New England often depended on local young men and women who used wage work to supplement income from what was still principally a rural, farm-based family economy. In the early part of the nineteenth century this pattern became commonplace. It was strongly prescribed culturally that whereas men might remain in the factory system upon marriage, women were expected to quit the factory and reenter the domestic sphere (see Haraven 1978; Lamphere 1987; and Prude 1983 for discussions focused on New England communities). The stage was set for women with children to be considered unfit for wage labor. Even though married women with children were chastised by some for their factory work in England and Europe (e.g., Jevons 1882; Jones 1894), they participated at much higher levels and generally were more accepted than in America. By 1840 immigrant families began arriving in the United States from Ireland, Germany, and elsewhere, effectively replacing the Yankee "factory girls," but it was during the 1880s and after, with the arrival of many immigrant women who would take work in the factories, that the public outcries from would-be reformers grew stronger.

We should also note that during the latter half of the nineteenth century there was a growing social activism, including the beginnings of a women's movement. This movement tended to be dominated by educated, middle-class women who were strongly maternalist in their orientation (e.g., see Ladd-Taylor 1994), although they advocated women's economic independence, suffrage, and other legal rights. The social construction of *womanhood* tended to be that of *motherhood*, regardless of whether it was the state, local politicians, the family physician, or women's organizations who were defining it. Working-class women, be they rural or urban, native-born or immigrant, were thus subject to a moral order and a prescribed set of roles that were narrowly defined and often at odds with economic realities.[3]

In addition to these three, many other categories of social identity or variables of measurement warrant similar attention (e.g., the rise of the medical profession at this time), but those just outlined suffice to provide a context for the material we present next. We should also mention that those pioneers in anthropology and human biology who were studying the formation and classification of races were not silent on issues of gender. There was considerable interest in male–female differences in anatomy, especially in the size and functioning of women's brains (see Gould 1981; Haraway 1989; Schiebinger 1993 for discussions). Understanding some of the subtext underlying these factors aids us in appreciating why certain variables and causal relations were essentialized in the manner and sequence in which they were proposed.

Historically, the blame for high infant mortality shifted from the notion of constitutional weakness in the poor and foreign-born to the individual mothers themselves and ultimately to the roles of poverty and of the state. These categories reflect different levels of appreciation of the problem and differing theoretical perspectives, each of which had implications for the successful reduction of infant mortality. That many of the categories were socially constructed and reflect values of the times makes them no less real, a priori, or no less significant in their relation to infant mortality. A systematic examination of these social and epidemiological transitions reveals the etiology of infant mortality and the steps taken to alleviate it. In our analysis we incorporate a number of variables, in addition to proportion foreign-born and levels of female employment, that reflect the broader interpretations that emerged historically as the complexities of the infant mortality problem were better understood.

Empirical Approaches: A Case Study from Massachusetts

The State of Massachusetts offers by far the best field in the United States for a careful study of the subject of infant mortality and woman's employment.

Aside from its comprehensive system of recording both vital and industrial statistics, its greatest industries are those which employ many women, namely, the manufacture of textiles and boots and shoes. It may also be said to be the best American example of a highly organized industrial district, and it therefore may be said to be not only representative of conditions for the industrial sections of the United

States, but is an index of the conditions which are becoming
increasingly predominant in this country.
                                    —Edward Bunnel Phelps, *Infant Mortality* (1912)

Massachusetts reflected the early development of the American factory
system, high levels of foreign immigration, and a well educated upper and
middle class. It was one of the first colonies to develop a vital registration
system in the 1600s. By the nineteenth century it was well endowed with
practitioners of the new scientific discourses of health, medicine, and statistics (see Rosenkrantz 1972 for discussion).

As early as the 1840s investigators in Massachusetts and elsewhere
were constructing explanations for the observed high rates of infant mortality (Shattuck et al. 1850). The association of these rates with the immigrant population and the poor was difficult to escape. Influenced by the literature largely from England, and from their own values on the role of
mothers, women's labor participation and literacy became emerging
issues. An example of the rhetoric coming across the Atlantic is the treatise
on Married Women in Factories in which Stanley Jevons states: "In this
article I . . . direct the reader's attention to one of the existing social evils,
which is unquestionably the cause of much of the infant mortality alluded
to, I mean the employment of child-bearing women away from the home"
(1882, 40).

Similar comments were ubiquitous in the United States as well. There
was a growing perception, supported by some empirical evidence from
both the United States and Europe, that infant mortality, as well as other
health and social problems, was worsening over time. To the reform-
minded this was a disturbing trend, prompting detailed examination of the
evidence. As the systematic collection of data proceeded from the mid-
nineteenth century onward, trends were readily apparent. Infant mortality
tended to rise slightly statewide from the 1850s to approximately the
1880s, and then declined slightly in each decade into the early 1900s (fig.
1). In urban-industrializing areas, the slope of the increase before 1880
tended to be steeper as compared to rural areas. Similarly, the changing
proportion of women employed in wage labor and the percentage of the
foreign-born population showed apparent patterns of association with
infant mortality. By the turn of the century, literacy (especially female),
proportion foreign-born, and female employment were becoming the
major factors of attention. The association of these three variables with
infant mortality was verified in a number of studies (e.g., Phelps 1912), but

researchers carefully evaluating the available data were well attuned to the fact that association (correlation) did not necessarily mean causation. Using basic statistical skills, students of the problem attempted to ascertain the most probable of the causes.[4]

Cross-Sectional Analyses—Bureau of Labor

The strategy for interpreting the pattern of association among the variables tended to break the data down by region or community and to create a series of data tables (cross-tabulations) in which it was hoped that the true causal relations would manifest themselves. This seldom happened. The data were still aggregated at a level that precluded direct observation of exactly which members of the community or which families were experiencing difficulty, losing infants and young children, or avoiding serious morbidity.

To aid in the interpretation of the cross-tabulation data, we can subject it to modern statistical techniques possibly to ascertain effects that were obscured by the earlier lack of inferential statistics. We do this first for Phelps's now classic study on the relationship between infant mortality and women's wage work in Massachusetts. Among the data he utilized were figures from the state census for the thirty-two cities in Massachusetts as of 1885 (he also included 1905). Both for the state as a whole and for the cities individually, he found that infant mortality had actually decreased after 1885, confirming impressions that the peak was reached somewhere in the years 1875–80 (Phelps 1912, 28–33). But the issue of effects of the foreign-born and female labor participation persisted.

By dividing the thirty-two cities by size and comparing the levels of infant mortality, female employment, and percentage foreign-born, we can readily observe the apparent associations that were cause for concern (fig. 2). Using the 1885 state census we reassessed the data on the thirty-two cities, following the steps and data categories to the best of our ability (see appendix). In this way we were assured of knowing exactly what the data represented whereas in the text of Phelps some ambiguities regarding variable definitions remained. Phelps (1912, 30–32) did not see many significant differences between the 1885 and the 1905 data, so we restricted our analysis to 1885. Our data appear consistent and comparable with Phelps's.

Using a logistic regression model with infant mortality rate (deaths <1 yr./1,000 births) as the dependent variable, we introduced Phelps's inde-

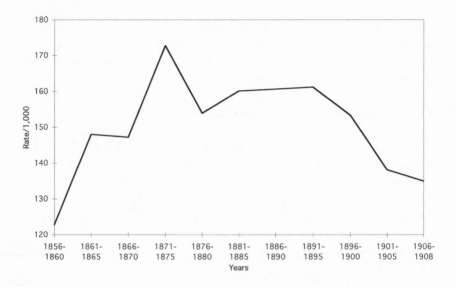

Fig. 1. Infant mortality in Massachusetts, 1856–1908

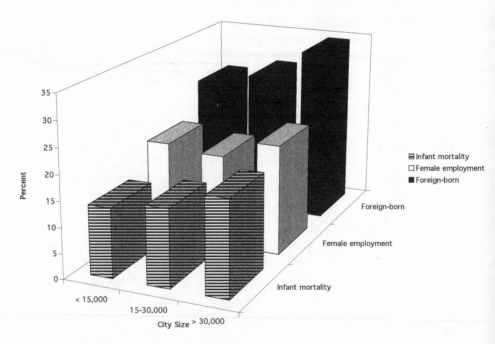

Fig. 2. Infant mortality, percentage foreign-born, and female employment, 1885

pendent variables of size of city, percentage foreign-born, and percentage of women aged greater than ten years in "gainful" occupations as well as those "illiterate."[5]

The results of this model provide some insights and also some alternatives to Phelps's more intuitive rendering of the results. Size (as measured by population/city) was most strongly associated, followed by percentage foreign-born, followed by females gainfully employed. Population size and females employed both entered with a $p < .05$ and the adjusted R^2 (explanatory value) was .68 (table 1). Percentage foreign-born approached significance and was a major confounder of females employed, changing the coefficient by more than 30 percent.

We interpret the results on percentage foreign-born to be indicative of an important effect and retain it in the final model. Illiteracy failed to enter significantly in any of the tests, while size always entered with significance. These results are confirmed by observation of the scatter plots of each variable on the infant mortality rate. Phelps's impressions were that size of cities and the proportion of women in extra-domestic work were related with "less regularity" (49) and that proportion foreign-born and illiteracy were "with fair uniformity coexistent with a high infant mortality rate" (48).

To discern these effects, Phelps looked at the cities in which women's labor participation was highest, and indeed, he found that infant mortality was also among the highest (1912, 33–49). But he was also able to identify communities in which extra-domestic work was relatively high, and in which the infant mortality rate was comparatively lower. By process of elimination eventually he was able to argue that cities in which textile trades predominated had both the highest female labor participation and the highest infant mortality rates. But they also had something else—the
and the lowest wages.

TABLE 1. Results of the Regression Analysis of Phelps's 32 cities in 1885

Dependent Variable	Independent Variable	R^2
IMR	a) pop*	68.4
	b) pctfb**	
	c) wom, emp*	

Note:
IMR = Infant mortality rate/1,000
a) = Population size of city
b) = Percentage foreign-born
c) = Women "gainfully" employed
*$p < .05$ **$p = .137$

lowest wages. Conversely, in the boot and shoe manufacturing cities, women's labor participation might still be relatively high but infant mortality comparatively low and wages comparatively high. This finding led Phelps to conclude that women's wage work per se was not the problem. By default, and with reference to studies in England and Wales, Phelps concluded that percentage foreign-born and, especially, the ignorance of mothers were responsible. This process of comparison between cities to identify the underlying cause of poverty's effect on infant mortality was a theme that would be repeated often.

To further complement Phelps's analysis and to consider less urbanized or industrialized parts of the state, we collected a second sample of data. On inspecting the vital rates in Massachusetts given in the *Annual Vital Statistics Report* (1917) we noted that infant mortality rates tended to be fairly high during the 1870s, and because 1875 provided a good state census with manufacturing figures, we decided to center the analysis on that year. Because Phelps and other researchers had already focused on Lowell, Fall River, and the other major textile centers of the northeast, we decided to direct our attention to a number of smaller communities located mainly in central and western Massachusetts. We included data from some of the larger centers for comparative purposes.

We selected twenty communities, each of which developed manufacturing industries during the latter half of the nineteenth century (table 2). Some of these towns were quite small (less than 2500 inhabitants) and were included to shed light on the roles that women's work and other factors might have played in what were essentially rural manufacturing villages. One town, Colrain, proved too small to provide data, so the sample was reduced to nineteen. Fall River, Lowell, Lawrence, and Springfield provided continuity with many of the previous studies on manufacturing cities. All communities were selected on the basis of representativeness of geographic location, size, and economic activity, but independently of their mortality rates.

In addition to population size and infant mortality rates, data were collected on a number of independent variables: population density, percentage foreign-born, males in manufacturing, females in manufacturing, illiteracy rate, average weekly wages, and a general fertility measure calculated as children aged less than 5 per woman aged 15 to 45. The rich documentation of vital statistics and census information for nineteenth-century Massachusetts makes it possible to refine these variables even more for certain time periods. However, the listed variables are sufficient for an initial examination of the association between women's work and infant and childhood mortality.

Given the small number of communities in this sample and the potential sampling and bias problems in using historical material, it was necessary to consider a set of simple regression equations that might optimize the available data. Three a priori models were selected to be tested, and a fourth, "best" model was determined post hoc from the completed regression results. In this way we were able to take a more inferential approach than Phelps could. Each model reflects a stage in the development of etiological thinking on infant mortality—from environmental causes (ca. 1850s), to foreign-born households and women's work (ca. 1880s), to conditions of poverty as reflected in low wages and employment (ca. 1900s). The models tested include an *ecological*, a *sociocultural*, and an *economic* interpretation (table 3). Each model uses a minimum set of the independent variables to account for the dependent variable (infant mortality rate) by town.

The ecological model is basically an epidemiological one, specifying population density and fertility as the important effects. Its argument is

TABLE 2. Population Size and Infant Mortality Rates for Communities Selected for Cross-Sectional Analysis

Town	Population	IMR
Adams	15,750	185.5
Agawam	2,248	108.0
Buckland	1,921	214.0
Chicopee	10,331	151.0
Conway	1,452	186.2
Deerfield	3,414	135.0
Fall River	45,340	250.0
Greenfield	3,540	100.5
Holyoke	16,260	208.4
Lawrence	34,907	232.0
Lowell	49,677	186.5
Montague	3,380	139.3
Northampton	11,108	150.0
Orange	2,497	186.2
Palmer	1,921	111.0
Pittsfield	12,267	140.3
Shelburne	1,590	178.5
Springfield	31,053	173.5
Ware	4,142	277.0

Note: IMR = Infant mortality rate/1,000

essentially that community and household "crowding" are the best predictors of high infant mortality. Pathogenicity and environmental effects are given preeminence as explanatory variables.

The sociocultural model proposes that illiteracy, which is considered a proxy for both the proportion of foreign-born and the educational attainment of all women, and the proportion of females engaged in manufacturing are sufficient to account for infant mortality. (Although we do not have a good proxy variable for each, we would also expect religious attitudes and ethnicity to be responsible for some aspects of differential child mortality.) Women's work and level of education are deemed causal in this model.

In the economic model, wages and the proportion of males in manufacturing are evaluated. This model tests the most important standard-of-living variables and might permit us to argue that it is the proportion of men dependent on wage earning that is important as an indicator of the level of poverty rather than the proportion of women working in manufacturing.

TABLE 3. Results of Three Regression Analyses of Infant Mortality in 19 Cities and Towns

Model	Dependent Variable	Independent Variable	R^2
Ecological	IMR	a) Density b) Fertility	7.7
Sociocultural	IMR	a) Fem, Mfg b) Illiteracy*	12.9
Economic	IMR	a) Male, Mfg* b) Wages*	42.3
"Best"	IMR	a) Male, Mfg* b) Wages* c) Illiteracy**	45.6

Note:
IMR = Three-year average centered on 1875
Density = Population/occupied dwellings, 1870
Fem, Mfg = Proportion females in manufacturing
Male, Mfg = Proportion males in manufacturing
Wages = Average weekly wage in manufacturing
Illiteracy = Foreign-Born and native nonliteratues in English
Fertility = Children < 5/women aged 15–46
*$p < .05$
**$p < .10$

Our interpretation of the ecological model is that it emphasizes and perhaps reifies the environmental crowding and "nature." The sociocultural model was constructed to hypothesize factors of gender and ethnicity and in this sense essentializes cultural factors, whereas the economic model foregrounds materialist variables. The models capture some of the playoffs of variables implicit in the work of Phelps and others but specifies them in a more analytical fashion.

Results of the regression using the ecological model were disappointing. Neither variable entered with significance or provided much explanatory power (table 3). We are concerned about the sensitivity of the density measure we used, because it expresses only overall community density as opposed to neighborhood density. Still, it is the only measure available to us at present. If it does capture some of the true effects of crowding, then this model is poor, indeed. It was necessary to control for absolute population size in order to estimate a density effect, but some size effect is no doubt operating in this sample, as well as in the 1885 series. For example, if we divide the sample into the towns with population under 10,000, 10,000 to 15,000, and over 15,000, then infant mortality rates show consistent increases: 163, 167, and 210, respectively.

The sociocultural model fared slightly better. Illiteracy had a significant inverse association with infant mortality, while the proportion of females in manufacturing contributed little to the R^2 and was not significant. Illiteracy in this case is acting most strongly no doubt as a proxy for the foreign-born, and the proportion of females actually in the work force is not a strong predictor of infant mortality.

The third model, the economic, produced substantially better results than the first two, with an R^2 of 42.3 percent. Both variables were significant and in the expected direction of association. The data and partial correlations also suggest that wages and proportion of males in manufacturing have independent effects on infant mortality (table 3).

The "best" model is a permutation of the economic model. Males in manufacturing and wages provide the best two-variable model. The best three-variable model also adds illiteracy. If two statistically outlying communities, Palmer and Ware, are eliminated ($n = 17$), then the R^2 in the best two-variable model is elevated to 65.5 percent. The best three-variable model (with illiteracy) is only marginally better at 66.6 percent.[6]

Taken together, the 1875 and 1885 analyses both support and contradict the findings of Phelps and others. Wages, and particularly *male wages,* seem to be more strongly associated with infant mortality than are ethnic-

ity (proportion foreign-born) and proportion of women working. Illiteracy, given Phelps's views, along with strong evidence from research in a
number of historical and development settings, might have been expected
to show stronger effects. It is clear that Phelps recognized that these factors were not fully independent of one another. He points in his conclusions to the conjunction of poverty, percentage foreign-born, and maternal ignorance as all tending to be present when infant mortality is high.
Our models depart from his in pointing to the strength of size of community and poverty in affording explanations. Phelps's and our interpretations both considered wages to be important, and neither has strong evidence for his hypothesis of maternal ignorance.

Community Analysis—Fall River, Massachusetts

Between 1875 and 1905, the infant mortality rate for the city of Fall River,
Massachusetts, declined from a high of 250 per thousand to approximately 175 per thousand. Still, this very high rate was of serious concern
to health professionals and government planners in 1905. A major component of volume 13 of the U.S. Bureau of Labor series was the case study
of Fall River, Massachusetts, written by Charles Verrill (1912). From this
study it is possible to infer certain effects of work in the cotton mills and
other conditions of the community at that time, effects that are obscured
by Phelps's cross-sectional approach.

Verrill and his colleagues collected data for the year 1908 on the city
of Fall River.[7] A total of 859 infants had died in their first year, and there
were 227 stillbirths. Of these totals, 580 live births and 165 stillbirths were
traced to their mothers and the mothers were interviewed for work habits,
feeding patterns, ethnicity, and so forth. In summarizing and reinterpret-
ing some of these data our purpose is to identify effects that might have
resulted directly from women's outside work and to suggest possible intervening variables of significance.

Verrill's report concluded that women who worked in the mills did not
suffer significantly higher rates of infant mortality than those who stayed
at home or worked at home. Those who worked in the mills throughout
their pregnancy accounted for 45.9 percent and 41.8 percent, respectively,
of the infant deaths and stillbirths in the sampled population. Of the
women working in the mills, only 83 (14.4 percent of all mothers experiencing infant loss) returned to their jobs before the death of their child.
Verrill notes, however, that those who did return to work in the mills after

childbirth experienced a considerably higher rate of infant loss owing to diarrheal infections than those who stayed at home (62.7 percent for workers versus 34.6 percent for those who stayed home, an 80 percent higher rate for factory workers).

Since the number returning to work was small, and since children whose mothers stayed at home tended to fare as poorly in most respects as those whose mothers worked, Verrill concluded that work in the mills did not constitute a significant risk over being at home. Instead he stated: "The causes of the excessive infant mortality in Fall River may be summed up in a sentence as the mother's ignorance of proper feeding, of proper care, and of the simplest requirements of hygiene. To this all other causes must be regarded as secondary" (1912, 74).

His conclusion was based on the strong evidence for gastrointestinal causes of death in both the at-home and the working population. Verrill's study is remarkable for the detailed information it obtained on feeding practices, living conditions, and work habits. He could demonstrate that the diarrheal infections were the result of early weaning and bottle feeding. But the study was also flawed in many aspects of its research design, given the original question. Its results can be reinterpreted by considering the following caveats.

Verrill never ascertained the proportion of the total infant mortality that was contributed by working women as opposed to nonworking women. A more accurate assessment of the contribution would have required the determination of the number of live births and infant deaths as a function of the women "at risk." Using the 1905 state census and 1910 federal census, we can estimate some of the necessary denominators. Verrill states that one-third of the estimated 13,000 mill workers were married women or widows. Extrapolating from the censuses and estimating the percentage of nonworking married women, it appears that the working married women accounted for an estimated 60 percent more deaths than their absolute numbers would suggest.

Verrill qualifies his observations at several points (1912, 110, 120 ff.) and notes that a perhaps not insignificant proportion of women at home had recently worked in the mills and may have been too weak or sick to return. Thus, some of the women at home may have been "working women." If so, the effect would be to elevate mortality rates for the "at-home" group and diminish the impact of the working women's group.

Because Verrill sampled only women who had lost children rather than all women having infants in 1908, the "at-home" population is perhaps also biased toward mothers who were more compromised in terms of health or who were relatively poorer, economically. This bias would also elevate mortality rates for the comparison (control) group and correspondingly lessen rates for working women.

That the major proximate cause of high infant mortality is related to feeding practices remains valid, and the results of Verrill's study are important for ascertaining causes of death for infants of both wage-working and at-home mothers and for an understanding of general levels of mortality. That women who returned to the mills while their children were alive had such high levels of infant mortality clearly indicates one potential outcome of women's working, regardless of the size of the population so affected. Verrill was able to demonstrate the increased dependency on artificial feeding among these women. His tendency to blame the women for their ignorance, however, should be considered more a reflection of class bias than a conclusion supported by his data.[8]

Discussion

What these examples suggest to us is that variations in infant mortality are not well accounted for by the proportion of women engaged in manufacturing, even though some effect is present. To what extent can we generalize from these results? We believe that the direct effects of nonhousehold work on infant and child health were exaggerated in the early literature. This is by no means a novel observation; many health reformers at the turn of the century were making similar arguments, including Phelps and Verrill. The proportion of women in wage work did show significant associations with infant mortality in the initial test (fig. 2) but not in the cross-sectional examples. This could be the result of a number of factors, not least of which is that there may be no effect. Alternatively, the measure may not be sensitive to the proportion of married women or women with dependent children, or the presence of an effect may be strongly associated with the types of work women were doing outside the home. Moreover, Abel and Folbre (1990) have shown that for some western Massachusetts communities, the census significantly underestimated the number of working women. Nor do we yet have a good sense of regional patterns; further work needs to be done in this area.

That wages and males in manufacturing do show significant associations is reassuring and expected (e.g., see U.S. Children's Bureau 1915, 1919). Studies from the earliest part of the twentieth century onward have noted the relationship between infant mortality and measures of poverty.

That there is a clear, inverse relationship between wages and infant mortality in this small sample is in keeping with other findings. The proportion of males in manufacturing is presumed to be sensitive to a number of factors related to control over food and other resources such as housing and sanitation.

Illiteracy in Massachusetts in the late 1800s was heavily influenced by the proportion of the foreign-born. The illiteracy variable should therefore be an indication of education and poverty, since most of the foreign-born population in the 1870s consisted of recent immigrants recruited to do low-level wage work in industrializing centers. Education is also known to be strongly associated with infant survival in both historical and contemporary populations. In the present test, however, we suspect education per se to be of little significance in explaining the variation.

Fall River

Reanalysis of Verrill's study of Fall River provides further insight. We believe that the data he presented do indicate some increased risk for women working outside the home during pregnancy, although the exact level of risk is difficult to estimate. Women working in the mills were at higher risk for infant loss, and a smaller fraction also contributed some additional mortality by returning to work while the child was still nursing. That these latter women also lost children was largely the result of premature weaning of the infant. We also believe there is a subtle but substantial, and largely unmeasurable, effect on infant mortality among the women at home that is also related to women's work. This effect resulted from at least two factors: (1) weak and debilitated women who desired or needed to work during pregnancy, but could not, and who were essentially homebound, were also more likely to lose a child; and (2) some of the at-home women no doubt fed their children artificially or weaned them so that they could take jobs in the mills as soon as possible due to economic necessity. Verrill's research design did not permit him to estimate how many at-home women this might include.

Phelps's and Verrill's views were that women's "ignorance" regarding the care and feeding of their children was far more important than whether or not they worked in the mills—the "culpability of mothers" interpretation. The detailed information collected and documented does, indeed, suggest strongly that feeding practices accounted proximately for a significant amount of infant mortality. In addition, the number of stillbirths appears to have been unnecessarily high and might reflect some undetected level of abortion and willful neglect (several fetuses were apparently well into the second trimester and some very close to full term, according to Verrill, although no specific figures were given). There was also a substantial proportion of newborns diagnosed with congenital "debility."

Taken together, the results of Verrill suggest that a proportion of the infant mortality experienced in Fall River in 1908 can be attributed to women's work outside the home. Why were so many infants fed artificially or weaned so young? We suspect that the requirement to work and earn a living was the overriding factor. While some small percentage of women no doubt practiced willful neglect, it is likely that most simply had no other options given their poverty and general state of health. During the early 1900s condensed milk and proprietary baby formulas were ubiquitous, fashionable, and heavily advertised as "better for baby." In unsanitary conditions, the risks of using these foods were considerable (Apple 1987, 1995; Levenstein 1983; Swedlund 1990). Dublin's (1916) later study of Fall River lends added support to this conclusion for Fall River.

Ignorance, Motherhood, and "Otherness"

As investigators inferred that a proportion of the foreign-born and women's wage work could be removed from the infant mortality equation, what was left as the residual? Ignorance remained, especially the ignorance of a subgroup created by coupling the extant variables, that is, the ignorance of foreign-born women. That there was in the progressive reformers' mission a goal of maternal education might at first imply a simple problem with a simple solution, but we suggest that a deeper meaning was present.

To properly contextualize the discourse on mothers' ignorance, it is necessary to provide a brief (if superficial) account of Victorian beliefs and attitudes toward race and gender and of the gradual transformation of those beliefs in England and North America. The Victorian Era coincided with the rise of evolutionism and the origins of anthropology. As social Darwinists (e.g., Galton) and, more importantly, the social evolutionists such as Herbert Spencer addressed issues of race and gender, many of the earlier moral teachings of the church were inscribed into evolutionary ideology, as were the status relationships between men and women and among the "races of mankind" (see Stocking 1987, chap. 6). Women's brains and the brains of the so-called savage races were arrested at an immature age, according to Spencer and others, and for this reason were incapable of the higher levels of reasoning possessed by white men. Yet women were also "instinctively"—by nature—mothers, caregivers, and protectors of home and hearth. Representations of the virtuous, responsible, and capable mother in opposition to the immature, fickle, and capricious young woman were a contradiction not easily dealt with but played out in many Victorian texts.

The historiography of this period reveals many attempts to place the so-called savage races and colonized states into an evolutionary scheme in which they were inferior to Europeans. But there were also peoples among the European ethnic groups and states who were believed to evince the remnants of savagery. As Stocking notes (1987, 235), distinctions between race and nation were considerably blurred. For the English there was a "close articulation, both experiential and ideological, between the domestic and the colonial spheres of otherness" (1987, 234). The so-called Celtic fringe held a station on the evolutionary scale well above that of the darker skinned "lowest races" but still well below the Anglo-Saxon middle and upper classes. The Irish were characterized in both scientific and popular literature as lacking the higher mental capacities possessed by their English neighbors. Many Victorians believed that the lowest classes in the urban centers were also innately of diminished capacity.

Conflation of race, ethnicity, and nationality was thus considerable, and so was confusion over the acquisition versus the inheritance of traits. Spencer was quite Lamarckian in his views, holding that progress was possible in the races (and women) through the inheritance of acquired characteristics (Stocking 1987, 222). Galton was not Lamarckian and was therefore a much stronger proponent of eugenic intervention (1987, 233). Despite the Victorians' confusion regarding heredity, it was widely held that habits could be or could become hereditary, and that once having done so they were manifested as "racial instinct" (1987, 236).

Thus, in the late-nineteenth-century United States, the term *ignorance* did not, we believe, imply simply a lack of education and a corresponding solution. While the notion encompassed the need for proper instruction—which reformers were prepared to provide—it also included notions of inherent deficiency that could not easily be remedied. A sense of these perceptions can be gleaned from the literature of the day. For example, when the Boston Board of Health reported on the sanitary condition of the city in 1870 it noted:

By comparing the deaths, by all and by selected diseases, occurring among given numbers of the various nationalities assembled together in our country, we might, to a certain extent, determine for each race its amount of innate healthfulness, its power of resistance to disease, and its degree of adaptability to our climate and institutions. (1875, 17–18)

and:

Our Irish inhabitants and their offspring, by consequence of their numbers, and of their morbid tendencies, exert a distinct influence upon our apparent sanitary condition. In the case of Boston, the influence thus exerted is so great that it becomes necessary to make allowances for this etiological factor, when attempting to make an estimate of our real sanitary condition compared with that of other cities. (1875, 180)

American physical anthropologists of this period were certainly invested in the view of racial and ethnic hierarchy, and their attempts to classify the human races typically divided Europeans into several regional as well as national types. As racialist perspectives on human variation gained momentum and "scientific" legitimacy during the Progressive Era (1890–1920), some scholars became associated with what would eventually be identified as the formal discipline of physical anthropology, with its own journal (*American Journal of Physical Anthropology*) and organization (American Association of Physical Anthropologists). The role of Aleš Hrdlička in forming the association and journal are well known (Spencer 1981). But also among those active in forming the discipline were some of America's best known and respected eugenicists, including Madison Grant, Henry Fairfield Osborn, and Charles Davenport, the first director of the Cold Spring Harbor Laboratory and the Eugenics Record Office (Stocking 1968; Kevles 1985).[9]

Most of the eugenicists' attention was focused on what came to be called the threat of "race suicide" through foreign immigration. But these men were also concerned with the quality of children born to immigrant parents in the United States, and they feared that too few children were being born of "native white" parentage. Their agenda for managing foreigners was two-pronged: limit immigration of those deemed less fit, and improve the health and survival of children born in the United States ("race betterment"). To this end, the American Academy of Medicine sponsored a national conference on infant mortality in 1909 that led to the establishment of the American Association for the Study and Prevention of Infant Mortality (AASPIM). Charles Davenport was a prominent figure in these associations, and AASPIM had a section on eugenics at each of its annual meetings thereafter (see Meckel 1991, 108–19; Klaus 1993, 38–42). The tenor of discussions within AASPIM was that by discouraging reproduction of the unfit and by encouraging the proper care of infants in their first year of life, both reductions in infant mortality and production of better babies could be accomplished.

The eugenicist project was by no means the only—or even the major—goal of AASPIM or the federally created Children's Bureau founded in 1912, but it was an important element of the reformist view and an arena in which physical anthropology was ideologically located, albeit tangentially. Most important for our purposes, however, is to foreground the fact that the development of an emphasis on mothers' education (particularly that of foreign-born mothers) was situated in these deliberations of the health reform movement. Lamarckian notions that "proper" maternal behavior could be learned, and that intellectual and behavioral traits deemed deficient in at least some of the foreign-born could be instilled, motivated the reformers to action. Ignorance and otherness were more profoundly associated with each other than some readings seem to imply. The results of the foregoing analyses must be considered in this light.

Conclusion

> The children of women engaged in industrial occupations suffer from
> the effects of maternal neglect. They are handicapped from the moment
> of birth in their struggle for existence, and have to contend not only
> against the inevitable perils of infancy, but also against perils due to
> their neglect by their mothers, and to the ignorance of those to whose
> care they are entrusted.
> —Hugh Jones, *The Perils and Protection of Infant Life,* 1894

Jones's beliefs seem to embody much of the late-nineteenth-century discourse on the problems of infant mortality and its causes. It encompasses women's work, ignorance, maternal neglect, and also the evolutionary rhetoric of the day complete with "Man's" natural struggle against a hostile world.

A central aim of this chapter has been to show how the social milieu and political economy of the times informed and influenced the scientific approaches undertaken. It also has been our intention to indicate that infant mortality was responsive to the efforts at abatement by early health reformers despite their political and social agendas. Indeed, advances in science and medicine always take place in a social and political context. Acknowledging these contexts historically helps us to understand better the successes and failures of the past. Can we expect less in the present? In our concluding remarks we would like to highlight some points of this chapter and then to briefly touch on some facets of this historical experience that seem to resonate well with efforts at the prevention of infant morbidity and mortality today.

First, the methodological: This research is presented from the shifting and unstable platforms of both positivist and interpretive perspectives. While some might well argue that these approaches are incompatible, it is not our purpose to reconcile them, but rather to recognize the tension that may exist between them and then to exploit their respective strengths for enlightenment on a complex historical question. One of the ultimate questions posed in science and politics is "What are you trying to prove?" And in vernacular usage this question almost always implies a suspicion of a political agenda, intentional distortion, or hiding of the truth. The methods employed in this chapter are aimed at enlarging the perimeter from which questions may be asked, and from which different kinds of answers may be derived.

The exercise in "recycling" earlier studies and old data has been useful to this end. It has assisted us in seeing how "objective" data collected for resolution of a question was strongly influenced by ideological underpinnings of the times. Evidence is presented to suggest how several aspects of the research problem were socially constructed. And yet, the imperfect data and models seem to have levels of validity and reliability that permitted, historically, a critiquing of old conclusions and tests of alternatives, and that can be useful in the rephrasing of questions now. Learning more regarding the background of the health researchers and reformers has aided in our understanding of their phrasings of the original questions. For example, as bureaucrats for the Department of Labor, it is not too surprising that Phelps and Verrill found little evidence of the effect of married women's factory work on the health of infants and children. Our reevaluation of the data and Dublin's (1916) follow-up study would suggest that effects were present and reflected a larger economic problem. Class, ethnicity, and occupation of the researchers were no doubt influential in the framing of most questions and answers, and we would argue that the emphasis on women's ignorance and ethnicity—in some respects—may have retarded the rate of the mortality transition by deflecting attention from public health measures, housing, and wages.[10]

The roles that anthropology and eugenics played in pursuing natural explanations of group difference and notions of intelligence may have fueled researchers' beliefs regarding infant mortality more than we may have previously assumed. Then, as now, the nature–nurture controversy found several arenas in which complex etiologies were reduced to simple, oppositional explanations. The pervasiveness of social Darwinist thought in turn-of-the-century America is easily lost sight of in the vital statistics and health reports of the period. A careful reading of the medical literature, biography, and historiography of the period, however, suggests a strong influence was present (see Hofstadter 1955).[11]

Substantively our purpose has been to evaluate the structure of infant mortality in Massachusetts in the late nineteenth and early twentieth centuries and to measure some of the associated variables. Despite the limited examples, the murkiness of the data, and the socially constructed ways in which groups and problems were defined, the models to explain infant mortality got improved, and so did the levels of actual deaths gradually become reduced. The identification of pathogenic pathways, particularly in the case of weanling diarrheas, was a major step in reducing proximate causalities. Improved water supplies, pasteurization, higher wages, and even home economics education were all responses to assessed needs, and no doubt all were of measurable value. The reformers, despite their class interests, accomplished a great deal in identifying problems and promoting change. The ultimate causalities of proportion foreign-born, maternal ignorance, women's wage work, and others slowly gave way to more systemic explanations relating to poverty and the conditions of working class life by the 1920s. Work conducted by the Children's Bureau and the modeling of infant mortality developed by Woodbury and associates (1926) were precursors to the contemporary standards for mortality prevention and epidemiological research.

Past and Present in Infant Mortality Research

We believe that there remains an issue of conflation of race/ethnicity, class, and gender in contemporary examples of infant mortality research, and it behooves us to be vigilant to the problem. Historical case studies can help us appreciate the problems and pitfalls. For example, in nineteenth- and early-twentieth-century studies of biological differences, the groups being compared might well have been, as they were for Phelps and Verrill (1912), Irish, Portuguese, and French Canadian. The arguments regarding their "ignorance" and "difference" carry a powerful message for today's researchers. The fact that "Colored" might include African-Americans, East Indians, and Filipinos in the same group is instructive to those investigators who would lump African Americans, Puerto Ricans, and "other Hispanics" into the same category for purposes of analysis today. In this way epidemiologists can mistakenly reify ethnicity and easily mask other underlying factors.[12]

By the other side of the same token, ethnicity can sometimes be very important in accounting for differences net of economic factors. Many studies have pointed to a consistent difference in "white" and "black" infant mortality rates in the United States. A recent examination of infant mortality among "white" and "black" college-educated parents showed that there were slight but significant differences in outcome, with the blacks having higher infant mortality (Schoendorf, Hogue, and Rowley 1992). The difference is apparently confined to low birth weight babies and less adequate perinatal care, and suggests that, even today, college-educated African Americans may not have access to the same quality of pre- and postnatal care as their Euro-American counterparts. This suggests to us that the understanding(s) that anthropology brings to issues of ethnicity can be important to contemporary health problems, but that understanding is very different from the racial constructions of the nineteenth and early twentieth centuries.

Preston and Haines's (1990) study of infant and childhood mortality in turn-of-the-century United States suggests that race is probably the single most important category in accounting for variation. Is this wrong given the foregoing discussions? Probably not. The design of the study and the availability of data forced the authors to impute some important variables relating to income, but the authors argue that race at this time in the United States worked like caste to isolate and restrict access to resources and adequate health care. So, even with improved estimates of wages and controls on occupation across geographic region we should expect to find race to be an important variable, but a far different one than that envisioned by nineteenth-century reformers. A great deal of caution is warranted in invoking ethnicity as explanation. Biological anthropologists have not presented an exemplary case in historical epidemiology.

Finally, we must add to this equation another dimension, the status "woman" in general and "working woman" in particular. That immigrant and minority women receive the lowest wages and fewest resources was true in the 1890s as it is in the 1990s. The difference is that in the 1890s the women were blamed for going to work and abandoning their children; in the 1990s the women are blamed for not working and staying at home to care for their children. History tells us that we have tried both accusations without much success. Now it seems time to do something about the real underlying problems—problems that were beginning to be well appreciated by the early 1900s.

Gender, ethnicity, and race are important categories in the equations of infant mortality then, not because they have some inherent biological explanatory power, but because they have tremendous social explanatory power, even net of income and class. The new physical anthropology should be, at least in part, about the documentation, explanation, and prevention of health differences in these groups. This calls for individuals trained in the biology of health and disease who also have a broader understanding of political economy, ethnicity, race, and gender than one normally associates with traditional biological anthropology programs. The new genetics will undoubtedly increase our catalog of debilitating inherited diseases and make great strides in our understanding of their etiology. Whether these findings will have any great significance in their geographic and ethnic distribution remains to be seen, but we know now that a significant proportion of ill health—be it in children or adults—is responsive to economic and environmental improvements. Recently, physical anthropologists have become increasingly aware of the important role we can play in the study of health in relation to class, ethnicity, and gender (e.g., see Crooks 1995). Let us proceed.

APPENDIX A. Massachusetts Infant Mortality Data

City	Population	Percentage Foreign-Born	Births per 1,000 Total Population[a]	Deaths under 1 Year per 1,000 Births[a]	Females Age 10 and Over	
					Percentage Engaged in Gainful Occupations[b]	Percentage Illiterate
Beverly	9,186	14.73	19.8	118.9	15.88	3.37
Boston	390,393	34.14	30.1	188.2	17.22	9.55
Brockton	20,783	19.40	23.6	146.9	18.83	4.04
Cambridge	59,658	32.16	28.9	172.3	15.24	9.58
Chelsea	25,709	25.60	25.1	166.9	12.63	3.03
Chicopee	11,516	39.79	31.1	176.1	32.52	21.37
Everett	5,825	20.86	33.6	131.9	9.37	2.49
Fall River	56,870	49.16	32.6	239.7	36.99	24.93
Fitchburg	15,375	23.98	31.2	134.3	17.56	9.59
Glouster	21,703	32.32	26.4	138.8	8.57	7.14
Haverhill	21,795	19.09	26.4	157.1	23.15	6.14
Holyoke	27,895	49.79	42.1	168.1	37.32	18.91
Lawrence	38,862	43.94	30.2	213.9	34.72	12.31
Lowell	64,107	40.37	29.1	222.5	37.69	12.88
Lynn	45,867	21.30	25.8	140.7	24.74	5.34
Malden	16,407	26.41	28.9	133.4	17.66	4.24
Marlboro	10,941	26.17	30.7	154.6	22.06	13.34
Medford	9,042	23.38	22.4	130.9	11.38	5.57
New Bedford	33,393	30.71	28.9	177.7	22.75	14.44
Newburyport	13,716	19.00	22.9	152.7	19.61	10.83
Newton	19,759	27.81	22.1	111.9	10.75	7.31
North Adams	12,540	27.04	42.3	115.1	22.39	9.68
Northampton	12,896	26.01	23.4	135.7	18.84	9.20
Pittsfield	14,466	23.32	24.6	144.8	19.54	5.72

Quincy	12,145	30.34	34.9	124.0	8.44	7.10
Salem	28,090	27.06	24.9	180.6	19.29	9.26
Somerville	29,971	25.02	26.3	154.3	11.56	5.91
Springfield	37,575	23.79	27.3	157.3	16.80	8.74
Taunton	23,674	27.75	27.8	140.5	18.55	9.04
Waltham	14,609	27.47	25.1	131.7	26.12	7.85
Woburn	11,750	30.00	32.1	127.0	12.67	10.71
Worcester	68,389	29.51	31.0	155.6	14.69	8.70

Source: U.S. Congress, 61st Cong. 2d sess., 1912, Senate Document 645, *Report on the Condition of Women and Child Wage-earners in the United States, in 19 Volumes, vol. 13, Infant Mortality and Its Relation to the Employment of Mothers*, U.S. Government Printing Office, Washington, DC, 28, 30–31.

[a] Average annual birth rate computed by dividing total number of births, 1881–90, by ten times population at Census of Massachusetts, 1885.

[b] Domestic service not included

NOTES

We would like to thank Andy Anderson and Alison Donta (Social and Demographic Research Institute, University of Massachusetts, Amherst) for consultation on the regression models. Susan Hautaniemi and Jane Kepp provided consultation and editorial assistance. We thank Alan Goodman and Thomas Leatherman for their editorial suggestions and also the participants of the Wenner-Gren Conference for their input—especially Barbara Bender, Arturo Escobar, Lynn Morgan, and Gavin Smith for specific suggestions and insights. Margaret Connors, Sheila Johansson and Richard Meckel provided several useful suggestions. The senior author would like to thank Marjorie Abel (University of Massachusetts), whose contributions to this paper are substantial. As colleague, collaborator, and friend she has generously shared her knowledge of anthropology, women's history, and the Progressive Era. Final revisions on this chapter were made possible by a Weatherhead Scholar-in-Residence Award at the School of American Research, Santa Fe, New Mexico. Some of the data presented here are a result of the project on "Mortality Change during Industrialization," National Science Foundation Grant 9224572.

1. A much more detailed discussion of this rationale and also of the treatment of race, class, and gender in relation to infant mortality in historical Massachusetts is found in Alan Swedlund, "'This Treasure Lost': Infant and Childhood Mortality in Massachusetts, 1830–1930" (ms., Department of Anthropology, University of Massachusetts, Amherst).

2. This is not to negate or ignore the evidence for genuine group differences in the distribution of certain genotypic risk factors, such as cystic fibrosis in northern Europeans or Tay-Sachs in Ashkenazi Jews.

3. As with other topics covered here, there is a substantial literature on the social construction of women's work and of motherhood in the late Victorian and Progressive Eras. We are indebted to Marjorie Abel for sharing her work and clarifying many questions that we had regarding this material (see Abel and Swedlund n.d. and Abel 1995).

4. The quality of their work can be very impressive even by today's epidemiological standards, especially the studies by the Bureau of Labor, the series of studies by the U.S. Children's Bureau (e.g., Duke 1915; Dempsey 1919), and the work of Woodbury and his associates (1926). A particularly relevant expression of concern for the problem was the publication of the volume *Infant Mortality and Its Relation to the Employment of Mothers* prepared for the U.S. Commissioner of Labor as part of a nineteen-volume study on woman and child wage earners in the United States. The two reports contained therein, written respectively by Phelps and Verrill (1912), form the focus for discussion.

5. Gainful employment was defined as Phelps did, excluding domestic service from the state census data. The logistic program is available in the STATA package. During regression diagnostics and goodness-of-fit tests, Boston was identified as a clear outlier—mostly due to population size—and thus was dropped from the analysis.

6. It should also be noted here that bivariate plots of the data used in the regression models indicated a somewhat nonlinear association between infant mortality and males in manufacturing. As the proportion of males approaches 30 percent the effect on the infant mortality rate appears to strengthen, and the association is exponential and positive thereafter. This nonlinear effect is not sufficient, however, to alter substantively the results or interpretation of the model(s). What this observation does perhaps bear on importantly are the rural–urban contrasts between some of these communities (see Swedlund 1990).

7. It should be noted here that while Verrill was the author of the report, agents Laura Keisker, M.D., Edith Shatto, and Frances Valentine actually conducted the fieldwork and no doubt were influential in writing the report. We thank Marjorie Abel for bringing this to our attention.

8. A later study of Fall River by Dublin (1916), based on data collected in 1913 by the Woman's Club of Fall River and the District Nursing Association of Fall River, pointed strongly to the effects of inadequate wages for both men and women as the principal factors involved, something that Verrill and Phelps had both alluded to but not seriously analyzed.

9. As Blakey (1987) notes, it was only after Grant and Davenport began to compete with Hrdlička for professional power that he began to oppose them.

10. Sheila Ryan Johansson (1996) has challenged us to consider whether the political economy and social milieu described here were instrumental in any way in affecting the course of the infant mortality transition—be it positive or negative—or whether these issues are simply anecdotal to the history of infant mortality intervention and have no direct, measurable impact. Indeed, this is an important and daunting question. To some readers this may not pose a substantive issue because the nature of the discourse(s) is the question, but to many social scientists and epidemiologists, measurable effect is the *bottom line.* It is our contention that attitudes of physicians, boards of health, and reformers in the Bureau of Labor and Children's Bureau *did* affect the course and rate of the mortality transition in both positive and negative ways. While this is an area in which care must be taken not to overgeneralize, examples of the ways the transition would have been retarded would include:

   a. Physicians' co-optation of obstetrics from midwives when their own practices were no more effective and quite possibly worse (see Kobrin 1966). Physicians' medicalizing and pathologizing of breastfeeding and collusion with the infant formula industry (see Apple 1987; Meckel 1991); and, some physicians' therapeutic heroics that proceeded well into this century (see Starr 1982; Warner 1986).
   b. The Massachusetts State Board of Health, officially founded in 1869, was preceded by some local boards and by the state legislature in outlawing certain unsanitary practices, such as the sale of contaminated or adulterated food, but there was little in the way of mechanisms for enforcement and there was much more concern about the behavior of some citizens, including the foreign-born, than there was active effort at sponsoring reform.

Even though studies on the benefits of pasteurization of milk were conducted in Boston as early as 1890, resistance from the dairy interests (and even from some physicians who believed that pasteurization destroyed the nutritional value of milk) prevented statewide pasteurization until 1928 (see Meckel 1991; Rosenkrantz 1972; Swedlund 1990).

c. As national and state reform efforts gained momentum at the turn of the century, the quality of advice dispensed by the medical and health communities was definitely improving. However, the Act of Congress creating the Children's Bureau (1912), for example, specified again that the primary role was information collecting and secondarily education. Moreover, policies at the national level were consistently noninterventionist in matters of wages, housing, and sanitation. By 1914 the Children's Bureau was publishing its popular brochure *Infant Care* and many pediatric physicians were also providing improved advice on child care, but at the same time the bureau was prevented from dispensing any advice on birth control even though it was apparently frequently sought (see Abel and Swedlund n.d.; Ladd-Taylor 1994). Diarrheal deaths were dropping significantly concurrent with the mother education movements of the Progressive Era, but the direct causal link is still quite difficult to establish (see Meckel 1991, 154–58). Despite the difficulties in making correct inferences on the impact of various attitudes and policies, we see this as an important arena for future research.

11. We wish to make our intent clear here. It is not our purpose to condemn individuals or to claim great insight into their specific intent. We leave that to the psycho-historians. We assume that most health reformers and medical practitioners of the times were motivated by a desire to do good and to be objective about the facts they observed. We wish to observe certain historical events from a late-twentieth-century perspective, but we do not wish to measure historical figures with a late-twentieth-century yardstick.

12. For discussions in which this is addressed see Hahn (1995, 113–26) and Farmer, Connors, and Simmons (1996).

REFERENCES

Abel, Marjorie R. 1995. Infant Mortality, Working Mothers and the Politics of Motherhood. Invited paper presented at the Northeastern Anthropological Association Meetings, Lake Placid, New York, April.

Abel, Marjorie R., and Nancy Folbre. 1990. A Methodology for Revising Estimates: Female Market Participation in the U.S. Before 1940. *Historical Methods* 23 (4): 167–76.

Abel, Marjorie R., and Alan Swedlund. n.d. The Study of Infant Mortality in the Progressive Era (m.s.). Department of Anthropology, University of Massachusetts, Amherst.

Apple, Rima D. 1987. *Mothers and Medicine: A Social History of Infant Feeding, 1890–1950.* Madison: University of Wisconsin Press.

Apple, Rima D. 1995. Constructing Mothers: Scientific Motherhood in the Nineteenth and Twentieth Centuries. *Social History of Medicine* 82:161–78.

Armstrong, David. 1986. The Invention of Infant Mortality. *Sociology of Health and Illness* 82:211–30.

Ball, Helen L., and Alan C. Swedlund. 1996. Poor Women and Bad Mothers: Placing the Blame for Turn-of-the-Century Infant Mortality. *Northeast Anthropology* 52:31–52.

Blakey, Michael L. 1987. Skull Doctors: Intrinsic Social and Political Bias in the History of American Physical Anthropology. *Critique of Anthropology* 72:7–35.

Boston Board of Health. 1875. *The Sanitary Condition of Boston: The Report of a Medical Commission.* Boston: Rockwell and Churchill Printers.

Crooks, Deborah L. 1995. American Children at Risk: Poverty and Its Consequences for Children's Health, Growth, and School Achievement. *Yearbook of Physical Anthropology* 38:57–86.

Dempsey, Mary V. 1919. Infant Mortality: Results of a Field Study in Brockton, Mass. Based on Births in One Year. Infant Mortality Series No. 9. Children's Bureau, U.S. Department of Labor. Washington: Government Printing Office.

Dublin, Luis. 1916. Infant Mortality in Fall River, Massachusetts: A Study of the Mortality among 833 Infants Born in June, July and August, 1913. *Publications of the American Statistical Association* 14:505–20.

Duke, Emma. 1915. Infant Mortality: Results of a Field Study in Johnston, Penn. Based on Births in One Calendar Year. Infant Mortality Series No. 15. Children's Bureau, U.S. Department of Labor. Washington, DC: Government Printing Office.

Dyhouse, Carol. 1978. Working-Class Mothers and Infant Mortality in England, 1895–1914. *Journal of Social History* 122:248–67.

Farmer, Paul, Margaret Connors, and Jamie Simmons, eds. 1996. *Women, Poverty and AIDS: Sex, Drugs and Structural Violence.* Monroe, ME: Common Courage Press.

Ginsberg, Caren A., and Alan C. Swedlund. 1986. Sex-Specific Mortality and Economic Opportunities: Massachusetts, 1860–1899. *Continuity and Change* 13:415–45.

Gould, Stephen J. 1981. *The Mismeasure of Man.* New York: W. W. Norton.

Hahn, Robert A. 1995. *Sickness and Healing: An Anthropological Perspective.* New Haven: Yale University Press.

Hamilton, E. G. 1909 Excessive Childbearing as a Factor in Infant Mortality. Transactions of the Conference on the Prevention of Infant Mortality, New Haven, CT.

Haraven, Tamara K. 1982. *Family Time and Industrial Time: The Relationship between the Family and Work in a New England Industrial Community.* Cambridge: Cambridge University Press.

Haraway, Donna J. 1989. *Primate Visions: Gender, Race, and Nature in the World of Modern Science.* New York: Routledge.

Hedger, Christine. 1908/1909. Address to the Academy of Medicine, 1908/9.

Hewitt, Margaret. 1958. *Wives and Mothers in Victorian Industry.* Westport, CT: Greenwood Press.

Hofstadter, Richard. 1955. *Social Darwinism in American Thought.* Boston: Beacon Press.

Jevons, Stanley. 1882. Married Women in Factories. *Contemporary Review* 37–53.

Johansson, Sheila R. 1987. Neglect, Abuse and Avoidable Death: Parental Investment and the Mortality of Infants and Children in the European Tradition. In *Child Abuse and Neglect: Biosocial Dimensions,* ed. R.J. Gelles and J. B. Lancaster. New York: Aldine.

Johansson, Sheila R. 1996. Personal communication.

Jones, Hugh R. 1894. The Perils and Protection of Infant Life. *Journal of the Royal Statistical Society* LVII:I 1–103.

Kevles, Daniel J. 1985. *In the Name of Eugenics: Genetics and the Uses of Human Heredity.* Cambridge: Harvard University Press. 1995 printing.

Klaus, Alisa. 1993. *Every Child a Lion: The Origins of Maternal and Infant Health Policy in the United States and France, 1890–1920.* Ithaca: Cornell University Press.

Knowlton, Charles L. 1845. The Autumnal Fevers of New England. *Boston Medical and Surgical Journal* 32:69–73.

Kobrin, Francis E. 1966. The American Midwife Controversy: A Crisis of Professionalization. *Bulletin of the History of Medicine* 40:350–63.

Kraut, Alan M. 1994. *Silent Travelers: Germs, Genes and the 'Immigrant Menace.'* Baltimore: Johns Hopkins.

Kunitz, Stephen J. 1994. *Disease and Social Diversity: The European Impact on the Health of Non-Europeans.* Oxford: Oxford University Press.

Ladd-Taylor, Molly. 1994. *Mother-Work: Women, Child Welfare, and the State, 1890–1930.* Urbana: University of Illinois Press.

Lamphere, Louise. 1987. *From Working Daughters to Working Mothers: Immigrant Women in a New England Industrial Community.* Ithaca: Cornell University Press.

Lentzner, Harold, and Gretchen Condran. 1985. Seasonal Patterns of Infant and Childhood Mortality in New York, Chicago and New Orleans. Presented at the Annual Meetings of the Population Association of America.

Levenstein, Harvey. 1983. 'Best for Babies' or 'Preventable Infanticide'? The Controversy over Artificial Feeding of Infants in America, 1880–1920. *Journal of American History* 701:75–94.

Massachusetts State Board of Health. 1879. Eleventh Annual Report. Public Document, 30. Boston: Band, Avery and Co.

Massachusetts State Registrar. 1918. 77th Annual Report on the Vital Statistics of Massachusetts for the year 1918.

Meckel, Richard A. 1991. *Save the Babies: American Public Health Reform and the Prevention of Infant Mortality, 1850–1929.* Baltimore: Johns Hopkins.

New York Milk Committee. 1912. *Infant Mortality and Milk Stations,* ed. P. van Ingen and P. E. Taylor. New York: New York Milk Committee.

Newman, George. 1907. *Infant Mortality: A Social Problem.* New York: E. P. Dutton and Co.

Phelps, Edward B. 1912. Infant Mortality and Its Relation to Woman's Employment: A Study of Massachusetts Statistics. Part 1. Report on Condition of Woman and Child Wage-Earners in the United States, vol. XIII. Washington, DC: Bureau of Labor.

Preston, Samuel, and Michael Haines. 1990. *Fatal Years: Child Mortality in Late Nineteenth-Century America.* Princeton, NJ: Princeton University Press.

Prude, Jonathan. 1983. *The Coming Industrial Order: Town and Factory Life in Rural Massachusetts, 1819–1860.* Cambridge: Cambridge University Press.

Roseberry, William. 1989. *Anthropologies and Histories: Essays in Culture, History and Political Economy.* New Brunswick: Rutgers University Press.

Rosenberg, Charles E. 1979. The Therapeutic Revolution: Medicine, Meaning, and Social Change in Nineteenth Century America. In *The Therapeutic Revolution: Essays in the Social History of American Medicine,* ed. M. Vogel and C. Rosenberg, 3–25. Philadelphia: University of Pennsylvania Press.

Rosenkrantz, Barbara G. 1972. *Public Health and the State: Changing Views in Massachusetts, 1842–1936.* Cambridge: Harvard University Press.

Scheper-Hughes, Nancy. 1992. *Death Without Weeping: The Violence of Everyday Life in Brazil.* Berkeley: University of California Press.

Schiebinger, Londa. 1993. *Nature's Body: Gender in the Making of Modern Science.* Boston: Beacon Press.

Schoendorf, K. C., C. J. Hogue, and D. Rowley. 1992. Mortality among Infants of Black as Compared with White College-Educated Parents. *New England Journal of Medicine* 32623:1522–26.

Scrimshaw, S. 1978. Infant Mortality and Behavior in the Regulation of Family Size. *Population and Development Review* 4:383–403.

Scrimshaw, S. 1984. Infanticide in Human Populations: Societal and Individual Concerns. In *Infanticide in Animals and Man,* ed. G. Hausfater and S. Hrdy. New York: Aldine.

Shattuck, Lemuel, et al. 1850. *Report on the Sanitary Commission of Massachusetts.* Reprint, 1948. Cambridge: Harvard University Press.

Spencer, Frank. 1981. The Rise of Academic Physical Anthropology in the United States, 1880–1980: An Historical Review. *American Journal of Physical Anthropology* 56:353–64.

Spencer, Herbert. 1876–96. *The Principles of Sociology.* 3 vols. New York 1898–99.

Starr, Paul. 1982. *The Social Transformation of American Medicine.* New York: Basic Books.

Stocking, George W., Jr. 1968. *Race, Culture and Evolution: Essays in the History of Anthropology.* New York: Free Press.

Stocking, George W., Jr. 1987. *Victorian Anthropology.* New York: Free Press.

Swedlund, Alan C. 1990. Infant Mortality in Massachusetts and the United States in the Nineteenth Century. In *Disease in Populations in Transition: Anthropo-*

logical and Epidemiological Perspectives, ed. A. Swedlund and G. Armelagos, 161–82. Westport, CT: Bergin and Garvey.

U.S. Children's Bureau. 1915. Infant Mortality Series No. 15. U.S. Department of Labor. Washington, DC: Government Printing Office. (See also Duke 1915.)

U.S. Children's Bureau. 1919. Infant Mortality Series No. 9. U.S. Department of Labor. Washington, DC: Government Printing Office. (See also Dempsey 1919.)

Verrill, Charles. 1912. Infant Mortality and Its Relation to the Employment of Mothers in Fall River, Mass. Part II. Report on Condition of Woman and Child Wage Earners in the United States, 13. U.S. Bureau of Labor. Washington, DC: Government Printing Office.

Warner, John H. 1986. *The Therapeutic Perspective: Medical Practice, Knowledge, and Identity in America, 1820–1885.* Cambridge: Harvard University Press.

Wise, P., and D. M. Pursley. 1992. Infant Mortality as a Social Mirror. *New England Journal of Medicine* 326:1558–59.

Wolf, Eric. 1982. *Europe and the People Without History.* Berkeley: University of California Press.

Woodbury, Robert. 1926. *Infant Mortality and Its Causes.* Baltimore: Williams and Wilkins. (Also published by the U.S. Children's Bureau as *Causal Factors in Infant Mortality: A Statistical Study Based on Investigations in Eight Cities. 1925.*)

Wright, Peter. 1987. The Social Construction of Babyhood: The Definition of Infant Care as a Medical Problem. In *Rethinking the Life Cycle,* ed. Alan Bryman, Bill Bytheway, Patricia Allatt, and Teresa Keil, 103–21. London: Macmillan.

Chapter 9

Unequal in Death as in Life: A Sociopolitical Analysis of the 1813 Mexico City Typhus Epidemic

Lourdes Márquez Morfín

Following the inherited influences of European and North American scientific traditions, Mexican physical anthropology was initially highly descriptive and deterministic. Until the 1960s the main goals of analysis of contemporary and past human biologies was to compare and classify.

By the end of the 1960s this approach had radically changed for some. At the same time that physical anthropologists in North America were turning toward ecological studies, researchers in Mexico, especially the teachers and students from the Escuela de Antropología de México, began to adopt a Marxist perspective. In place of prior descriptive and deterministic approaches, these new studies began to emphasize how humans are social beings with biologies imbedded in social, political, economic, and ideological structures, as well as physical environments and genetic structures (Dickinson and Murguia 1982; Peña 1982; Sandoval 1982). As a result of this movement, Mexican physical anthropologists participated with cultural anthropologists in a critical discussion on the objectives of physical anthropology and the relevance of general anthropological concepts to their work.

As part of this theoretical perspective, several bioanthropologists began to explore the biological consequences of urbanization, particularly among Native Mexican populations (see Murguia 1981). Following this theme, I initiated studies of patterns of health and illness among distinct ethnic groups in Mexico City in the nineteenth century in relationship to sociopolitical and economic conditions (Márquez 1984). As an example of this approach, in this chapter I focus on the Mexico City typhus epidemic of 1813.[1] Specific questions addressed concern the spatial distribution of ethnic groups and deaths in relationship to sanitary conditions and public health policies (Márquez 1984).

Epidemics are revealing subjects for bioanthropological investigation because they present opportunities to evaluate the determinants and conditioning factors that govern who gets sick and who recovers. Following Frenk et al. (1994, 31), this study relies upon a model of health that considers four basic determinate levels: (1) a systemic level of population, genome, environment, and social organization; (2) a societal level, including structural determinants of social stratification, occupational structure, and redistribution mechanisms; (3) an institutional/household level that includes more proximate factors such as working conditions, living conditions, life-style, and health-care systems; and (4) the individual level of health status.

The perspective of the study might best be called social epidemiological in that the focus is on the interrelation of social, economic, and political factors in determining the expression and rate of disease (i.e., morbidity rate), and the number of deaths due to that disease (i.e., lethality rate: the percentage of sick people who die).

Material and Methods

The primary sources upon which this study is based are located in the historical archives of Mexico City.[2] I used the census of 1811 as a basis for the socioeconomic research. Parochial registers were used to obtain information on baptisms, deaths, and marriages for the period from 1800 to 1839 (fig. 1). The morbidity and mortality rates of 1813, in particular, were obtained for each one of the thirty-two wards of the civil jurisdiction. Lists of sick and dead people during the epidemic, which were made by order of the city government in 1813, were used to construct mortality and lethality rates. Maps pertaining to the distribution of sewage systems, drains, pavement types, and garbage collection provided information on the geography of sanitary conditions. The narratives of people of the period were used in order to gain a sense of the atmosphere and the conditions of life of the inhabitants of the city (map 1).

The City and Its Inhabitants.   During the first half of the nineteenth century, Mexico City was one of the most heavily populated cities of the continent. Nearly 165,000 people of different ethnic groups—Spaniards, Indians, Creoles, mestizos, and mulattos—lived there (Humboldt 1984).

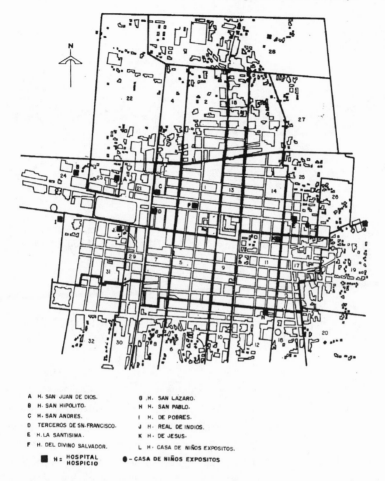

A   H· SAN JUAN DE DIOS.
B   H· SAN HIPOLITO.
C   H· SAN ANDRES.
D   TERCEROS DE SN·FRANCISCO·
E   H·LA SANTISIMA·
F   H· DEL DIVINO SALVADOR.

G   ·H· SAN LAZARO.
H   H· SAN PABLO.
I   H· DE POBRES.
J   H· REAL DE INDIOS.
K   H· DE JESUS·
L   H· CASA DE NIÑOS EXPOSITOS.

■ H= HOSPITAL HOSPICIO   ●=CASA DE NIÑOS EXPOSITOS

Map 1.   Mexico City wards and locations of hospitals, 1813

Increasingly, these groups were less distinguished by their "racial" origins and more by their social and economic positions. Inhabitants lived in different wards of the city in accord with their income and social status (Báez Macías 1969, 60–69).

The map of the wards (map 1) helps to visualize the size of the city, its limits, and the density of urbanization, and it provides a reference point to understand the mortality and morbidity that took place in each sector. Urbanization and services were very heterogeneous. The part surrounding the Main Plaza was the best built and endowed with services: lighting,

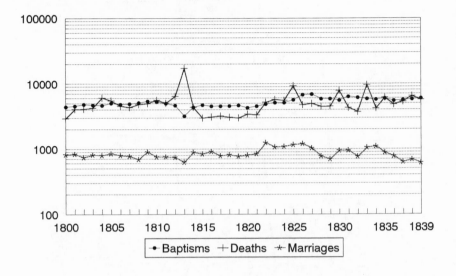

Fig. 1.   Baptisms, deaths, and marriages, Mexico City, 1800–1839.
(From Maldonado 1976.)

water, stone pavement, drainage, and garbage collection. In the heart of
the city we also find differences in the quality of the housing. Houses in the
central area tended to have two to three levels with upper areas used as living quarters and lower levels sometimes used for storage and corrals
(Moreno Toscano 1974, 1978, 1981). The robust construction of the central area diminished as one moved to the outskirts, giving way to humble
dwellings and shanties in the slums of the outskirts.

The people with the best economic resources lived in the central part
of the capital; a high percentage of them were peninsular Spaniards and
Creoles. The outskirts were the areas housing the Indians, who were often
employed in service/roles such as city sweepers, water carriers, or itinerant
vendors. The intermediate part was inhabited by artisans: blacksmiths,
leather workers, tailors, jewelers, and carpenters.

The inhabitants of the city suffered from the time of the conquest and
even before from hunger, destruction, and sicknesses. They were immuno-
logically defenseless against most European-derived pathogens, and they
suffered from other factors caused by social inequality. From the begin-

ning, smallpox and measles decimated the Indian population to an unprecedented level. Poor nutrition, the absolute lack of sanitation, and demanding work contributed to the severe course of diseases such as typhus and typhoid. This set of conditions did not change by the nineteenth century.

Mortality Rate. Certain years stand out as having excessive deaths during the first half of the nineteenth century (fig. 1). Excessive mortality in 1804 was caused by an influenza outbreak. In 1813 the number of deaths grew dramatically to 17,267. This may be an underrecorded number according to other sources, but, nonetheless, it represents the highest mortality rate of the period. During the period from 1814 to 1821 the deaths dropped and continued at approximately 3,000/year. In 1825 smallpox attacked again and caused the raw annual death count to rise from an average of about 4,500 in the four previous years to 7,600. In 1833 cholera arrived in Mexico and accounted for almost 10,000 deaths. Starting from that year, annual deaths oscillated between 4,000 and 6,000 (Maldonado 1976).

Morbidity and Lethality Rates in 1813.   An epidemiological study is one that attempts to account for the distribution of diseases in terms of age, sex, race, geography, occupation, and so on (MacMahon and Pugh 1978, 1). In research on epidemics, as well as historical demographic research on parishes in Mexico, mortality rates have been obtained by sex and age. Obtaining mortality rates by ethnic group is more complex, especially since some of the documental sources do not provide ethnic identification and/or the reliability of these data are questionable (see Morner 1961). The study of the demographic process by socioeconomic group in the periods prior to this century is difficult. Upon what criteria, for example, are social groupings to be defined? Are these criteria faithfully recorded?

In the case of the lists made by the Town Council of the city in 1813, we found information about the number of sick and dead in each ward.[3] In order to obtain incidence, that is, how many people out of the total population of each ward became sick during a period of time, I used the census of 1811, which was the closest to the date of the epidemic.

Mexico City was very heterogeneous in respect to its social, political, and economic composition. Nevertheless, in general terms, differential locations within Mexico City were occupied by distinct groups.

Ethnic Group.   Mexican society of that period can be considered a "society of castes" in progressive transition toward a society of classes. Cardoso (1977) maintains that societies of castes and societies of classes are not mutually exclusive categories, and the racial differentiation corresponds to economic and social differences. The biological factors, however, were not primary for this differentiation. For example, "in the exporting and administrative sector there was a predominance of peninsular born and the creoles predominated among landowners and industrialists."[4] The Indians were occupied in services or in the area of production related to agricultural labor.

Occupation.   Arnold (1979) proposes that economic factors are only one criterion for evaluating social groups. If the Mexican elite were patriarchal, plutocratic, and oligarchical, as suggested by Ladd (1984), one should begin research on occupational categories. In this respect, the excellent work of González Angulo (1983) on artisans in Mexico City and their spatial distribution in 1811 provides a starting place. Information on other occupations is not as systematized as that for the artisans, however, a variety of sources provide key data points and insights (Kicza 1986; Ladd 1984; Lira 1983; Toscano 1974, 1978, 1981).

Residence Location.   Residence location is of prime importance because morbidity statistics are recorded by ward. Therefore, our first analysis relates each one of the variables to spatial location. We then put emphasis on the presentation of the percentages of population by wards, ethnic groups, sex, and occupation. Urbanization, services, and equipment of each ward, in particular drinking water, drainage, stone pavement, and garbage collection, are aspects of fundamental importance in the study of morbidity, especially when the epidemic being analyzed is related to sanitary conditions (Guzmán 1988, 39; Cabrera 1988, 21).

Results

The devastation caused by the 1813 epidemic, known at that time as "mysterious fever," has not been fully evaluated, despite the excellent work of Donald Cooper (1980). The armed conflict for independence led to a reduction in food production, as well as countryside abandonment, hoarding, scarcity, inflation, and enormous migration to the city of people without work and with few economic resources. These people arrived to house themselves in the most miserable places and occupied themselves with any kind of work, which only aggravated the situation. The town council did not have the resources to carry out their functions adequately, and there were great deficiencies in the cleaning of the streets, drainage, canals, and carts for garbage collection. The bankruptcy of the city government made it impossible to help the sick. There were not enough doctors and no financial support to aid the poor people.

The epidemic was especially cruel to the poor. In the outskirts of the city, thousands of deaths were caused by a disease that found favorable grounds in deplorably unsanitary conditions of life. There were several factors that converged to cause and elevate morbidity. Unsanitary conditions, specifically the lack of systems for collection of garbage, the placement of the large garbage dumps, the arrival in the city of sick people who stayed in the wards near the entrance to the city, the location of hospitals, and the unhealthy state of the areas of commercialization of food, are principal elements that explain the differential morbidity in the city (map 2).

The highest rates of morbidity were recorded in wards 25, 26, 20, and 18, situated on the east side of the city, where the entire population apparently got sick. Morbidity in those places is related to their sanitary conditions, as well as the fact that they are zones of entrance into the city. The eastern zone was the place of residence of unskilled, unemployed, and underemployed laborers. In that part of the city there were no streets, but rather paths and alleys, and a canal ran toward the area from Saint Ann's Parish. A huge garbage dump existed where waste was deposited by the garbage wagons of the city. Side by side, perishable foods were sold and distributed. Migrants with scarce resources established themselves on the city's eastern outskirts, where they could find a hut to sleep in, and next to the San Lazaro hospital, which was described as "the dungeon more terrible and repugnant than the prisons of the coast." (González Obregon 1979, 139).

High rates of morbidity (66 percent or greater) were found in wards 27, 19, and 17, also on the eastern side of the city, and wards 21, 23, 24, and 8. These rates seem to relate to zones of access to the city (south side entrance of San Cosme; and the "garita de la Piedad" at zone 8). Morbidity rates decreased to 10 to 30 percent in wards surrounding the central zone of the capital, and the morbidity rate near the Main Plaza was the lowest of all.

The typhus lethality rate was around 20 percent in all groups and in periods of epidemics it rose to 23 percent. It is high in the adult groups.

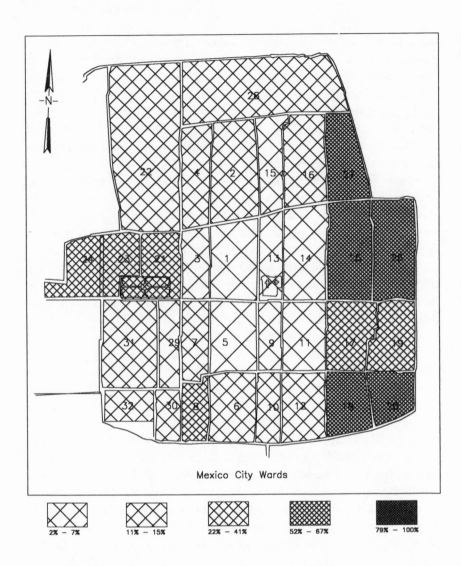

Mexico City Wards

2% – 7%   11% – 15%   22% – 41%   52% – 67%   79% – 100%

Map 2. Frequency of sick individuals, typhus epidemic, 1813. (From AGN, Epidemias, vol. 9, exp. 11, 1813.)

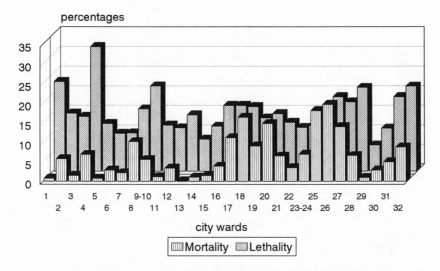

Fig. 2.   General mortality and lethality rates by typhus in Mexico City
in 1813 (distribution in the 32 wards)

The information recorded for the Mexico City population in 1813 (fig. 2,
map 3) reveals a mortality rate between 0.8 percent and 19.7 percent,
which is not high.

The results obtained until now indicate that the epidemic of 1813 was
an attack of typhus combined with other diseases such as typhoid. Typhus
was an endemic disease that attacked young adults. It is an infectious disease, for which the rat, which breeds in unsanitary conditions, is the reser-
voir, and the flea and the louse are the arthropoidal vectors.

The epidemic of 1813 appears to have been due to the convergence of
infectious diseases. The distribution of the epidemic among the population
reveals social inequalities. In that year, from April to August, the poor
outcasts, the vagrants, the poor, the apprenticed of the city, in one word
the "rabble" of the period, as these people were called by the elite, suffered
the rigors imposed by the poor situation (fig. 3). The resources of the city
council were channeled, when it was possible, to works of urbanization
and an infrastructure of the central areas of the capital, where the people
of the highest social and economic position lived.

The differences in the lethality rate among wards may be explained by
the location of the hospital and cemeteries, places where the numbers of
deaths caused by the epidemic were better recorded. That seems evident to

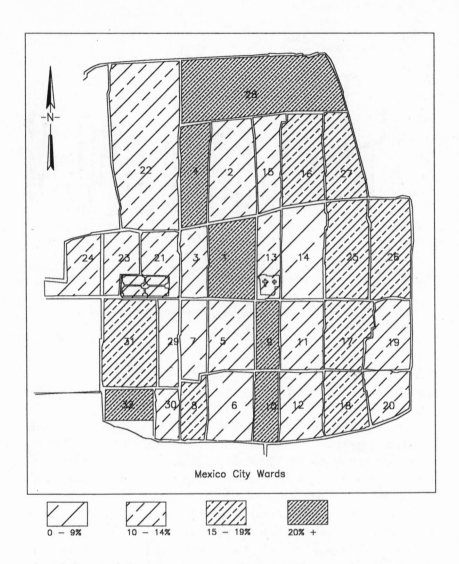

0 – 9%   10 – 14%   15 – 19%   20% +

Map 3.   Lethality rate, typhus epidemic, 1813. (From AGN, *Epidemias, vol. 9, exp. 11, 1813.*)

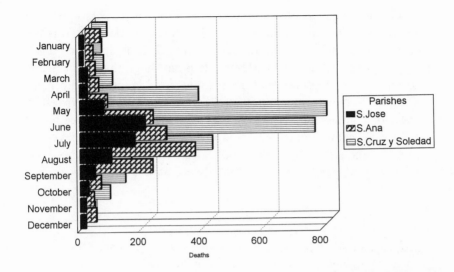

Fig. 3.   Length and seasonality of the typhus epidemic in Mexico City, 1813. (From Maldonado 1976.)

me in the central wards, which recorded a very low morbidity and a slightly higher lethality rate. On the other hand, perhaps there is an immunological influence on the population of better resources, who, due to less contact with sick people, lacked the antibodies that help one to recuperate.

Conclusion

The dynamics of morbidity and mortality are complex, and understanding these dynamics is made more problematical by inexact statistics. Yet, this study of the Mexico City epidemic of 1813 suggests strongly how epidemics discriminate against the poor. Understanding the geography of disease in colonial times, especially in relationship to both proximate ecological factors such as sanitation and more global political factors such as ethnic relations and migration rates provides an interesting comparison to demographic issues today.

In this chapter I have applied a theoretical approach that emphasizes the social determinants of health, including economic structure, political institutions, science and technology, and culture and ideology. It is perhaps not unexpected that a more socially and politically informed bioanthropology has developed in Mexico. It is my hope that this ongoing research provides an example of the advantages of a more social perspective applied to bioanthropological research. It is also gratifying that some of my North American colleagues are beginning to discover the importance of political-economic factors in their analysis of the human condition. As Morgan says (this vol., chap. 17), perhaps in this generation some of the theoretical leads will come from Mexico and South America.

NOTES

The data upon which this paper is based are from Márquez (1994).

1. Exanthematic typhus, petechial fever or "tabardillo" to the Spaniards, or "metlatzahuatl" to the Indians, was a disease endemic to New Spain. It continued to take many lives in later centuries.

2. Archivo General de la Nación, Archivo Histórico de la Ciudad de México, Archivo Histórico de la Secretaría de Salubridad y Asistencia.

3. AGN, *Epidemias,* 9 (11): 1918

4. Villoro (cited in Cardoso 1977). See also Arnold (1979, 281–310) on the social, economic, and political status of the bureaucracy of Mexico City between 1808 and 1822.

REFERENCES

Archivo General de la Nación (AGN).

Archivo Histórico de la Ciudad de México (AHCM).

Archivo Histórico de la Sría. de Salubridad y Asistencia (AHSA).

Arnold, Linda. 1979. Social, Economic, and Political Status in the México City Central Bureaucracy: 1808–1822. In *El trabajo y los trabajadores en la historia de México,* ed. Elsa C. Frost, Michael Meyer, and Josefina Vazquez, 281–310. Tucson: University of Arizona Press.

Báez Macías, Eduardo. 1967. Planos y censos de la ciudad de México, 1753. *Boletin del Archivo General de la Nación* 7:209–484.

Báez Macías, Eduardo. 1969. Ordenaneas para el establecimiento de Alcaldes de Barrio en la Nueva España. Ciudad de México y San Luis Potosi. *Boletin del Archivo General de la Nación* 10 (1–2): 51–125.

Cabrera, Gustavo. 1988. Mortalidad salud y problación. In *La mortalidad en México: niveles, tendencias y determinantes,* ed. Mario Bronfman and José Gómez de León, México: El Colegio de México.

Cardoso, Ciro. 1977. México en el siglo XIX (1821–1910) Historia económica y de la estructura social, *Cuadernos de trabajo* No. 16, Departamento de Investigaciones Históricas, México, INAH.

Cooper, Donald. 1980. *Las epidemias en la ciudad de México, 1761–1812.* México: IMSS (Col. Salud y Seguridad Social, Serie Historia).

Dickinson, Federico, and Raul Murguia. 1982. Consideraciones en trono al objecto de estudio de la antropologia ficica. *Estudios de Antropologia Biologica, Coloqui de Antropologia Juan Comas* 1:51–64.

Frenk, Julio, Jose L. Bovadilla, Claudio Stern, Tomas Fejka, and Rafael Lozano. 1991. Elements for a Theory of the Health Transition. *Health Transitions Review* 1(1):21–38.

González Angulo, Jorge. 1983. *Artesanado y ciudad a finales del Siglo XVIII.* México: F.C.E.-S.E.P.

González Obregon, Luis. 1979. *México Viejo.* México: Promeria.

Guzmán, José Miguel. 1988. Mortalidad infantil y diferenciación socioeconómica en America Latina, 1960–1980. In *La mortalidad en México: Niveles, tendencias y determinantes,* ed. Mario Bronfman and José Gómez de León, México: El Colegio de México.

Humboldt, Alejandro de. 1984. Ensayo Politico sobre el reino de la Nueva España (1811), México, Porrúa ("Sepan cuántos . . . ," 39).

Jimenez Ornelas, Rene y Alberto Minujin Zmud. 1982. Mortalidad infantil y clases sociales. *Memorias de la segunda reunión nacional sobre la investigacion demogréfica en México.* México: CONACYT.

Kicza, John. 1986. *Empresarios coloniales. Familias y negocios en la ciudad de México durante los borbones.* México: F.C.E.

Ladd, Doris. 1984. *La nobleza mexicana en la época de la Independencia, 1780–1826.* México: F.C.E.

Lira, Andres. 1983. *Comunidades indígenas frente a la ciudad de México. Tenochtitlan y Tlatelolco sus pueblos y barrios, 1812–1919.* México: CONACYT.

Maldonado, Celia. 1976. *Estadisticas vitales de la ciudad de México.* México: INAH.

Márquez Morfín, Lourdes. 1982a. *Playa del Carmen: Una población de la costa oriental en el Postclásico (un estudio osteológico).* (Col. Científica 119) México: INAH.

Márquez Morfín, Lourdes. 1982b. Distribución de la estatura en colecciones mayas prehispánicas, *Estudios de Antropología Biológica II, Coloquio de Antropología Física, Juan Comas,* 253–69.

Márquez Morfín, Lourdes. 1984. *Sociedad colonial y enfermedad. Un ensayo de osteopatología diferencial,* Col. Científica 136. México: INAH.

Márquez Morfín, Lourdes. 1994. *La desigualdad ante la muerte en la ciudad de México. El tifo y el colera, México, Siglo XXI.*

McMahon, Brian, and Thomas Pugh. 1978. *Principios y métodos de epidemiologia.* México: La Prensa Médica Mexicana.

Moreno Toscano, Alejandra. 1971. El paisaje rural y las ciudades, dos perspectivas de la Geografía Histórica. *Historia Mexicana* 21:242–68.

Moreno Toscano, Alejandra. 1974. Migraciones hacia la ciudad de México durante el siglo XIX: perspectivas en investigación, *Investigaciones sobre la historia de la ciudad de México, I*, 1–26 (Cuadernos de trabajo). Mexico: DIH-INAH.

Moreno Toscano, Alejandra. 1978. *Cuidad de México. Ensayo de construcción de una historia*, 11–20 (Col. Científica 61). México: INAH.

Moreno Toscano, Alejandra. 1981. Los trabajadores y el proyecto de industrialización, 1820–1867, *La clase obrera en la historia de México, México, Ed. Siglo XXI*, 303–10. Mexico: UNAM.

Morner, Magnus. 1961. *El mestizaje en la historia de Ibero-America.* Instituto Panamericano de Geografía e Historia.

Murguia, Raul. 1981. *Diferenciacion social de la Proporcionalidad Corporal.* Tesis Inedita, Escuela Nacional de Antropologia e Historia.

Peña, Florencia. 1982. Hacia la Construccion de un Marco Teorico Para la Antropologia Fisica. In *Estudios de Antropologia Biologica, Coloquio de Antropologia Juan Comas* 1:65–74.

Sandoval, A. Alfonso. 1982. Hacia una Historia Geneologica de la Antropologia Fisica. *Estudios de Antropologia Biologica, Coloqui de Antropologia Juan Comas* 1:25–49.

Suárez, H. Eugenio. 1945. Epidemiología del tifo exantémico en Chile, *Primera reunión interamericana del tifo.* México: Secretaría de Salubridad y Asistencia e Instituto de Asuntos Interamericanos.

PART 3

Case Studies and Examples: Contemporary Populations

Chapter 10

Illness, Social Relations, and Household Production and Reproduction in the Andes of Southern Peru

Thomas L. Leatherman

The central theme of this volume is that integrating perspectives from anthropological political economy and human adaptability provides a useful starting point for new biocultural perspectives on the human condition. The Andes provides an ideal place to address an integration of perspectives, because there is a corpus of work in both ecological and political-economic perspectives, and sharp distinctions can be drawn between the two (Starn 1991, 1994). Important work in human adaptability and biocultural anthropology was carried out in the 1960s using an ecological approach (e.g., Baker and Little 1976; Thomas 1973). Recent biocultural research, however, has attempted to integrate political-economic perspectives into human adaptability studies and draw attention to issues of poverty, social relations, and health in shaping Andean biology (e.g., Carey 1990; Leatherman 1996; Leatherman et al. 1986; Leonard and Thomas 1988; Luerssen 1994; Thomas 1997; Thomas et al. 1988). The contrasting biocultural approaches represented in these studies provide a clear example for assessing the implications of changing research perspectives.

This chapter has two objectives. The first is to illustrate how integrating political-economic perspectives into a biocultural approach can lead to different questions, analyses, and interpretations about the human condition. This objective is achieved through a comparison of two research projects in the southern Peruvian Andes. The first, under the direction of Paul Baker in the 1960s in the District of Nuñoa, focused on human ecology and adaptation to a high altitude environment (Baker and Little 1976). The second was under the direction of R. Brooke Thomas, a member of the original Nuñoa research team. It was carried out in the early 1980s in the same district as the earlier research and examined the consequences and responses to illness among small-scale farmers (Thomas et al. 1988). The second objective is to summarize key features and findings of the later Nuñoa project to provide an example of biocultural research that attempted to integrate perspectives from anthropological political economy and human adaptability. It examines the interactions between illness and household economy in three locales in the District of Nuñoa, and how differences in patterns of illness, coping responses, and outcomes are shaped by the particular social relations of rural producers in the three sites.

Changing Biocultural Perspectives: A Tale of Two Projects

Orin Starn (1991) has attacked ethnographic and biocultural studies from the 1970s in the Andes as "missing the revolution," the revolt of *Sendero Luminoso* (Shining Path) which came to dominate the political landscape in Peru during the 1980s and into the 1990s. He argued that the ecologically oriented community studies in the 1970s tended to erect analytical boundaries around the populations and cultures being researched to the neglect of interregional and national processes. Starn's critique of ecological anthropology in the 1960s and 1970s is not new, but rather, made specific to the Andean context. Ecological approaches have been repeatedly criticized for emphasizing the single case study of functional adaptation within a bounded, self-regulating ecosystem (Wolf 1982, 17). While Starn omits reference to work by North American scholars that are exceptions to this gloss on Andean scholarship, his general critique of much of Andean research is probably fair. Indeed, research from this era was concerned with the uniqueness of the physical landscape (e.g., the vertical ecology, "harsh" climate, and limiting constraints of high altitude hypoxia) to the exclusion of broader sociopolitical and economic interactions. Andean society and economy were seen to exhibit dual themes of complementarity (e.g., integration of complementing ecoproduction zones as in Murra's [1984] vertical archipelago model) and cooperation (e.g., formalized systems of cooperative labor exchange such as *ayni* reciprocity and *minka* communal work relations). These foci in both biological and cultural research helped reify the notions of successful adaptation and resilience in Andean populations, and the continuity of tradition over novel responses to changing conditions.

Early expectations in mountain ecology and high altitude biology research were that broad adaptive patterns would be discerned through cross-population and cross-cultural comparisons of the Andes with other highland systems (e.g., the Himalayas and Ethiopian highlands). Yet, similarity in adaptive pattern was less than expected. Also, in spite of the constancy and presumed forcefulness of hypobaric hypoxia as an environmental stressor, relatively little evidence was found for genetic adaptations. The reason for both of these results was that each region and each population had a distinctly different history, a rather obvious and important feature, but one never really discussed in interpretations of high altitude biology.

Influenced by political-economic theoretical perspectives in cultural anthropology, Andean ethnography and history in the 1970s and early 1980s increasingly emphasized the political unrest, exploitation, and poverty which were so much a part of the Andean reality (e.g., Collins 1991; Orlove 1977; Roseberry 1983; Smith 1989). They drew attention to the marginalizing effects of centuries of domination, the 150 years of international wool trade, the more recent market penetration and monetization of rural economies, and a failed agrarian reform. Andean history was really a number of histories of how particular social and economic formations in particular environmental settings intersected with a range of broad external political and economic forces. This transformation in thinking about Andean peoples provides a context for viewing similar shifts in biocultural research on human biology and behavior.

Early Nuñoa Research (1960s)

It was within the "ecological-biocultural" approach criticized by Starn that important research on human ecology and high altitude biology was carried out in the 1960s and 1970s. One of the most successful and significant projects was carried out in the District of Nuñoa (Puno) in the southern Peruvian Andes by Paul Baker and students (Baker [1996] provides a personal history of the development of this research). Results of the research were published in *Man in the Andes* (Baker and Little 1976) and reflected the researchers' dominant focus on high altitude human biology, but also the breadth of an ecological orientation. These studies provided a view of population biology and biobehavioral responses to environmental stress for a single region which was rare in biological and biocultural research. Besides documenting in some detail ontogenetic and physiological responses to hypobaric hypoxia and cold, information was collected on a range of biosocial parameters including population demography, biological reproduction, nutrition, growth and development, energy flow, and general sociocultural characteristics.

The development of an ecological model in this research was pivotal to the broadening of frameworks in biological anthropology and human adaptability studies (see Thomas, this vol., chap. 2, for a discussion of changing models in human adaptability research). Yet, like other ecological models, it conceived of the local population and ecosystem as a closed, self-regulating system with goals of maintaining internal homeostasis in the face of multiple stresses emanating primarily from the physical environment. The focus was on detailing adaptation in what was assumed to be a relatively homogeneous native population. Hypobaric hypoxia provided a stressor that culture (i.e., technology) could not buffer, and therefore might reasonably provide a context for population-level genetic adaptations. The selection of problem and population was purposeful and reflected key interests in human biology and environmental physiology in identifying adaptations to extreme environments. The nature of the problem, research design, and methodologies meant that broader interregional and international contexts and local variation in economy and class were not key considerations in the research.

Later Nuñoa Research (1980s)

A restudy of the Nuñoa population provided the opportunity for comparisons across two decades of significant social and economic changes. Were the agrarian reform policies of the early 1970s, the expanded market and transportation systems, and an increased number of schools and health clinics accompanied by improvements in health and nutrition? Or did these changes have a negligible or negative impact, and why? It also provided an opportunity to see how a biocultural approach that integrates anthropological political economy with human adaptability might lead to different interpretations of Andean biology and adaptations. Were physical environmental factors such as hypoxia and cold dominant forces shaping human biology, or was biological variation (e.g., health, nutrition, and growth) better explained by examining variation in social relations in rural households? Thus, our research questions and approach differed substantially from the earlier studies. We focused on problems of social origin—poverty, illness, and undernutrition—and examined the relationships between illness, work, production, and household economy; specifically, the vulnerability to illness and its impacts on household economies.

The approach we developed expanded the traditional ecological framework to explicitly assess local conditions as a product of interaction with larger (global, national, regional) historical forces. We examined human biology (i.e., health and nutrition) as a product of social relations through which people access fundamental resources and through which labor is mobilized and appropriated. We emphasized human agency in shaping the local environmental contexts and in coping with illness as it impacted their lives and livelihood. Because individuals and households are embedded in different webs of social relations, their illness experiences, coping options, and outcomes were expected to vary widely. What is good for one individual, household, and class may often be detrimental to another. Thus, we were concerned less with population-level analysis, and more with variation in social relations and health within and between communities in the region. We were concerned less with evaluating the net benefit of a specific response, and rather with examining a "coping process" that recognizes how past behaviors might structure present actions, and how current responses might structure the future by contributing new problems and altering contexts for response.

This shift in perspective necessarily altered our views on both environment and adaptation. The Andean environment has often been characterized by its physical properties as a multiple stress environment that was harsh, unproductive, and generally marginal for human populations. Yet this marginal environment provided rich and diverse productive options in the past (Murra 1984). In this sense, the environmental conditions of the rural Andean populations with whom we (and earlier researchers) worked had as much to do with changes in control over the means of production and the organization of the labor process as with its physical extremes (recognizing of course that hypoxia is not a social product). Specifying that adaptive capabilities of rural producers are largely determined by access to and control over productive resources and labor locates coping responses within local political economies. Thus, political-economic conditions not only shape the unequal distribution of illness within the community, but they also shape its effects on household economies by influencing the coping process.

Summary

The point of this comparison of the two Nuñoa projects is to illustrate how a shift in perspective that in many ways is a logical progression in theory and approach (Thomas, this vol., chap. 2) can lead to fairly dramatic departures in the sorts of questions generated and in the very conception of the nature of Andean human–environment interaction. By recognizing that environments are products of human action, and hence both social and historical, we shift our gaze from the apparent overpowering effect of extreme stressors such as hypobaric hypoxia to problems such as nutrition and illness. Moreover, this avoids the all too common tendency to "naturalize" social phenomena such as poverty, illness, and "modernization." By recognizing that human agents are embedded in complex webs of social relations, the potentially homogenizing effect of a population approach is clearer. Members of a population experience the environment differently and act on this experience with different goals, options, and constraints on their action. This, in turn, leads us to examine variation in experience and constraints among individuals, and the local and external forces that shape this variation. It also directs us to follow the consequences of action to the creation of new problems and contexts for future response.

Perspectives on Health and Household Economy in Nuñoa

The perspective outlined above was developed in a two-year (1983–85) field study in the District of Nuñoa (Puno) in highland Peru (Thomas et al. 1988). The primary objectives of the research were to evaluate the impact of illness on household work and production, and to examine consequences and responses to this impact. While considerable attention had been given to documenting the health status of peasant populations and the conditions contributing to poor health, little emphasis had been placed on the consequences of poor health to the material and social well-being of these groups. A major premise in this research was that illness is a catalyst as well as a symptom of poverty, vulnerability, and change. Particularly in a production system that relies on critical inputs of strenuous human labor, any factor such as illness that reduces labor power might have negative impacts on household production and reproduction. Thus, two conceptual and analytical themes run through our approach and analysis. One is a focus on the *vulnerability* of rural producers to illness and its impacts. The second is a focus on the links between *illness, household production, and reproduction.*

Vulnerability crosscuts issues of exposure to problems, coping capabilities, and resiliency to persist (e.g., achieve social reproduction) in the face of perturbations (Chambers 1989, Dow 1992, Watts and Bohle 1993). Those with greatest exposure to stress and weakest coping capacities will suffer the greatest consequences and have the most difficulty rebounding. In this sense the poor are usually among the most vulnerable. However, a more nuanced understanding of vulnerability requires an examination of different aspects of social relations that underlie poverty and how they affect not only levels of illness, but also coping capacities and the outcomes of poor health on the economic and social functioning of the household. For example, levels of illness might be equally distributed among two households, but the impacts of illness on production might be greater in one over the other because they were unable to get extra help, or were forced to delay planting or harvests. The resource base of the two households may in turn determine how resilient they are to these impacts, as one household with stored wealth in terms of land, animals, or other material assets can persist and even recover losses in the long run while another might be devastated.

Rural households in the Andes engage in a variety of production activities to achieve reproduction, which for rural producers refers to "the perpetual generation or acquisition of the products required for a domestic unit to continue its capacity as a unit of production and reproduction" (Luerssen 1991, 10). This entails reproducing the means of work (e.g., land, tools, seed) as well as the labor force (i.e., health maintenance and biological reproduction). Poor health then forms a crucial link between household production and reproduction. "The inability to guarantee normal levels of consumption might result in declining nutrition or lowered health standards of household members; the lowered quality of labor power reproduction might subsequently affect the productive capacity of the household in the next cycle" (Deere 1990, 267). Of particular interest is the point at which the resilience of households to the consequences of illness is sufficiently constrained to mark a transformation from a functioning production unit to one unable to maintain levels of reproduction and health, what Deere (1990) calls household disintegration. "The consequences of disintegration could include lowered nutrition levels accompanied by higher morbidity and mortality rates, outmigration of family members, fewer years of schooling, or even the inability of a household to continue as primary producers" (Luerssen 1991, 14). In this sense, our focus on vulnerability to illness and its impacts on household economy is about the reproduction of poverty and poor health shaped by the social relations through which individuals access the material means of production and labor, and their articulation in the local cash economy.

Research Design and Methods

Our research design called for an expanded scope of data collection into the social and economic arena. We maintained the same rigorous use of methods from field biology as characterized the work by Baker and colleagues (1976) and collected much comparable information on growth, nutrition, demography, and other biobehavioral parameters to facilitate comparisons with the earlier findings and assess changes that had occurred over the ensuing fifteen years. We gathered additional information on the economy, demography, and activity patterns of households along with measures of diet, nutrition, and health. Information on health status and perceptions of health included two-week and longer recalls of illness events, symptomatology, and workdays lost to illness. Household economic relations were characterized by access to land and labor, and artic- ulation with the wage economy, as well as by material conditions and pos- sessions in the household (see Leatherman 1992, 1994, 1996 for a more complete description of research methodology).

Information on these domains was gathered seasonally in three com- munities in the District, including a farming *ayllu,* an alpaca herding coop- erative, and a semi-urban town. An initial sample of 140 households in the first survey was followed by subsamples of 104 and 65 households in two subsequent surveys. A brief description of the communities is provided later. They have been described in greater detail in earlier publications (Leatherman 1994, 1996).

The farming *ayllu* (3950 meters) is a small community of 25 families surrounded on all sides by state-administered cooperatives (formerly by haciendas). Household economies are based on farming and limited herd- ing, and supplemented by wage labor and small-scale commodity produc- tion. The alpaca herding cooperative (4400 to 5000 meters) was formed from the lands of three haciendas and consists of 25 households. Each household receives a small salary and usufruct rights to land for farming and raising private herds (*waqcha*) in exchange for their care of coopera- tive herds. The semi-urban town (4000 meters; population 4000) is the market center and administrative capital of the district, and has the only secondary school and health clinic in the district. While some farming is reported by most households, all (except for a few large landholders) relied on wage labor, and 60 percent of the households reported wage work as their chief source of income. One-half of these households had permanent jobs and half performed temporary wage work. Twenty-two percent of town households were landless, and only 16 percent owned private lands. The majority obtained small plots (less than one hectare) through rents or usufruct rights from community lands or *empressas* where they worked.

Contexts of Vulnerability

The vulnerability of Andean peoples in southern Peru is rooted in a history of conquest and colonization, hacienda domination, and pro-urban industrialization policies of the last forty years (Alberti 1981; Morner 1985). The earlier Nuñoa research in the 1960s encountered a reality shaped by patron–client relations, agrarian stagnation, and poverty. Important changes in the decade prior to our research, especially the implementation of agrarian reform policies and increased capitalization of rural economies, altered the social relations of rural producers but not the stagnation or poverty. These changes were experienced differently and with different implications for levels of vulnerability in the three communities we studied.

An agrarian reform was instituted in the early 1970s in an effort to redress inequities in the land base among the rural peasantry, but in effect it replaced haciendas with even larger cooperatives that employed fewer people. In the District of Nuñoa, three cooperatives controlled 60 percent of the land and employed about 25 percent of the rural population (Luerssen 1994). While households that obtained membership in the newly formed cooperatives benefited, other households formerly linked to haciendas through sharecropping arrangements became landless. The town doubled in size between 1960 and 1980, in part as a result of post-reform landlessness. Town residents with communal land rights and members of the *ayllu* received no new land in the transition. Also, cooperatives discontinued informal rent-for-work or sharecropping arrangements through which some of these households had accessed additional land and resources like dung for fuel and ichu grass for roofs from the former haciendas. Thus, while secure access to land for farming and herding benefited members of the alpaca herding cooperative, access to land and resources for town and *ayllu* households remained the same or decreased following the reform.

Increased capitalization of the regional rural economy was accompanied by growth in the number of markets, transportation systems, and the commoditization of goods and labor. Purchased goods increasingly replaced basic needs formerly produced in the household, and this heightened the vulnerability to price fluctuations and inflation, especially in the town where the majority of food was purchased. Increasingly, small-scale producers with limited access to land worked in the local wage market or migrated to larger towns in search of work. Yet, the level of income most households could obtain through wage work was usually inadequate to meet daily basic needs. Those with permanent jobs obtained regular and marginally adequate incomes, while those involved in temporary wage work obtained neither steady incomes nor a living wage. For households in the *ayllu* and especially in the town, outmigration for wage work and the necessity to take temporary jobs when they were available led to conflicts in the availability and scheduling of household labor to meet other production needs (Leatherman, Thomas, and Luerssen 1989; Leatherman 1996). Also, labor reciprocity was diminished under the relations of a wage market (Leatherman 1996; see also Brown 1987; Erasmus 1956). This was especially the case in the town because most available workers were landless or near landless, and thus had little incentive to engage in reciprocal agricultural work. Access to nonhousehold labor was based on cash payments, and cash exchanges were even common between close kin not residing in the same household. In the *ayllu* and cooperative, cash payments were also common, but stronger kinship ties and a stronger moral economy meant that these households could rely on extended kin networks in times of need (e.g., illness) to a greater degree than in the town.

Thus the different social relations that structured access to production inputs, labor, and the wage economy provided rural producers in these three locales with different levels of basic needs, nutrition, and health; different coping capabilities under the impact of illness; and different degrees of resiliency to withstand the consequences of illness on the production process. The following section relates these levels of vulnerability to the health status, coping capacities, and outcomes of illness on household production and reproduction in the three communities.

Household Health, Production, and Reproduction

Diet, Nutrition, and Illness

The social and economic marginality of rural producers in the southern Andes and changing patterns of vulnerability are reflected in diet, nutrition, and health status. Previous dietary surveys at the regional and local level (Ferroni 1982; Gursky 1969; Picon-Reategui 1976) suggested marginal nutriture and the potential for undernutrition in large segments of the Nuñoan population. Leatherman (1994) compared findings from the 1960s and 1980s on dietary diversity in the three communities, and on economic variation in dietary diversity in the town. In earlier studies by Gursky (1969), the farming *ayllu* and the town had the most diverse diets and the cooperative the least. In the 1980s, the total diversity of foods consumed (based on food items consumed by at least 20 percent of the households in at least one locale) increased by 22 percent in the town and 43 percent in the cooperative, but decreased by 11 percent in the *ayllu*. In all communities, there was a replacement of higher quality highland grains with rice and noodles, and in the town and cooperative there was an increase in nonlocal vegetables (tomatoes, cabbage, carrots) and other processed foods. Cooperative households were also able to store more foods for longer periods than either the town or *ayllu*. They had on hand six foodstuffs that would endure at least one month, compared to two in the ayllu and none in the town. Ready access to markets made storage less important to town households but for rural households adequate storage meant better food security and fewer costly trips to markets. In the case of the *ayllu*, households with few stored items often avoided trips to markets by purchasing foods from a traveling vendor but at greatly inflated prices.

Overall, the data on dietary diversity and storage suggest that the dietary diversity among cooperative and town households had increased, while dietary diversity among community households remained unchanged or decreased. For the two rural sites, this was a reversal of positions from the pre-reform study by Gursky (1969). While dietary diversity in the town increased, there was significant variation between households of different economic status. A rough ranking of dietary adequacy among the three locales found the poorer town households and *ayllu* households at the bottom, followed by the herding cooperative households and wealthier town households (Leatherman 1994). Leonard and Thomas (1988), using food-weighing methods and dietary recall in a subsample of town households, found that dietary breadth and quality (including caloric consumption) had not improved since the 1960s, and that significantly lower caloric intakes occurred among poorer households seasonally. Similarly, comparisons of growth between school-aged children in the mid-1960s and early 1980s illustrated no secular increase in height (Leatherman, Carey, and Thomas 1995), which would be expected if nutritional and health conditions had improved.

A conservative estimate of nutritional status suggests that 57 percent of the children sampled in the three communities were at risk for undernutrition ($Z \leq -2.0$) and that up to 20 percent of the children may suffer from chronic undernutrition ($Z \leq -3.0$) (table 1). The greatest degree of stunting (low height for age) was found among the poor farming community, which was also the lowest in altitude (3850 m), and the least stunting was evident among children in the wealthier herding cooperative, which was the highest in altitude (4200–4800 m). Thus, at a local level, social and economic status and not altitude determined degrees of stunting. Also, height, weight, triceps skinfolds, and upper arm circumference were significantly greater (t-test, $p < .02$ or greater for all) among individuals of higher economic status in the town. If we assume that the assessments of dietary diversity are associated with nutritional status, then we can conclude that nutrition has improved in the herding cooperative but has deteriorated in the *ayllu*. Nutrition in the town has not improved, although individual and household variation in nutritional status may have changed with shifts in the regional and local economy.

Household health surveys found substantial illness events, symptomatic complaints, and related disruption to work activities in the three communities. Respiratory problems were the leading cause of illness for each measure. On the average, 37 percent of the individuals reported suffering from a health problem during the previous two-week period. More individuals from the farming *ayllu* reported illness events (44.8 percent) than from the town (36.1 percent) or cooperative (30.7 percent). On the average, adult males and females reported 18 percent and 25 percent of symptoms mentioned in the questionnaire respectively, while children (<18 years) reported about 7 percent, regardless of sex or age.

A more "functional" measure of illness used in the morbidity surveys was an assessment of workdays lost due to illness over the previous two-week period (table 2). Eighty percent of the households reported some level of work disruption due to illness among adult members in at least one of the three seasonal health surveys. On the average for any given survey, almost 60 percent of the households surveyed reported disruption to the work of at least one adult member, and this amounted to a loss of 4 to 5 workdays of the two-week recall period. Similar to the morbidity analysis, families from the farming *ayllu* reported greater degrees of work disruption due to illness. When "days lost" were standardized for the entire sample (transformed into Z-scores), these differences were significant among the three communities ($p < .05$). Based on annual estimates of work lost, households in the *ayllu* lose about one-third more workdays than semi-urban families and two-thirds more than the herding families from the cooperative (table 2). Within each site, adult women are at greater risk for disruptive effects of illness than men.

TABLE 1.　Nutritional Rankings of Children Based on *Z*-score Categories for Height for Age in Three Sites in the District of Nuñoa[a]

Nutritional Rank	Town		Community		Cooperative		District	
	N	%	N	%	N	%	N	%
Normal ($Z \geq -1.99$)	72	45.9	11	26.8	20	45.5	103	42.6
Stunted ($Z = -2.0$ to -2.99)	56	35.6	17	41.5	17	38.6	90	37.2
Severely Stunted ($Z \leq -3.00$)	29	18.5	13	31.7	7	15.9	49	20.2
Sample Size (N)	157		41		44		242	

[a]Average of measures taken during three household health surveys

TABLE 2.　Illness Work Disruption Among Adults from a Town, Community, and Cooperative[a]

Illness Measure	Town		Community		Cooperative	
	M	F	M	F	M	F
Households (N)	43		18		18	
Percent households with ill members	62		54		55	
Individuals (N)	32	53	17	23	17	27
Percent symptoms reported	16.8	22.7	20.6	30.3	15.3	20.7
Percent adults with work lost	13.5	28.9	20.5	22.5	10.2	20.7
Median days lost/ sick adult	3.6	4.9	5.7	7.9	3.3	3.1
Annual days lost/ household[b]	40.3		75.9		27.1	

[a]Adapted from Leatherman 1994. Values averaged across three survey periods.
[b]Average for all households in the sample, combining work lost in males and females.

Among the entire sample of households, economic rankings were significantly associated with symptomatology indices ($r = .27$, $p < .05$), although not with days lost. While these associations reflect an expected relationship between material conditions and health, they do not indicate what aspects of local social relations might underlie vulnerability to illness in each community. In the *ayllu* and cooperative, the key factors structuring wealth and health are ownership of herds and access to land. For example, *ayllu* households planting more fields in grain report fewer illness symptoms ($p < .05$). Grain is planted to feed cows and horses that are not pastured, and both represent a significant economic value. Also, cows produce milk for cheese, which is consumed in the household and is a valued commodity for sale in the town. Conversely, *ayllu* households performing more temporary wage work (an indication of less access to land and herds) suffer more workdays lost to illness ($p < .05$).

Compared with the rural communities, levels of illness among town households have more to do with sources of monetary income through wage work and commercial ventures. Households with a steady source of income (e.g., with permanent jobs or a business) report significantly fewer illness symptoms and fewer days of work lost than households with irregular incomes ($p < .05$) (Leatherman 1998). Poorer families relying on different combinations of small-scale farming, temporary wage work, and commodity production for their income reported about 8 percent more symptoms ($p < .002$) and over twice the days of adult work lost per two-week period ($p < .03$). No significant differences in illness were found between farmers and nonfarmers among the poor. This is in contrast to work in the same town from 1987 to 1988 (four years later and under more severe economic conditions) by Susan Luerssen (1994) where variation in health status was found between poor farming and poor nonfarming households. In her study the poor farming households ate twice the value of local cultigens and meat as nonfarming households, and reported only one-third the median work days lost over six-month (8 vs. 24 days) and one-month (1 vs. 3 days) recall periods. In 1986 a reallocation of lands from cooperatives to agrarian communities (called *Rimanakuy*) occurred in response to civil unrest, and by the time of her research, 10 percent more townspeople had access to communal lands than in the early 1980s. Also, real wages had dropped as market goods were undergoing triple-digit inflation. These changes in local social relations in the town likely accentuated the importance of farming in health status of poorer semi-urban households.

Effects of Illness on Household Production and Reproduction

The information on "functional morbidity" (days lost) illustrates the potential impact of illness on work and hence production. We evaluated the effects of illness on household production primarily in terms of farming because small-scale farming production was the most widely practiced activity and we considered it to be a critical practice in the reproduction of Andean households. A total of 64 households from the three communities were followed through the annual cycle of production, measuring levels of illness, household and nonhousehold labor utilized, production inputs (e.g., seed and fertilizers) and harvest outputs of the production process. Subsequently, households were divided into three levels of illness based on prevalence and severity of illness events during the three surveys. The three levels represented: (1) mild to moderate illness of short duration, (2) more severe acute problems and mildly disruptive chronic problems, and (3) moderate to severe chronic problems (table 3). We found a steady increase in the person-workdays per field cultivated as illness categories became more incapacitating, but found significant changes in production levels only in the case of chronic illness. Compared with healthy households, those with chronically ill members planted 48 percent fewer fields overall, and 57 percent fewer fields in potatoes. They harvested 23 percent fewer pounds of potatoes, but worked 31 percent more person-days per field (*masa*) to plant, weed, and harvest their potato crops (Leatherman 1992).

Illness is most likely to impact production when it coincides with periods of high labor demands. Acute problems are not so problematic if they do not overlap with critical production periods or if they can be contained over the short run. Chronic problems, on the other hand, always overlap with critical production periods, even if the severity of impairment may be less than in many acute cases. Thus it was important for households with illness, and especially those with chronically sick members, to gain access to nonhousehold workers if they were to complete agricultural tasks in a timely manner (i.e., within seasonal windows of opportunity) and especially to respond to emergency situations (e.g., flooding of fields by heavy rains). In the increasingly monetized economy, reciprocal labor had diminished, and for most households access to nonhousehold labor during seasonally constrained production periods was dependent on their ability and willingness to hire workers for cash or a cut of the harvest. Whether or not households utilized outside help in times of illness or planted fewer fields using available family labor depended on the social relations through which they accessed land and engaged in income-generating activities.

Town households with chronically ill members often planted fewer fields ($r = .41$, $p < .05$; correlation between "work days lost" and fields planted). They had limited control over the basic productive resources (usufruct rights or rented land) and were economically dependent on multiple economic activities. Access to reciprocal labor was very limited in the town, and the vast majority of exchanges were based on cash (Leatherman 1996). In fact we observed fathers and sons, and siblings, demanding cash payments for help in times of need. Thus, many chose to plant fewer fields with available household labor and thus maintain some level of production to supplement wage or commercial activities which often comprised a major portion of their income. Other households that normally planted one to two fields of potatoes on land they rented for cash or labor, and that were unable to meet the labor or monetary obligations (e.g., due to illness) to acquire the land, chose not to plant crops that year. Also, those who obtained land in usufruct for planting had to fulfill communal work obligations or pay a fine for every communal workday missed. A disabling ill-

TABLE 3.   Levels of Illness and Measures of Farming Production in Households from Nuñoa District[a]

Production Measure	Levels of Illness[b]						Percentage Change Level 1–3[c]
	Level 1 AM-M		Level 2 AS-CM		Level 3 CM-S		
	Mean	(s.d.)	Mean	(s.d.)	Mean	(s.d.)	
Total fields planted	5.2	(3.1)	4.6	(3.6)	2.7	(2.3)	−48
Potato fields planted	2.1	(1.2)	1.9	(1.2)	0.9	(0.5)	−57
Workdays/ potato field	13.1	(5.4)	15.9	(11.0)	17.2	(7.5)	−31
Yields[d]/ Potato field	16.5	(9.6)	17.9	(8.8)	12.8	(9.3)	−23
Households (N)	24		26		14		

[a]Adapted from Leatherman 1992; combines data from three communities.
[b]AM-M (Acute Mild-to-Moderate); AS-CM (Acute Severe-to-Chronic Mild); CM-S (Chronic Moderate-to-Severe)
[c]All changes significant at $p < .01$ (t-test)
[d]Measured in Arrobas (about 25 lbs.)

ness of even moderate duration then could effectively erase access to communal land.

Households with consistent and predictable access to land (e.g., landowners in town, members of the rural community and cooperative) did not significantly reduce the number of fields planted, but had lower yields per field than their healthy counterparts ($r = -.71$ in the *ayllu*, and $r = -.54$ in the cooperative, $p < .05$; correlations between "workdays lost" and yield per field). For the majority of these households, labor was less constrained and farming production was a larger component of food security. Reducing the number of fields in production was not considered an option by most. Members of the cooperative maintained the highest levels of production primarily because they had a steady wage and thus available cash to hire help, and because they engaged in more reciprocal labor exchanges. Particularly older households in the cooperative had access to reciprocal labor from younger members. This is because membership in the cooperative for younger families requires sponsorship by an established family, thus building social obligations of aid to the older household in times of need. *Ayllu* households had less cash available to hire non-household labor but somewhat predictable though limited access to reciprocal labor because of the extended kin structure of the *ayllu*. As one individual said, he had no option but to help a sick brother in his fields or suffer social sanctions from the rest of the community. Also, the control over their own labor was less constrained than in the town where economic strategies were often based on three to five income-generating activities, or in the cooperative where obligations to herds took priority.

In every community, therefore, illness led to production losses but to different degrees and with different implications for levels of household reproduction. Despite lower yields in *ayllu* and cooperative households experiencing illness, their net production was higher than those in the town who reduced the number of fields in cultivation. While reduced production means less surplus and perhaps missed opportunities, for those with already limited access to land and labor and without a steady source of income, it translates into reduced attainment of basic needs and lower levels of nutrition. This implied a redefining of basic needs for the household, and, thus, increased risk of future illness. Over time this can lead to what Deere (1990) characterized as household disintegration. For some, this process was a slow spiral downward in household economic and biological well-being, while for others it happened in the space of a single year. The unfortunate reality was that individuals at greatest risk of illness were the least able to cope with its impacts and thus were at greatest risk to negative economic consequences. It is among these groups that irreversible changes in productive capabilities and diminished levels of reproduction increase their marginality.

Discussion: Illness, Vulnerability, and Exploitation

One theme emphasized in this research is how vulnerability in Nuñoan households is closely linked to increased poverty and illness, and to reduced coping capacities and resilience. The results of our investigations illustrate that the poor experience more illness, have fewer means to cope with its impacts, and hence suffer greater consequences to production and reproduction. They also show limited resiliency to prevent these consequences from reproducing more poverty and poor health in the future.

A second theme was to examine how illness can play a critical role in the perpetuation of poverty and poor health through its effects on household production and reproduction. Clearly, illness can and does affect household reproduction by reducing production and intensifying demands on household labor, through monetary expenses in treating illness and hiring help, and in constraining the ability to meet social and labor obligations through which one maintains access to basic means of production. Heightened levels of undernutrition, illness, infant mortality, and growth impairment are symptoms of reduced levels of basic needs that partially defines incomplete reproduction.

A more developed analysis of vulnerability and of linkages between illness, production, and household reproduction must examine how social relations of rural producers underlie poverty, coping responses, and the consequences of illness on household economies. As described in the case of small-scale farmers, individuals, and households make different decisions about how to deal with the impact of illness on production depending on the social relations through which they access land and labor, articulate with the wage market, or carry out a range of other economic activities. Illness also alters the context and may heighten the vulnerability to potentially exploitative social relations.

One of the most obvious consequences of illness on the production process is diminished labor power of the household. Hiring extra workers provides one means to replace lost labor power in illness, but this further reduces the size and/or value of the harvest retained by the household.

Intensifying the utilization of family labor is another, yet this in turn exploits family members' time and energy. While this may be the only feasible alternative or efficient use of funds and labor, this is time that cannot be spent in other economic activities, school, visiting, or community work projects and ritual activities. This diminishes the long-term earning potential of household members (e.g., from too few years of education), as well as the social networks and resources of the household.

Illness is a time of vulnerability in which a variety of debts and obligations can occur. When too sick to work, individuals often take out loans in order to meet immediate basic needs, hire laborers, or to purchase treatments. The market price for a particular product can vary widely by season, and to repay these loans, they might be forced into selling their products at low market value. Farmers might borrow seed that must be repaid immediately after harvest, and some reported that after repaying seed and providing a portion of the harvest to workers they employed and to landowners in sharecropping arrangements, they had little left for household consumption. Herders are often forced to pledge a portion of their future wool production at a set price, which may fall well below market value at the time of shearing. At times of emergency, households may be forced into quick sales of animals or products to meet immediate basic needs of the household or obtain treatments for an ill member. Whenever households are forced to sell their own goods at low prices and purchase others at inflated prices, a surplus transfer takes place via poor terms of trade. Aware of these transfers, many opt to produce at whatever level they can with the labor and seed they possess or can purchase, and to avoid loans or obligations that put them in a heightened position of vulnerability.

Many households obtain land through rents in labor, cash, or kind, which entails a direct extraction of surplus labor value of the farmer by the landowner. If the impacts of illness reduce the production on this land, the asymmetrical aspects of this sort of relation are magnified. One can further invest in the production process by hiring labor, but given the scarce cash flows and the general unpredictability of production outcomes (e.g., due to irregular rainfall and crop disease) many households experiencing illness choose not to make the payments necessary to access land. The consequence of this decision is to rely on wage work for meeting the requirements of household reproduction. Yet, typical wages paid for temporary unskilled labor are lower than what is needed to meet basic household needs. In this sense, farming subsidizes the low wage as much as wage work subsidizes household subsistence production. Households in this position (i.e., relying on temporary unskilled wage work for the majority of their income) experienced the greatest levels of illness and malnutrition in the district. Outmigration of some household members (and hence lowered consumption needs and occasional remittances) provided one avenue to persist at lowered levels of reproduction. Sending children to work in other households was another.

Deere (1990) states that levels of household reproduction depend upon levels of production and surplus extraction. In this sense, illness is linked to household reproduction by diminished levels of production, and by altering the contexts of surplus extraction and exploitation. Because illness often introduces a heightened level of vulnerability into an already vulnerable situation, it provides a particularly sharp lens through which to view not only structural inequalities but the reproduction of a number of conditions that perpetuate the inequality and vulnerability of many Andean households.

Conclusion: The Relevance of a Biocultural Perspective

In this chapter, I have argued that building a new biocultural approach in anthropology is essential for understanding the ways in which the interaction of large-scale forces and local environments shapes the contexts for human biology and health. The approach combines perspectives from human adaptability and political economy to examine the vulnerability of Andean households to the consequences of illness on household economies. It focuses on social relations that shape both the access to basic production resources and the coping capacities to deal with problems of illness that can threaten household production and reproduction. Illness emerges not only as a product of poverty, but as an integral part of the reproduction of poverty and poor health that persists among rural producers in the Andes. In a broader sense, this highlights the critical role of human biology in the process of human–environment interaction.

In building new biocultural perspectives we need to highlight the tensions in the dialectic between coping and exploitation, between the resilience that biological plasticity can provide and the consequences of impaired biology on the ability to deal with everyday realities. Perspectives from human adaptability have provided rich detail and keen insights into the strategies of response by agents dealing with the everyday problems in local environments, and on the ways biology affects and is affected by human–environment interactions. Yet, adaptability perspectives for the most part have not addressed the underlying social relations that structure local conditions and biological variation. Nor have they imagined a full range of responses that might include resistance and system transformation as well as adjustment and accommodation. The critical role of human agents' capacities to cope with conditions of change, to resist forces of exploitation in their lives, and to actively engage their environment in systemic transformation must also be central to our perspective. In order to achieve this, we need to understand local conditions within their more fully developed global histories. We need to understand that strategies of response fit these histories and that they may have distinctly different impacts on segments of what might appear to be homogeneous populations. Hence local conditions, experience of stress, and capacity to cope are not community-wide experiences but are intricately tied to the social relations of individuals, households, and classes.

The key issue is what relevance a biocultural approach enmeshing adaptability and political-economic perspectives has for addressing the social and biological impacts of the global conditions that will dominate our concerns in the twenty-first century, conditions ranging from environmental degradation to political unrest, from ethnic genocide to persistent poverty, malnutrition, and disease. A biocultural approach that examines how political-economic processes affect people's lives, and how people mediate these effects through their actions, can only help further our understanding of the human impacts of change. Such an approach provides for biological anthropology a way to link a long-term interest and conviction of viewing environments as prime movers in human adaptation with a politically, historically, and socially rich contextualization of human–environment interactions. Moreover, it provides an opportunity for making biology relevant to the rest of anthropology and the broader anthropological study of the human condition.

REFERENCES

Alberti, G. 1981. *Basic Needs in the Context of Social Change: The Case of Peru.* Paris: Organization for Economic Cooperation and Development.

Baker, P. T. 1996. Adventures in Human Population Biology. *Annual Reviews of Anthropology* 25:1–18.

Baker, Paul T., and Michael A. Little, eds. 1976. *Man in the Andes: A Multidisciplinary Study of High-Altitude Quechua.* Stroudsburg, PA: Dowden, Hutchinson and Ross, Inc.

Brown, Paul F. 1987. Population Growth and the Disappearance of Reciprocal Labor in a Highland Peruvian Community. *Research in Economic Anthropology* 8:201–24.

Carey, J. W. 1990. Social System Effects on Local Level Morbidity and Adaptation in the Rural Peruvian Andes. *Medical Anthropology Quarterly* 4:266–95.

Chambers, R. 1989. Vulnerability, Coping and Policy. *IDS Bulletin* 20:1–7.

Collins, J. 1991. *Unseasonal Migrations: The Effects of Rural Labor Scarcity in Peru.* Princeton: Princeton University Press.

Deere, C. D. 1990. *Household and Class Relations: Peasants and Landlords in Northern Peru.* Berkeley: University of California Press.

Dow, Kirstin. 1992. Exploring Differences in Our Common Future(s): The Meaning of Vulnerability to Global Environmental Change. *Geoform* 23 (3): 417–36.

Erasmus, Charles J. 1956. Culture, Structure and Process: The Occurrence and Disappearance of Reciprocal Farm Labor. *Southwestern Journal of Anthropology* 12:444–69.

Ferroni, M. A. 1982. Food Habits and the Apparent Nature and Extent of Dietary Nutritional Deficiencies in the Peruvian Andes. *Archives Latinoamericanos de Nutricion* 32 (4): 850–66.

Gursky, M. 1969. *A Dietary Survey of Three Peruvian Highland Communities.* M.A. thesis, Pennsylvania State University, University Park.

Leatherman, T. L. 1992. Illness as Lifestyle Change. *MASCA Research Papers in Science and Archeology* 9:83–89.

Leatherman, T. L. 1994. Health Implications of Changing Agrarian Economies in the Southern Andes. *Human Organization* 53 (4): 371–80.

Leatherman, T. L. 1996. A Biocultural Perspective on Health and Household Economy in Southern Peru. *Medical Anthropology Quarterly* 10 (4): 476–95.

Leatherman, T. L. 1998. Changing Biocultural Perspectives on Health in the Andes. *Social Science and Medicine* 47 (8): 1031–41.

Leatherman, T., J. Carey, and R. B. Thomas. 1995. Socioeconomic Change and Patterns of Growth in the Andes. *American Journal of Physical Anthropology* 97 (3): 307–22.

Leatherman, T. L., J. Susan Luerssen, L. B. Markowitz, and R. B. Thomas. 1986. Illness and Political Economy: An Andean Dialectic. *Cultural Survival Quarterly* 10 (3): 19–21.

Leatherman, T. L., R. B.Thomas, and J. S. Luerssen. 1989. Challenges to Seasonal Strategies of Rural Producers: Uncertainty and Conflict in the Adaptive Process. *MASCA Research Papers in Science and Archeology* 5:9–20.

Leonard, W. R., and R. B. Thomas. 1988. Changing Dietary Patterns in the Peruvian Andes. *Ecology of Food and Nutrition* 21:245–63.

Luerssen, J. S. 1991. *Household Reproduction and Illness in a Highland Peruvian Town.* Ph.D. dissertation, University of Massachusetts, Amherst.

Luerssen, J. S. 1994. Landlessness, Health and the Failures of Reform in the Peruvian Highlands. *Human Organization* 53 (4): 380–87.

Morner, M. 1985. *The Andean Past.* New York: Columbia University Press.

Murra, J. 1984. Andean Societies. *Annual Review of Anthropology* 13:119–41.

Orlove, B. S. 1977. *Alpacas, Sheep and Men.* New York: Academic Press.

Picon-Reategui, Emilio. 1976. Nutrition. In *Man in the Andes,* ed. Paul T. Baker and Michael Little, 208–36. Stroudsburg, PA: Dowden, Hutchinson, and Ross.

Roseberry, W. 1983. *Coffee and Capitalism in the Venezuelan Andes.* Austin: University of Texas Press.

Smith, G. 1989. *Livelihood and Resistance: Peasants and the Politics of Land in Peru.* Berkeley: University of California Press.

Starn, O. 1991. Missing the Revolution: Anthropologists and the War in Peru. *Cultural Anthropology* 6 (1): 63–91.

Starn, O. 1994. Rethinking the Politics of Anthropology: The Case of the Andes. *Current Anthropology* 35 (1): 13–38.

Thomas, R. B. 1973. Human Adaptation to a High Andean Energy Flow System. Occasional Papers in Anthropology, No. 7. Pennsylvania State University, University Park.

Thomas, R. B. 1997. Wandering to the Edge of Adaptability: Adjustment of Andean People to Change. In *Human Adaptability, Past, Present and Future,* ed. S. J. Ulijasek and R. Huss-Ashmore, 126–56. Oxford: Oxford University Press.

Thomas, R. B., T. L. Leatherman, J. W. Carey, and J. D. Haas. 1988. Consequences and Responses to Illness among Small Scale Farmers: A Research Design. In *Capacity for Work in the Tropics,* ed. K. J. Collins and D. F. Roberts, 249–76. New York: Cambridge University Press.

Watts, M., and H. G. Bohle. 1993. The Space of Vulnerability: The Causal Structure of Hunger and Famine. *Progress in Human Geography* 17 (1): 43–67.

Wolf, Eric. 1982. *Europe and the People Without History.* Berkeley: University of California Press.

Chapter 11

On the (Un)Natural History of the Tupí-Mondé Indians: Bioanthropology and Change in the Brazilian Amazon

Ricardo V. Santos and Carlos E. A. Coimbra Jr.

Over the past decades, the Amazon Basin has been the scene of drastic social, economic, and environmental changes. For Amerindian peoples, the rapid and abrupt contact with national societies and the resulting socioeconomic changes are often associated with disruptive processes in various aspects of traditional life. This is particularly the case in semi-isolated groups which still rely on traditional means of subsistence. Among the immediate consequences of contact, even at present, are population decimation due to epidemics of infectious diseases, alterations of birth and mortality rates, and disruption of subsistence activities. In addition to the high social and biological costs incurred in the short run, native populations have had to cope with long-term changes. As a result, such factors as demographic structure, nutritional and health status, subsistence base, and settlement patterns are often greatly affected. These long-term modifications take place as native groups become part of, and interact more frequently with, the complex structure of national socioeconomic systems.

There are three objectives for this chapter. First, we argue that, despite the rapid rate of change in Amazonia, bioanthropology has yet to systematically investigate the interplay between socioeconomic transformation and human biology in the region. This is true even though native Amazonian peoples have been the focus of intensive bioanthropological research throughout the past forty years. Second, we present a case study of the Tupí-Mondé from the Brazilian southwestern Amazon, through which some of the links between environmental and socioeconomic changes and physical well-being are considered. Third, we argue that the explanatory power of bioanthropological research in Amazonia and else-

269

where will greatly benefit when its practitioners start paying more attention to the political-economic dynamics which affect the populations under study.

Human Biological Research on Native Amazonian Peoples

Since the 1960s, there has been a major effort toward better understanding various aspects of the human biology of native Amazonian populations. Research has mainly focused on population genetics and epidemiology. Framed within the neo-Darwinian evolutionary perspective, the former has mainly focused on the mechanisms involved in the production and maintenance of genetic variability (Neel 1970, 1994; Salzano and Callegari-Jacques 1988), with special emphasis on (1) population structure and natural selection, (2) the rate of genetic diversification, and (3) the response of genetic systems to a rapidly changing environment. These concerns reflect interest in models of genetic microdifferentiation under certain demographic conditions—small population size and the village fusion–fission pattern—conditions under which the human species likely evolved. As pointed out recently by one of the leading figures in this line of research:

> In the late 1950s I began to devote considerable thought to the question of just how to study the operation of natural selection in our species . . . I found it impressive and depressing how little solid data there was relating specific genes to specific traits of selective advantage and disadvantage . . . To understand ourselves, and how the conditions regulating survival and reproduction had changed, we must understand the biology of precivilized man much better . . . These concerns about the operation of natural selection very quickly merged with fascination with the question of human origins and evolution that most humans share in one form or another . . . It also became clear that, with respect to a significant study, it was now or never; the relative few remaining primitive populations of the world were so rapidly being disrupted that ours was almost surely the last generation to encounter any of them in a *relatively* undisturbed condition. (Neel 1994, 118–20)

Researchers sought to study small-scale, preindustrial societies in relative isolation, their choices falling on those supposedly little affected by external historical and political processes.

pop. genetics - focused on the mechanism of genetic variability
- genetic microdifferentiation

The general thesis behind the [research] program was that, on the assumption that these peoples represented the best approximation available to the conditions under which human variability arose, a system type of analysis oriented toward a number of specific questions might provide valuable insights into problems of human evolution and variability . . . the groups under study are certainly much closer in their breeding structure to hunter-gatherers than to modern man; thus they permit cautious inferences about human breeding structure prior to large-scale and complex agriculture. (Neel 1970, 815)

From the perspective of population genetics, there has not been a search for genetic adaptation per se, in the classical sense of reproductive advantage in particular environmental circumstances. Instead, the focus has been on population structure and the application of methodologically sophisticated biometric analyses to elucidate genetic processes at the microevolutionary level. These studies have been important in revealing the role of random processes (e.g., genetic drift and founder effect) as related to high levels of interpopulation genetic variability. The major human biology projects were carried out among the Xavánte, Makiritáre, Yanomámi, and Kayapó (Salzano and Callegari-Jacques 1988).

Epidemiological research is a second field that has received attention in human biology projects. Much of the literature on this topic is concerned with: (1) the characterization of levels of morbidity through cross-sectional biomedical surveys; (2) clinical and immunological studies in "virgin soil" populations; and (3) the elucidation of the role of population size as an intervening factor in the persistence of specific pathogens in small-scale populations (Coimbra 1995; Salzano and Callegari-Jacques 1988).

The genetic and epidemiological studies on native Amazonian populations have reached a remarkable degree of methodological and theoretical sophistication. On the basis of specific case studies, researchers have been able to generate important theoretical formulations. To maintain this perspective, the focus has been upon recently contacted and/or semi-isolated populations. This has involved an emphasis on categories such as "isolated," "pristine," "primitive," "unacculturated," "undisturbed," and "virgin soil" that permeate much of the bioanthropological literature in Amazonia from the 1960s onward.

Frontier Expansion toward Southwestern Amazonia
and Tupí-Mondé Peoples

The Tupí-Mondé include some seven small-scale groups living on reservations located in the Brazilian states of Rondônia and Mato Grosso, in the southwestern Amazon region (fig. 1). The Tupí-Mondé speak languages classified within the Tupí linguistic stock, Mondé family. This chapter deals with sociocultural and bioanthropological data from three of the four Tupí-Mondé groups whose reservations are within the Aripuanã Indian Park: the Gavião, Suruí, and Zoró. These are societies that experienced contact[1] with Brazilian national society as a result of frontier expansion at different periods in the twentieth century.[2]

Like most extant native Amazonian populations, the Tupí-Mondé are upland forest dwellers whose traditional subsistence is based on shifting horticulture, complemented by hunting, fishing, and gathering (Brunelli 1989; Coimbra 1989; Santos 1991). The Aripuanã region is rolling country, crossed by small water courses, and mostly covered by interfluvial upland forest. Traditionally, Tupí-Mondé societies are nonstratified from a socioeconomic standpoint, the main differentiation being along gender and age lines. Villages in precontact periods were constituted of no more than a few hundred individuals, living in large palm thatched longhouses with no internal partitions and inhabited by extended families. The Tupí-Mondé were semi-nomadic, as villagers would regularly move to new sites when garden productivity and the availability of forest products declined.

The history of Tupí-Mondé peoples is poorly documented. As far as is known, early travelers did not reach what is today the Aripuanã area. More recently, some effort has been made to compile ethnohistorical information (Menéndez 1981/1982, 1984/1985; Meireles 1984; Brunelli 1989); systematic archaeological research in the Aripuanã area is yet to be carried out. Notwithstanding, recent studies have suggested that the Tupí-Mondé have long been influenced by Western expansion in the Amazon Basin (Meireles 1984; Brunelli 1989; Coimbra 1989). There is evidence that they descend from the Tupí-Kawahíb, groups which would have reached the forests of Rondônia and northern Mato Grosso coming from the Tapajós, fleeing from intensified intertribal warfare associated with the arrival of Europeans centuries ago (Nimuendajú 1948; Menéndez 1981/1982, 1984/1985).

The Aripuanã region remained relatively isolated for most of the colonial period. Although the Portuguese reached southwestern Amazonia as

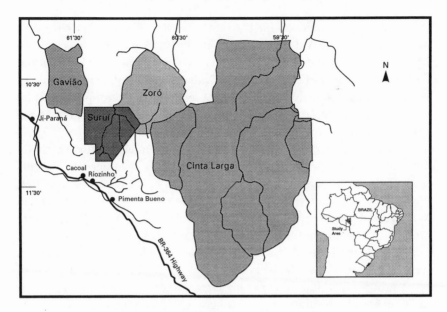

Fig. 1. Map showing Tupí-Mondé territories

early as the eighteenth century, the occupation was confined to the margins of the major rivers—Madeira, Mamoré, and Guaporé—away from Tupí-Mondé territories. Those early expeditions aimed at expanding and securing the borders of the territories claimed by the Portuguese Crown, locating gold deposits, and establishing commercial routes. Native groups living along those rivers were the ones that experienced the most disruptive consequences—epidemics, enslavement, social disruption—in this early phase of European expansion into the region (Davidson 1970; Meireles 1984; Hemming 1987; Coimbra 1989).

The relative isolation of Tupí-Mondé groups started breaking down at the end of the nineteenth century. Due to the expanded demand for rubber in the world market, the frontier penetrated inland along the tributaries of the large rivers (Weinstein 1983; Hemming 1987). During that period, the Amazon region witnessed a sudden rush of landless peasants from northeast Brazil who came to work in the extraction of natural rubber. The rubber trade and industry dominated the Amazonian regional economy, and as the frontier was pushed further inland, the isolation of native upland forest dwellers, like the Tupí-Mondé, became threatened

(Davidson 1970; Meireles 1984; Coimbra 1989). Researchers have estimated that over thirty different native groups were annihilated as the rubber enterprise expanded into Rondônia (Ribeiro 1956). The persecution, deliberate killing, and enslavement of Indians were routine in those days. It was through these violent means that several native groups became an essential part of the regional economy, their labor force supporting the rubber extraction enterprise.

Changes accelerated in the first half of the twentieth century (Meireles 1984; Hemming 1987; Coimbra 1989; Santos 1991). Two significant events took place during this period: the construction of the telegraph lines that crossed Tupí-Mondé territories and a second rubber boom during World War II. Several hundred kilometers of Rondônia and Mato Grosso were crossed by expeditions that, between 1907 and 1914, constructed telegraph lines connecting Mato Grosso to Amazonas (Rondon 1946). The workers went deep into the forest and made firsthand contact with a number of isolated groups. The lines opened up large unexplored areas to Brazilian national society, resulting in the extinction of a number of native groups (Ribeiro 1956). With regard to the Amazonian rubber industry, it had been greatly affected in the early part of the century when large plantations were established in Malaysia by the British. The Amazonian rubber economy regained impetus during World War II as supplies from Malaysia could not reach the allies because of the Japanese occupation. It was during this second boom that new waves of Northeastern Brazilian workers were recruited and penetrated deep into the forest, reaching a number of still semi-isolated groups. The contact of the Gavião dates to this period.

The second half of this century witnessed a sharp acceleration in Western penetration toward southwestern Amazonia (Davis 1977; Mueller 1980; Meireles 1984; Becker 1987; Hemming 1987; Brunelli 1989; Coimbra 1989; Santos 1991). Starting in the 1960s, government efforts aimed at occupying and integrating the region into the Brazilian national context. National and international capital, mainly through loans provided by the World Bank, has been channeled to the region. The "development" effort resulted in the opening of highways and the establishment of large colonization and mining projects. These were the conditions needed for the onset of the largest migratory movement in Amazonian history.

The population of Rondônia increased from 37,173 in 1950 to 492,810 in 1980, that is, 1,228 percent in thirty years (IBGE 1981a). Most of the growth took place due to migration in the 1970s, when the population increased 333 percent. Such a huge influx of migrants changed the nature of the nearly century-long contact that local native groups had maintained with Brazilian nationals. Up to that period, the still semi-isolated Amerindian groups were used to fighting with rubber-tappers who periodically invaded their territories, and they could still retreat to unoccupied areas. As Rondônia and northern Mato Grosso became increasingly occupied by non-Indians, several Tupí-Mondé groups, including the Suruí and Zoró, were forced to come into permanent contact with Brazilian national society and, shortly after, to participate in the regional economic system.

Intensive migration has also come along with accelerated deforestation. Data from satellite images indicate that the rates of forest area cleared from 1975 to 1988 increased from 0.6 to 12.0 percent in Amazonia (Mahar 1989). The increase in rates of deforestation was highest in southwestern Amazonia, where Rondônia is located. As seen in figure 2, population increases in Rondônia came along with a sharp increase in rates of deforestation, particularly from the late 1970s onward.

Massive migration brought about serious land tenure problems. The colonization process was not well coordinated, so that by the mid-1970s approximately 80 percent of the families that arrived in Rondônia had no titles to plots in the colonization projects (Mueller 1980). The situation did not improve in the following years, as the Brazilian government was unable to settle the vast majority of migrants in the 1980s. The rapid pace of migration, coupled with the inefficiency of the public sector to manage land occupation, led to squatting on public lands and invasion of Indian territories, which directly affected the Gavião, Suruí, and Zoró (Meireles 1984; Brunelli 1989; Coimbra 1989; Santos 1991).

According to Sawyer (1992), the net effect of "development" in southwestern Amazonia was the migration of poverty from elsewhere in Brazil to the countryside and towns of Rondônia and northern Mato Grosso. The vast majority of the population in these regions lacks electricity, piped water, sewerage, and other basic infrastructure. Indeed, due in part to the extremely high rates of population growth, the public health situation prevailing in Rondônia is chaotic, as a number of infectious and parasitic diseases, including hepatitis, leishmaniasis, leprosy, and malaria, are highly endemic and the health system is unable to cope with the demands (Coimbra 1989; Santos 1991; Sawyer 1992). The example of malaria is illustrative. Data from the Brazilian Ministry of Health indicate that, of the 168,639 positive blood smears for Brazil in 1980, 59,178 (35.1 percent)

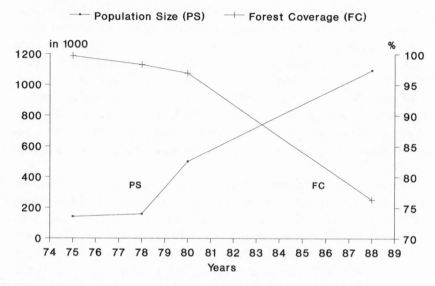

Fig. 2.   Population and deforestation trends in Rondônia, Brazil. (Data from Mahar 1992; IBGE 1978, 1990.)

were from Rondônia (IBGE 1981b, 163), where less than 1 percent of the country's population resides. Although health problems are serious at the regional level, they are even critical among native populations, who are extremely marginalized within the broader context of the Brazilian regional social system.

Frontier Expansion and Its Impacts on Tupí-Mondé Peoples

Native populations from southwestern Amazonia experienced increased mortality due to the spread of infectious and parasitic diseases long before the establishment of permanent contact with Brazilian national society (Ribeiro 1956; Caspar 1957; Davis 1977; Meireles 1984; Hemming 1987; Brunelli 1989; Coimbra 1989; Santos 1991). This implies that European penetration impacted on native peoples well prior to their incorporation into the regional economic system. Caspar (1957), for instance, described a measles epidemic which broke out in the first half of this century among the Tuparí, a neighboring tribe to the Tupí-Mondé, and which led to the annihilation of the entire population before the establishment of permanent contact. The French anthropologist Claude Lévi-Strauss, who traveled in Mato Grosso and Rondônia in the 1930s, provided in his *Tristes Tropiques* a compelling description of a visit to a relatively isolated Tupí settlement in the Aripuanã area. He wrote:

> In all there were six women, seven men, and one of them only an adolescent, and three little girls who seemed to be one, two, and three years of age; it was no doubt one of the smallest groups who could be imagined as managing to survive . . . Two members of the groups were afflicted with paralysis of the lower limbs: a young woman went about on two sticks, and a man, also young, dragged himself along the ground like a legless cripple . . . I wondered if poliomyelitis or some other virus had affected them, even before they had had time to establish lasting contact with civilization. (Lévi-Strauss 1974, 346)

Tupí-Mondé peoples faced massive depopulation as they experienced contact with Brazilian national society. A succession of measles, tuberculosis, and flu epidemics in the late 1960s and early 1970s killed 75 percent of the Suruí (Meireles 1984; Coimbra 1989). Chiappino (1975), a Red Cross physician who worked among the Suruí a few years after contact, reported that about 60 percent of the population had tuberculosis. Brunelli (1989) estimated that the Zoró numbered between 1,000 and 1,500 individuals distributed into several local groups in the immediate precontact period. This figure is almost five times higher than the Zoró population of 1990. It has been argued that, due to pronounced depopulation, the current composition of the Tupí-Mondé, which consists of seven groups, is a simplification of a more complex ethnic configuration which once existed in the Aripuanã area (Coimbra 1989).

Socioeconomic changes which followed contact resulted in changes in the Tupí-Mondé subsistence system. Their subsistence was based on small, mobile settlements of less than a hundred individuals. Permanent contact brought about sedentism and life in much larger villages, resulting in greater pressure upon natural resources which could no longer be alleviated by migration. At present, the Tupí-Mondé face the challenge of providing for food and shelter to a rapidly expanding population. The Suruí, for instance, have increased from 250 in 1979 to 401 in 1988 (Coimbra 1989), a rate of growth per annum of approximately 4.3 per 1,000. If this growth rate is maintained, the Suruí will double in population every sixteen years.

New modes of production became part of the Tupí-Mondé economy shortly after contact. The trend toward early articulation with the regional market economy has its roots in the "pacification" process. The contact of isolated groups in Brazil, as conducted by the National Indian Foundation (FUNAI), follows well-defined steps.[3] Initially, the natives are offered gifts as signs of the willingness of the "pacification" team to engage in peaceful interactions. As the work of "pacification" succeeds, the Indians tend to abandon their original village site and to move close to FUNAI outposts, where the distribution of industrial goods continues for some time, along with the provision of some basic health care. Hence dependence is fostered from the very first moment. In the long run, however, native groups are largely left on their own to obtain the products to which they gradually become accustomed. This is a strong stimulus toward participation within the regional market economy. Tupí-Mondé groups, to a lesser or greater extent, have gone through this process. At present, the Gavião and Zoró rely on rubber-tapping as their major cash income activity; others, like the Suruí, have diversified their economy, including coffee farming and logging (Brunelli 1989; Coimbra 1989; Santos 1991).

Cash income activities have come along with the curtailment of traditional subsistence practices, which are no longer scheduled according to the Tupí-Mondé agricultural calendar. The Suruí case provides a clear example of this trend. In the late 1970s and early 1980s, the southern portion of the Suruí reservation was invaded by colonists who started a coffee plantation. When the squatters were expelled in 1982 and 1983, the Indians occupied the coffee plantation, aiming at achieving economic independence. Coffee farming is a time- and energy-demanding work that requires continuous weeding in addition to investments in harvesting, sacking, and transportation. As a result, the Suruí were left with little time to work on their traditional gardens. Although some money was made from the selling of coffee, it was mostly channeled toward the purchase of status consumer goods, such as watches, sunglasses, and clothing, instead of food items and other basic needs once provided by their traditional subsistence economy (Coimbra 1989; Santos 1991).

Tupí-Mondé reservations are surrounded by colonization projects and/or large agribusiness enterprises. As already mentioned, the occupation of southwestern Amazonia has come along with rapid deforestation, to a point where, at present, Indian reservations are true islands of forest within large deforested landscapes. Logging is an important economic activity in Rondônia and Mato Grosso, so that local entrepreneurs exert pressure to exploit natural resources on the reservations. Uneven economic exchange has marked the relationships between Indians and local entrepreneurs, as the former often receive for the products extracted from their reservations prices well below the actual market values (Coimbra 1989; Santos 1991).

Alterations in housing patterns and village arrangements reflect the dynamics of socioeconomic changes in Tupí-Mondé societies. Nuclearization of the household unit is noticeable in all villages. Instead of the traditional communal houses inhabited by extended families, now the nuclear family is the most common arrangement. Families live in wooden or brick houses which to a large extent emulate the local rural Brazilian housing style. Different reasons account for the nuclearization process. The Zoró, for instance, abandoned their traditional "malocas" as they were converted en masse to Christianity by missionaries shortly after contact (Brunelli 1989). For the Suruí, coffee farming and logging have provided large amounts of cash, leading to intragroup socioeconomic differentiation in a previously egalitarian society (Coimbra 1989; Santos 1991).

Tupí-Mondé Health and Nutrition

This section aims at contextualizing specific aspects of Tupí-Mondé physical well-being as they relate to the political-economic reality of southwestern Amazonia. First, we will point out that the timing of biological disruption is closely related to trends in frontier expansion. Second, data will be provided to demonstrate that Tupí-Mondé health and nutritional conditions are poor, even when compared to the lowest socioeconomic strata of the Brazilian population. Third, we will argue that the introduction of new modes of production in Tupí-Mondé reservations has come with the emergence of specific epidemiological problems (i.e., an outbreak of a serious fungal disease called paracoccidioidomycosis). Fourth, we will show that the trend toward intragroup socioeconomic differentiation noticeable in some Tupí-Mondé groups is reflected at the biological level, as revealed by child growth patterns and adult anthropometrics.

Dental Enamel Defects: History from Their Mouths

Contact was a socially and biologically stressful experience for the Tupí-Mondé (Brunelli 1989; Coimbra 1989; Santos 1991). With the exception of broad estimates of population decline, however, bioanthropologists have few means to gain insights into the impacts of frontier expansion upon Amerindian groups like the Tupí-Mondé. As already mentioned, information that could potentially provide a diachronic perspective, including detailed archaeological, ethnohistoric, and demographic data, is meager, if not to say nonexistent, for the Aripuanã region.

The analysis of developmental defects in dental enamel (DDE) has proven to be an excellent means of gaining a diachronic view of Tupí-Mondé health status (Santos 1991). Enamel defects are regarded as epidemiological indicators of physiological disruption during times of tooth development (Goodman and Rose 1990). The rationale is that enamel formation may be affected by physiological imbalances, yielding an "accurate, prompt and permanent record" (Sarnat and Schour 1941, 1989) of chronological development during certain periods of the individual's life (Goodman and Rose 1990).

DDE frequencies by decade of enamel formation for the Gavião, Suruí, and Zoró are shown in figure 3.[4] For each of the groups, there is a peak for hypoplasia concentration: in the 1930s through 1950s for the Gavião, in the 1970s for the Suruí, and also in the 1970s for the Zoró. Interestingly enough, these peaks coincide with the contact periods of each of the three groups,[5] when they experienced the highest levels of biological disruption mostly due to disease epidemics. Hence the analysis of temporal variation in DDE expression reveals that the expansion of the Brazilian demographic and economic frontier toward southwestern Amazonia brought the Tupí-Mondé into its sphere of influence in a stressful way (Santos 1991).

Researchers have long debated the issue of the health status of traditional peoples with minimal or no contact with Western societies and the impacts of subsequent changes upon their health. Wirsing (1985), for instance, argued that unacculturated traditional societies are well-adapted to their environments, enjoying adequate health and nutrition. Such well-being would result from a combination of geographic isolation, nomadic or semi-nomadic life-style, knowledge of the environment, subsistence practices, and dietary diversity. Opposed to this picture, changes brought about by interethnic contact would lead to the disruption of traditional subsistence practices, resulting in deprived health and nutritional conditions.

DDE data reveal that such a dichotomous view is at best an oversimplification in the case of the Tupí-Mondé. The diachronic perspective attained by the analyses of hypoplasia frequencies suggests that pre- and postcontact frequencies are comparable. As can be seen in figure 3, DDE

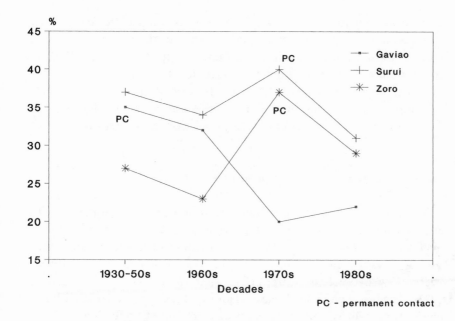

Fig. 3.   Frequencies of dental enamel defects in Tupí-Mondé anterior dentition according to decade of enamel formation. (Reproduced from Santos 1991.)

frequencies for the Suruí and Zoró in postcontact decades (i.e., 1980s) approach precontact levels (i.e., 1930s through 1950s, and 1960s). For the Gavião, there were too few old individuals (60 years of age or older), so that hypoplasia data could not be collected for precontact periods.

   A political-economic perspective is helpful in clarifying the issue of precontact vis-à-vis postcontact levels of physiological disruption. As detailed earlier in this paper, it is unlikely that, at least since the turn of this century, native populations from southwestern Amazonia have been in complete isolation from outside influences. Nonautochthonous diseases, often in epidemic form, have certainly reached the native populations of the region, even those still uncontacted. Such understanding leads to a rethinking of the conventional dichotomy between uncontacted "versus" contacted groups. As evaluated by enamel defects, the first half of this century was a stressful time for the Tupí-Mondé. At least in part, high levels of physiological disruption in the decades preceding contact may be explained as a consequence of the process of frontier expansion toward

Tupí-Mondé territories, which has led to a crescendo of direct and indirect stressful interactions between native peoples and the newcomers. These findings warn against generalizations that the Tupí-Mondé were living in equilibrium with their environment in precontact periods. As pointed out by Swedlund and Armelagos (1990), this historic perspective must replace the simplistic notion of groups either in isolation or not, and it deemphasizes the single-step concept of pristine populations becoming acculturated ones.

Tupí-Mondé Health: How Marginalization Is Reinforced

At present, the health and nutritional conditions of Tupí-Mondé peoples are extremely precarious, reflecting structural inadequacies in food production, sanitation, and health care. A number of infectious and parasitic diseases are endemic in the Aripuanã area (Coimbra et al. 1985a, 1985b, 1996a, 1996b; Coimbra 1989; Coimbra and Santos 1991; Santos 1991). The list of endemic diseases is long and includes malaria, leishmaniasis, tuberculosis, intestinal parasitism, pyoderma infection, scabies, gastroenteritis, upper respiratory infections and sexually transmitted diseases. Protein-energy malnutrition and anemia are common nutritional disorders on Tupí-Mondé reservations (Santos 1991, 1993; Santos and Coimbra 1991).

The determinants of Tupí-Mondé poor health and nutritional status are complex, but it seems that departure from their traditional adaptive system has worsened the situation. Due to intrinsic ecological conditions, the combination of hunting-gathering with horticulture as widely practiced by native Amazonians is adaptive only under conditions of high mobility. The Tupí-Mondé have abandoned their semi-nomadic way of life and are now living in larger permanent settlements, resulting in greater pressure upon natural resources. Some of the consequences may be shortened fallow, decreased agricultural and hunting/fishing potential, and soil degradation. Food production is affected under such conditions. Although quantitative data are not available, anthropologists working with the Tupí-Mondé have reported a downward trend in the diversity of their diet over time (Coimbra 1989). Reduced mobility also results in environmental pollution. Sanitary conditions are now precarious in all Tupí-Mondé villages, as none have latrines or any kind of sewerage disposal system. Defecation takes place in the bushes close to the villages, where domestic garbage is also thrown. Even if community size is small, the environment becomes increasingly polluted with the accumulation of waste. These are favorable conditions for the spread of water-borne diseases (and gastroenteritis in particular), which are known to be major health problems in Tupí-Mondé villages (Coimbra et al. 1985b; Coimbra 1989; Santos et al. 1991).

The inadequate provision of health services further compromises the biological well-being of Tupí-Mondé peoples. Living in the ecological and social environment of the frontier, where the transmission of several diseases is rampant, native populations of southwestern Amazonia are offered few ways to cope with the situation (Coimbra 1989; Santos 1991). Infrastructure and personnel are major constraints in the provision of health services, as infirmaries at the reservations are seldom operating. A consequence is that vaccination is always behind schedule and the long-term treatment of some diseases, such as tuberculosis and malaria, is not properly provided. It is not uncommon to see medication stocks deteriorating due to inappropriate storage. Because of problems of interethnic confrontation and the lack of appropriate infrastructure, there is a high turnover of health assistants at the reservation infirmaries.

These structural inadequacies may be seen as part of a larger process which forces native populations into permanent interaction with a dominant political-economic system, but which does not provide the populations with the adequate means to cope with the new conditions. The end result is that, at the tribal level, one sees reproduced the health and nutritional conditions that characterize the poor segments of the national society (Coimbra 1989; Santos 1991, 1993). Figure 4 shows that undernutrition and anemia are highly prevalent among the Tupí-Mondé. The epidemiology of protein-energy malnutrition is particularly illustrative. Anthropometric surveys conducted in 1990 and 1991 revealed rates of stunting of 38.0 percent, 57.7 percent, and 63.5 percent for Gavião, Suruí, and Zoró children 0 to 10.9 years of age, respectively, averaging 55.4 percent for the three groups (Santos 1991; Santos and Coimbra 1991). A recent nationwide survey showed that the prevalence of stunting in Brazilian children 0 to 5 years of age is 15.4 percent, reaching 27.6 percent for those living in extreme poverty (Monteiro, Benício, and Gouveia 1992). The highest rates of chronic undernutrition were observed in the impoverished northern (23.0 percent) and northeastern (27.3 percent) portions of the country. Hence the level of chronic undernutrition for Tupí-Mondé children, as evaluated by anthropometric parameters, is at least twice that of the most underprivileged segment of the Brazilian population.

Cash Cropping and the Production of a Disease

Paracoccidioidomycosis, regarded as the major systemic fungal disease in Latin America, is caused by the fungus *Paracoccidioides brasiliensis,* a free-living saprophytical microorganism of the soil. When infecting humans, *P. brasiliensis* produces a primary pulmonary infection that may spread to other organs. The disease can be fatal if not treated (Rippon 1982). Between 1983 and 1990, approximately fifteen cases of paracoccidioidomycosis were reported for the Suruí (Coimbra et al. 1994).

Detailed epidemiological investigation has provided support for the hypothesis that the outbreak of paracoccidioidomycosis among the Suruí is associated with changes in the group's subsistence practices, and with the adoption of coffee farming in particular. Considerable evidence supports this hypothesis (Coimbra et al. 1994): (1) the appearance of the first cases of the mycosis coincided with the transition to coffee farming; (2) the disease has not been reported for neighboring Tupí-Mondé groups (i.e., the Gavião and Zoró), none of which engage in coffee farming; and (3) paracoccidioidomycosis is known to be associated with agricultural activities in endemic areas of Latin America (Rippon 1982).

The results of immunological tests show that paracoccidioidin sensitivity prevalence rates are significantly higher for the Suruí compared to the two other Tupí-Mondé groups (Coimbra et al. 1994). Overall, nearly half of the Suruí sample has been exposed to *P. brasiliensis* (43.8 percent), compared to 14.9 percent of the Zoró and 6.4 percent of the Gavião.

The mechanisms that have increased the likelihood of exposure of the Suruí to the fungus are not yet completely clear. There are reasons to believe that the adoption of agricultural practices involving weeding (i.e., coffee farming) has favored the transmission of *P. brasiliensis,* the reason being a greater contact with contaminated soil dust particles. The Tupí-Mondé subsistence system—slash and burn agriculture—does not require weeding; instead, it utilizes fire in order to clean the land for planting. This practice minimizes contact with soil dust. Coffee farming, on the other hand, involves a labor-intensive crop that requires year-round weeding in Amazonia due to the rapid pace of secondary succession. Instead of using the hoe, the Suruí weed with machetes, which leads to an even closer contact with the ground as people have to bend forward in order to reach the weeds. At present, Suruí villages are surrounded by coffee plantations where there is plenty of exposed soil. At sunset, clouds of dust are easily seen over the villages (Coimbra et al. 1994). Previous research on the epi-

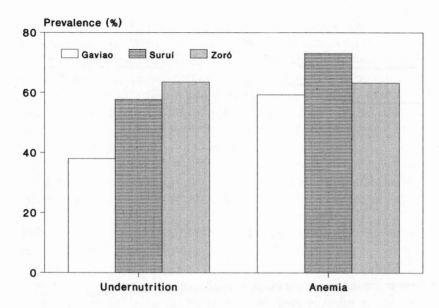

Fig. 4.   Rates of low height for age (below –2 SD from NCHS medians) and anemia in Tupí-Mondé children 0–10 years of age. (Reproduced from Santos 1991.)

demiology of paracoccidioidomycosis has shown that it is more prevalent among rural workers engaged in intensive agriculture. In the study conducted in Paracotos, Venezuela, in one of the few cases when P. brasiliensis was isolated from soil samples, the population was mostly involved in coffee farming. In this study, Albornoz (1971) detected a high rate (greater than 50 percent) of positivity to paracoccidioidin.

Hence the epidemiology of paracoccidioidomycosis in the Aripuanã area seems to be related to the ongoing process of environmental and socioeconomic changes taking place at the regional level. It provides an interesting example pointing to the emergence of an infectious disease in association with the increasing economic articulation of the Tupí-Mondé, and the Suruí in particular, with the market economy.

Socioeconomic Differentiation and Body Morphology

Coffee farming and logging generated large cash income for the Suruí society. As shown by Coimbra (1989), the incoming money was concentrated in the hands of a few leaders, their close kin, and their political supporters. Cash concentration led to a breakdown in Suruí traditional egalitarian organization. Hierarchization affected social life, village spatial organization, and household composition; it also influenced access to medical services and food. In a situation of widespread scarcity, the economically better-off families, or those with close ties to the political leaders, were able to afford private medical services in town and the purchase of industrial food items. Anthropometric surveys carried out in 1987 and 1988 yielded data demonstrating that the children of the economically better-off Suruí families were less nutritionally deprived (Coimbra 1989). The results indicated a positive association between socioeconomic status and anthropometric indicators of nutritional status.

Socioeconomic differentiation has also influenced the body morphology of Suruí adults. Mean Z-score values and 95 percent confidence intervals for four anthropometric parameters are presented by socioeconomic tertials for Suruí adults in figure 5. Anthropometric data were transformed into z-score values in order to combine the male and female samples. An index of socioeconomic status (SES) was derived in order to characterize quantitatively the process of differentiation within Suruí society (Santos and Coimbra 1996); it is based on five variables related to the characteristics of the household as well as type and number of personal belongings, ownership of "status" items, clothing, and presence of furniture and a gas stove in the house. The "typical" Suruí individual of high SES lives in a brick house instead of in the traditional longhouse, consumes a great deal of imported food and status consumer goods, owns some cattle, and no longer engages in traditional subsistence practices (e.g., hunting, fishing, land clearing). Suruí males and females of high SES tend to be highly sedentary. Those individuals of highest SES (category III) consistently present higher mean values for weight, body mass index, and sum of skinfold thickness, but not for stature.

The findings for the Suruí suggest that the differentiation in body morphology is associated with the uneven surplus accumulation of cash in a previously egalitarian society. Moreover, the process seems to be a recent one, as the lack of differences in stature indicates that the factors influencing Suruí anthropometrics have not been operating long enough to affect the long-term dynamics of linear growth. The major differences were noticed for those anthropometric parameters (i.e., weight, body mass index, and sum of skinfold thickness) more closely related to fat accumu-

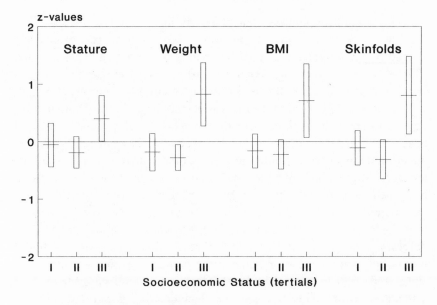

Fig. 5.   Mean Z-score mean values and 95 percent confidence intervals for stature, weight, body mass index, and sum of skinfold thicknesses in Tupí-Mondé adults according to categories of socioeconomic status, sexes combined. (Adapted from Santos and Coimbra 1996.)

lation. Changes in diet and in levels of physical activity are possibly the two major biological factors influencing Suruí body composition.

Tupí-Mondé (Un)Natural History

This chapter has briefly outlined the history of southwestern Amazonia over this past century, emphasizing its close intersections with global and regional political-economic processes. The history of Amerindian peoples from this region has been extensively shaped by the expansion of the Brazilian economic and demographic frontier into their territories. Starting in the late nineteenth century, the frontier expanded toward Rondônia and northern Mato Grosso as the demand for natural rubber increased in the world market; more recently, the "development" effort has aimed at occupying and integrating these regions into the contemporary Brazilian political economy.

The bioanthropological data presented in this chapter indicate that the human biology of the Tupí-Mondé peoples has been extensively shaped by the political and economic reality of southwestern Amazonia. This is what we imply by *unnatural* history. Arguing for a biological anthropology with a political economic orientation, Singer (1992, 2) writes, "the very physical shape of nature, including of course human biology, . . . has been deeply influenced by a long history of human activity and hierarchical social structures, that is to say, by the changing political economy of human society." That is, analytical models that *naturalize* the reality under study which overlook macrostructural processes, are likely to have their heuristic value limited. We share this perspective. In this chapter, major connections between micro- and macrostructural processes have been unraveled through the Tupí-Mondé case study: analyses of developmental defects of dental enamel reveal that these peoples suffered biologically with Western expansion. Their poor health and nutritional status reflect their marginality within the regional social system; their articulation with the regional economy included the adoption of new patterns of environmental exploitation that have enhanced the likelihood of exposure to pathogens; and cash income has led to socioeconomic and nutritional stratification in previously nonhierarchical societies. These examples show that the impacts of frontier expansion transcend temporal boundaries, as they influenced Tupí-Mondé precontact, contact, and postcontact social dynamics and biology.

As stressed earlier in the paper, research on the human biology of native Amazonian populations carried out over the past three decades has been extremely productive and relevant to the discipline of biological anthropology as a whole (Salzano and Callegari-Jacques 1988; Neel 1970, 1994). The conclusions drawn from specific studies, such as those carried out among the Xavánte and Yanomámi, have had theoretical implications that go far beyond the regional level. It has also been pointed out that a major feature of this research agenda has been its primary, yet not exclusive, interest in semi-isolated or recently contacted Indian groups.

At present, there is an urgent need to expand the traditional focus of human biological research in Amazonia so as to start developing analytical schemes relevant to the issue of change. This concern has already been made explicit in writings on Amazonian archaeology, ethnohistory, and ethnography (Posey 1994; Roosevelt 1994b; Whitehead 1994).[6] Bioanthropologists have yet to fully recognize the impacts of Western occupation upon the lives of native Amazonian peoples. By realizing the importance of local and global factors, bioanthropologists would be in a better position to unravel, and possibly incorporate into their models, social, economic, and historic aspects which shape the biological diversity of native Amazonians.

This may be obvious when dealing with the health and nutritional outcomes of contact and acculturation, as we did in this paper. But the linkages are not as well defined in other fields of interest to bioanthropologists, such as population genetics. Recent publications on the underlying causes of genetic diversity within some lowland South American linguistic stocks bear on that issue. Callegari-Jacques and Salzano (1989) suggested that the greater genetic diversity observed in Tupí speaking groups when compared to the Kárib could be explained by the smaller population size of the former, which could have favored the action of stochastic factors. Aguiar (1991) took a different perspective and argued that, in order to explain the differences between the two stocks, ethnohistoric information has to be taken into consideration. In Aguiar's alternative model, the recent history of the Tupí and Kárib, including depopulation, isolation, and intertribal relations, plays an important role in shaping between- and within-group biological differentiation.

In conclusion, bioanthropological research in Amazonia and elsewhere will certainly strengthen its analytical models when closer attention is paid to the interplay between local/global histories and human biology. In adopting a historical attitude, bioanthropologists will constantly remind themselves that the populations under study operate within larger contexts and that the interrelationships cannot be disregarded in their theoretical considerations.

NOTES

We would like to thank Alan Goodman, Emilio Moran, and Nancy Flowers for their helpful comments on this chapter which originated as a paper. We also benefited from the stimulating debates that took place during the Wenner-Gren symposium "Political-Economic Perspectives in Biological Anthropology: Building a Biocultural Synthesis" (Cabo San Lucas, Mexico, 1992), where this paper was originally presented. Funding for research on the Tupí-Mondé was provided by the Wenner-Gren Foundation, the John D. and Catherine T. MacArthur Foundation, the "Conselho Nacional de Desenvolvimento Científico e Tecnológico" (Brazil), and "Fundação Oswaldo Cruz."

    1. Contact experience refers to the period when official or nonofficial efforts are made to bring native populations into continuous interaction with Brazilian

national society. It invariably results in the sedentism of Indian groups and the onset of reservation life. Brazilian law guarantees the Indians the right to use of lands they inhabit, although land ownership is granted to the Union. At present, the Tupí-Mondé live in federally demarcated reservations administrated by FUNAI, the Brazilian National Indian Foundation, whose duties involve providing educational services, health care, and overall administration of community development projects.

2. Of the Tupí-Mondé groups herein considered, the Gavião was the first to enter into permanent contact with Brazilian national society, back in the 1940s and 1950s. Initial contacts were established with rubber-tappers, for whom the Indians worked for several years. With the establishment of their reservation in the 1970s (the "Area Indígena Igarapé Lourdes" with 185,000 hectares), the Gavião were freed from direct exploitation by local rubber-tappers and merchants. At present, the Gavião population is approximately 288 individuals. The Suruí and Zoró were brought into contact with Brazilian national society as the frontier expanded toward southwestern Amazonia in the 1960s and 1970s. The Suruí were contacted by FUNAI pacification teams in 1969, when the group was still living in autonomous villages relatively far away from major Brazilian settlements. Suruí contact was associated with the expansion of colonization in Rondônia. Presently, the Suruí number approximately 494 individuals, living in the "Area Indígena Sete the Setembro," with 220,000 hectares. Finally, the Zoró were contacted by FUNAI in 1977, also as an outcome of colonization expansion. Presently, they live in the "Area Indígena Zoró," with 430,000 hectares. Their total population is close to 215 individuals.

3. The "pacification" procedure as practiced today has its roots in the early part of this century, when it was devised by Cândido Mariano Rondon, himself an army official with Indian ancestry who traveled extensively in central Brazil constructing telegraph lines. Rondon made first contact with a number of groups. In order to attract the Indians into contact, they are offered gifts (mirrors, machetes, knives, shotguns, ammunition, etc.) by FUNAI agents. The expectation is that the gifts will be taken as signs of willingness to interact peacefully. Often already experiencing the effects of epidemics and with their territory encroached upon by the advance of the frontier, the Indians end up accepting "peaceful" contact.

4. Details of DDE analyses for the Tupí-Mondé may be found in Santos (1991), who followed the methodology described in Goodman et al. (1987). Information was collected on the distribution and kind of DDE on the labial surface of the anterior permanent dentition in 231 Tupí-Mondé individuals of both sexes and all ages.

5. The Suruí constitute an exception to this pattern, as they were contacted in the late 1960s (i.e., 1969), while the DDE data show a peak for hypoplasia concentration in the 1970s. It should be pointed out that epidemics struck the community mostly in the early 1970s, when the Suruí population came to live close to FUNAI's outpost in search of assistance (Coimbra 1989; Santos 1991).

6. A recent edited volume on Amazonian native populations brings several contributions that deal with the issue of change (Roosevelt 1994a). For example, Roosevelt (1994b, 1) argues that "the results of the past twenty years of research in

the area [Amazonia] reveal significant changes in human societies and their conditions of life . . . , but the implications of these changes have not yet been incorporated into Amazonia anthropology." For Whitehead (1994, 33), "there has been a deep alteration in both the scale and complexity of those societies, such that modern Amerindian groups are an uncertain guide as to how Amazonian peoples may have lived in the past." Finally, Posey (1994, 271) points out that "modern indigenous societies probably bear little resemblance to their precontact antecedents. Drastic depopulation due to European diseases and dominance left only remnants of aboriginal societies."

REFERENCES

Aguiar, F. F. 1991. Ethnohistory, Intertribal Relationships, and Genetic Diversity among Amazonian Indians. *Human Biology* 63:743–62.

Albornoz, B. 1971. Isolation of *Paracoccidioides brasiliensis* from Rural Soil in Venezuela. *Sabouraudia* 9:248–53.

Becker, B. K. 1987. Estratégia do Estado e povoamento espontâneo na expansão da fronteira agrícola em Rondônia: interação e conflito. In *Homem e Natureza na Amazônia,* ed. G. Kohlhepp and A. Schrader, 237–52. Tübingen: Geographisches Inst.

Brunelli, G. 1989. *De Los Espiritus a los Microbios: Salud e Cambio entre los Zoró de la Amazonía Brasileña.* Quito: Ediciones Abya-Yaa.

Callegari-Jacques, S., and F. M. Salzano. 1989. Genetic Variation within Two Linguistic Amerindian Groups: Relationships to Geography and Population Size. *American Journal of Physical Anthropology* 79:313–20.

Caspar, F. 1957. A aculturação da tribo Tupari. *Revista de Antropologia* 5:145–71.

Chiappino, J. 1975. The Brazilian Indigenous Problem and Policy: The Aripuanã Park. Document no. 19. Copenhagen, International Work Group for Indigenous Affairs (IWGIA)/ Geneva, Information Center for Indigenous Affairs in the Amazon Region.

Coimbra, C. E. A., Jr. 1989. From Shifting Cultivation to Coffee Farming: The Impact of Change on the Health and Ecology of the Suruí in the Brazilian Amazon. Ph.D. diss., Indiana University, Bloomington.

Coimbra, C. E. A., Jr. 1995. Epidemiologic Factors and Human Adaptation in Amazonia. In *Indigenous Peoples and the Future of Amazonia,* ed. L. Sponsel, 167–81. Tucson: University of Arizona Press.

Coimbra, C. E. A., Jr., R. V. Santos, and R. Tanus. 1985a. Estudos epidemiológicos entre grupos indígenas de Rondônia. I. Piodermites e portadores inaparentes de Staphylococcus sp. na boca e nariz entre os Suruí e Karitiána. *Revista do Instituto de Medicina Tropical de São Paulo* 27:13–19.

Coimbra, C. E. A., Jr., R. V. Santos, R. Tanus, and T. M. Inham. 1985b. Estudos epidemiológicos entre grupos indígenas de Rondônia. II. Bactérias enteropatogênicas e gastrenterites entre os Suruí e Karitiána. *Revista da Fundação SESP* 30:111–19.

Coimbra, C. E. A., Jr., and R. V. Santos. 1991. Avaliação do estado nutricional num contexto de mudanças sócio-econômicas: o grupo indígena Suruí do estado de Rondônia. *Cadernos de Saúde Pública* 7:538–62.

Coimbra, C. E. A., Jr., B. Wanke, R. V. Santos, A. C. F. Valle, and R. L. Costa. 1994. Histoplasmin and Paracoccidioidin Sensitivity in Tupí-Mondé Peoples from the Brazilian Amazonia. *Annals of Tropical Medicine and Parasitology* 88:197–207.

Coimbra, C. E. A., Jr., R. V. Santos, N. M. Flowers, C. F. Yoshida, M. L. Baptista, and A. C. F. Valle. 1996a. Hepatitis B Epidemiology and Cultural Practices in Amerindian Populations of Amazonia: The Tupí-Mondé and the Xavánte of Rondônia and Mato Grosso. *Social Science and Medicine* 42:1738–43.

Coimbra, C. E. A., Jr., R. V. Santos, and A. C. F. Valle. 1996b. Cutaneous Leishmaniasis in Tupí-Mondé Amerindians from the Brazilian Amazonia. *Acta Tropica* 61:201–11.

Davidson, D. M. 1970. Rivers and Empire: The Madeira Route and the Incorporation of the Brazilian Far West. Ph.D. diss., Yale University, New Haven.

Davis, S. H. 1977. *Victims of the Miracle.* Cambridge: Cambridge University Press.

Goodman, A. H., L. H. Allen, G. P. Hernandez, A. Amador, L. V. Arriola, A. Chávez, and G. H. Pelto. 1987. Prevalence and Age at Development of Enamel Hypoplasia in Mexican Children. *American Journal of Physical Anthropology* 72:7–19.

Goodman, A. H., and J. C. Rose. 1990. Assessment of Systemic Physiological Perturbations from Dental Enamel Hypoplasias and Associated Histological Structures. *Yearbook of Physical Anthropology* 33:59–110.

Hemming, J. 1987. *Amazon Frontier: The Defeat of the Brazilian Indians.* London: Macmillan.

IBGE (Instituto Brasileiro de Geografia e Estatística). 1978. *Anuário Estatístico do Brasil.* Rio de Janeiro: IBGE.

IBGE (Instituto Brasileiro de Geografia e Estatística). 1981a. Sinopse Preliminar do Censo Demográfico. IX. Recenseamento Geral do Brasil-1980. Rondônia-Roraima-Amapá. Rio de Janeiro: IBGE.

IBGE (Instituto Brasileiro de Geografia e Estatística). 1981b. Anuário Estatístico do Brasil. Volume 42. Rio de Janeiro: IBGE.

IBGE (Instituto Brasileiro de Geografia e Estatística). 1990. Anuário Estatístico do Brasil. Rio de Janeiro: IBGE.

Lévi-Strauss, C. 1974. *Tristes Tropiques.* New York: Atheneum.

Mahar, D. 1989. *Government Policies and Deforestation in Brazil's Amazon Region.* Washington, DC: World Bank.

Meireles, D. M. 1984. Populações Indígenas e a Ocupação Histórica de Rondônia. Unpublished manuscript, Cuaibá, Depart. de História, Universidade Federal de Mato Grosso.

Menéndez, M. 1981/1982. Uma contribuição para a etnohistória da área Tapajós-Madeira. *Revista do Museu Paulista*, n.s., 28:289–388.

Menéndez, M. 1984/1985. Contribuição ao estudo das relações tribais na área Tapajós-Madeira. *Revista de Antropologia* 27/28:271–86.

Monteiro, C. A., M. H. A. Benício, and N. C. Gouveia. 1992. Saúde e nutrição das crianças brasileiras no final da década de 80. In *Perfil Estatístico de Crianças e Mães no Brasil: Aspetos de Saúde e Nutrição no Brasil, 1989,* 19–42. Rio de Janeiro: IBGE/UNICEF/INAN.

Mueller, C. 1980. Frontier Based Agricultural Expansion: The Case of Rondônia. In *Land, People and Planning in Contemporary Amazonia,* ed. F. Barbira-Scazzocchio, 141–53. Cambridge: University of Cambridge, Centre of Latin American Studies.

Neel, J. V. 1970. Lessons from a "Primitive" People. *Science* 170:815–22.

Neel, J. V. 1994. *Physician to the Gene Pool: Genetic Lessons and Other Stories.* New York: John Wiley and Sons.

Nimuendajú, C. 1948. The Cawahib, Parintintin and Their Neighbors. In *Handbook of South American Indians,* ed. J. Steward, vol. 3, 283–97. Washington, DC: Government Printing Office.

Posey, D. A. 1994. Environmental and Social Implications of Pre- and Postcontact Situations of Brazilian Indians: The Kayapó and a New Amazonian Synthesis. In *Amazonian Indians from Prehistory to the Present,* ed. A. C. Roosevelt, 271–86. Tucson: University of Arizona Press.

Ribeiro, D. 1956. Convívio e contaminação. Efeitos dissociativos da depopulação provocada por epidemias em grupos indígenas. *Sociologia* 18:3–50.

Rippon, J. W. 1982. *Medical Mycology: The Pathogenic Fungi and the Pathogenic Actinomycetes.* Philadelphia: W. B. Saunders.

Rondon, C. M. S. 1946. Indios do Brasil: Centro, Noroeste e Sul de Mato Grosso, vol 1. Rio de Janeiro: Conselho Nacional de Proteção aos Indios.

Roosevelt, A. C., ed. 1994a. *Amazonian Indians from Prehistory to the Present.* Tucson: University of Arizona Press.

Roosevelt, A. C. 1994b. Amazonian Anthropology: Strategy for a New Synthesis. In *Amazonian Indians from Prehistory to the Present,* ed. A. C. Roosevelt, 1–29. Tucson: University of Arizona Press.

Salzano, F. M., and S. Callegari-Jacques. 1988. *South American Indians: A Case Study in Evolution.* Oxford: Clarendon Press.

Santos, R. V. 1991. Coping with Change in Native Amazonia: A Bioanthropological Study of the Gavião, Suruí, and Zoró, Tupí-Mondé Speaking Societies from Brazil. Ph.D. diss., Indiana University, Bloomington.

Santos, R.V. 1993. Crescimento físico e estado nutricional de populações indígenas brasileiras. *Cadernos de Saúde Pública* 9 (sup. 1): 46–57.

Santos, R. V., and C. E. A. Coimbra Jr. 1991. Socioeconomic Transition and the Physical Growth of Tupí-Mondé Amerindian Children of the Aripuanã Park, Brazilian Amazon. *Human Biology* 63:795–820.

Santos, R. V., and C. E. A. Coimbra Jr. 1996. Socioeconomic Differentiation and Body Morphology in the Suruí Indians from the Brazilian Amazonia. *Current Anthropology* 37:851–56.

Santos, R. V., A. C. Linhares, and C. E. A. Coimbra Jr. 1991. Estudos epidemiológicos entre grupos indígenas de Rondônia. IV. Inquérito sorológico para rotavirus entre os Suruí e Karitiána. *Revista de Saúde Pública* 25:230–32.

Sarnat, B. G., and I. Schour. 1941. Enamel Hypoplasia (Chronologic Enamel

Aplasia) in Relation to Systemic Disease: A Chronologic, Morphologic and Etiologic Classification. *Journal of the American Dental Association* 28:1989–2000.

Sawyer, D. R. 1992. Malaria and the Environment. Working Paper series, no. 13. Brasília: Instituto Sociedade, População e Natureza.

Singer, M. 1992. Farewell to Adaptationism: Unnatural Selection and the Politics of Biology. *Medical Anthropology Quarterly* 10:496–515.

Swedlund, A. C., and G. J. Armelagos. 1990. Introduction. In *Disease in Populations in Transition: Anthropological and Epidemiological Perspectives,* ed. A. C. Swedlund and G. J. Armelagos, 1–15. New York: Bergin and Garvey.

Weinstein, B. 1983. *The Amazon Rubber Boom.* Stanford: Stanford University Press.

Whitehead, N. L. 1994. The Ancient Amerindian Polities of the Amazon, the Orinoco, and the Atlantic Coast: A Preliminary Analysis of Their Passage from Antiquity to Extinction. In *Amazonian Indians from Prehistory to the Present,* ed. A. C. Roosevelt, 33–53. Tucson: University of Arizona Press.

Wirsing, R. 1985. The Health of Traditional Societies and the Effects of Acculturation. *Current Anthropology* 26:303–22.

Chapter 12

The Political Ecology of Population Increase and Malnutrition in Southern Honduras

Billie R. DeWalt

During the last two decades, Kathleen DeWalt, a variety of collaborators, and I have engaged in four major projects that have investigated the links between agricultural production and food consumption and nutrition. In addition to the topical interest of our research, there are several research strategies and themes that we have followed in our work.

First, our research has had a *policy emphasis.* That is, we have tried to focus our studies on issues and debates concerning appropriate and effective food and agricultural policies. Our work has been done in conjunction with government agencies, nongovernmental organizations, and/or bilateral or multilateral aid organizations that have had improvement of food and agricultural systems as their goal.

Second, we have attempted to utilize a *political ecology approach;* that is, blending political-economic and human ecological perspectives in the research process. Political-economic analyses have traditionally emphasized the tension between the state and the market, or the interaction of the pursuit of wealth and the pursuit of power as a means of organizing human society (e.g., Gilpin 1987, 11). The ecological effects of these processes have been of little concern (Redclift 1984, 1987). Human ecological analysis adds the dimension of focusing attention on demographic trends, environmental concerns, and issues related to human health and nutrition. A political ecology approach tries to combine the strengths of the two approaches to determine the dynamic interaction and potential contradictions among social, political, and economic processes; human health, nutrition, and demography; and the use and abuse of natural resources (see also Stonich 1993; Stonich and DeWalt 1996).

Finally, we have emphasized *microlevel/macrolevel linkages*. It is apparent that if we are considering political ecological processes, we have to pay attention to long-term historical trends, as well as to the interactions between local, regional, national, and international phenomena. There are thus three dimensions of microlevel and macrolevel linkages that must be contemplated (see DeWalt and Pelto 1985). The spatial dimension involves the size and "geographic" location of units. The time dimension involves attempting to sort out processes best seen in the short term from those that are better detected through diachronic analyses. The causal dimension involves determining proximate, functional, historical, and ultimate processes (Daly and Wilson 1983).

The following case study of southern Honduras will illustrate the use of these perspectives and themes. I will then close with conclusions about how these can be used to construct one variant of a biocultural synthesis within anthropology.

Honduras and Southern Honduras

Honduras is an especially important country in which to examine linkages between agricultural production and food consumption and nutrition. The country is one in which 60 percent of the population is directly involved in agriculture and where agriculture accounted for 83 percent of the value of merchandise exports in 1987. Honduras is the second poorest country in the Western Hemisphere, population growth averaged 3.4 percent per year during the 1980s, and food production per capita has declined substantially (World Bank 1992, 224, 268). The nation is characterized by extreme inequality of wealth,[1] and national nutrition surveys have estimated that 70 percent of children suffer from undernutrition (see SAPLAN 1981).

The south of Honduras is located in tropical dry and subtropical moist forest zones. The part of the south that lies adjacent to the Gulf of Fonseca is covered by a band of mangrove and marsh grass. Beyond the mangrove forests lies one of the few extensive plains on the Pacific coast of Central America. This savanna gives way to steep foothills that quickly become the jagged mountain ranges that form a broad base to the northeast and comprise much of the region (approximately 62 percent). Although these volcanic mountains rarely reach altitudes of more than 1,600 meters, they are exceedingly rugged and form myriad, isolated valleys. Thus, the whole region is characterized by sheer slopes, erratic precipitation patterns, and erosive soils. As a result, agriculture is very precarious and the area is exceedingly vulnerable to environmental degradation (USAID 1982; Stonich 1986).

Research in southern Honduras began in 1981 as part of the International Sorghum and Millet Collaborative Research Program (INTSORMIL) and, under other auspices, has continued to the present (see B. DeWalt and K. DeWalt 1982; Stonich 1991, 1993; DeWalt, Stonich, and Hamilton 1993; Stonich and DeWalt 1996; DeWalt, Vergne, and Hardin 1996). INTSORMIL is one of a series of long-term projects of the Agency for International Development to involve U.S. agricultural universities in collaborative research with institutions in developing countries in order to improve the production, marketing, and use of important food commodities.[2] Sorghum and millet were chosen for emphasis because they are grown as food crops in some of the poorest countries in the world. Anthropologists and sociologists from the University of Kentucky carried out most of the socioeconomic research within the INTSORMIL project; the majority of the project's funds have been spent on agronomic, plant breeding, entomological, and other agricultural research (see Reeves, DeWalt, and DeWalt 1987; B. DeWalt 1989).

Although sorghum and millet are grown for food primarily in Africa and Asia, farmers in drought-prone areas of Central America and Haiti also grow sorghum as a food crop.[3] In order to contribute to the agricultural research in Central America, we decided to study the food and agricultural systems of several communities on the drought-prone Pacific coast of Honduras. Our local-level research focused on three agrarian reform communities located on the narrow coastal plain and on six communities located in two ecological zones in the highlands of southern Honduras. In addition, our work also included a regional historical emphasis.

A Political Economy of the South

To understand the factors affecting people and communities, it is essential to understand the political economy of the region. Southern Honduras experienced a substantial expansion of commercial agriculture in the years immediately following World War II. At that time, the Honduran state became an active agent of development, creating a variety of state institutions and agencies to expand government services, modernize the country's financial system, and undertake infrastructural projects.

The period of intensified public sector investments between 1945 and

1975 coincided with temporary high world market prices for primary commodities like cotton, coffee, and cattle. With the infrastructural development, landowners and investors found it profitable to expand production
for the global market.

The Cotton Boom.   It was cotton cultivation that first transformed traditional social patterns of production in southern Honduras (Stares 1972,
35; White 1977; Durham 1979, 119; Boyer 1983, 91). In the late 1940s and
1950s, people from El Salvador began commercial cultivation of cotton in
Honduras.[4]

The major social effect of the cotton boom was to increase inequalities
in access to land. Large landowners revoked peasant tenancy or sharecropping rights, raised rental rates exorbitantly, and evicted peasants
forcibly from national land or from land of undetermined tenure (Durham
1979; Boyer 1983, 94). Increased cotton cultivation thus displaced many
poor farmers from the most suitable agricultural lands in the south. The
long staple cotton grown in the region, however, provided a substantial
number of seasonal jobs during the harvest season because it was picked
by hand.

Commercial production of cotton is dependent on the heavy use of
chemical inputs (especially insecticides and fertilizers). The indiscriminate
use of pesticides in the cotton growing regions remains one of the most
pervasive environmental contamination and human health problems in
Honduras and throughout Central America. The land and water contamination from pesticides, as well as high levels of pesticide residues in food
supplies, have had substantial effects on human health (USAID 1982;
Williams 1986; Leonard 1987). In addition, the increasing costs of pesticides, along with wildly fluctuating prices for cotton on the world market,
led many commercial farmers to search for alternative crops.

The Cattle Boom.   The expansion of the cattle industry has probably had
the most extensive and devastating environmental and social impacts on
the region (DeWalt 1985). Between 1960 and 1983, 57 percent of the total
loan funds allocated by the World Bank for agriculture and rural development in Central America supported the production of beef for export.
During that same period, Honduras obtained 51 percent of the total
World Bank funds disbursed in Central America—of which 34 percent
were for livestock projects (calculated from table 4–1 in Jarvis 1986, 124).

These programs were all channeled into the region through the large landowners, merchants, and industrialists who made up the elites of the countries (DeWalt 1985; Stonich and DeWalt 1989). In a context of declining agricultural commodity prices, high labor costs, unreliable rainfall, and international and national support for livestock, landowners reallocated their land from cotton and/or grain cultivation to pasture for cattle. Cattle appealed to landowners in Honduras because it could be produced with very little labor. With just two or three hired hands and extensive pasture it is possible to manage a herd of several hundred cattle. In Honduras, land reform programs ironically also encouraged the expansion of pasture for livestock. Landowners who feared expropriation of unutilized fallow and forest land fenced it and planted pasture as a way of establishing use of the land without substantially increasing labor inputs (DeWalt and DeWalt 1982, 69; Jarvis 1986, 157).

The expansion of pasture caused extensive changes in land use patterns in Honduras and the other Central American countries during the 1960s and 1970s. Expansion took place not only in the lowlands and foothills where cattle raising traditionally occurred, but also in the highlands where many of the wealthier peasant farmers also began investing in cattle production (Durham 1979; Boyer 1983; DeWalt 1985; Stonich 1986). Increased livestock production in the lowlands and the highlands also accelerated the expulsion of peasants from national and private lands (White 1977, 126–56; Stonich 1986, 139–43). Between 1952 and 1974, pasture in the southern region increased from 41.9 percent of the land to 61.1 percent. Precipitous declines occurred in both fallow land and the amount of land in forest.

These same trends occurred throughout the country. Many of the best lands in the country are used for pasture. The Central Bank estimated in August 1988 that 48 percent of the valley lands in Honduras—covering 31 principal valleys—is in pasture. Of this, 22 percent is located in the southern part of the country (USAID 1990, 10). Deforestation to plant pasture means that Honduras is losing its soils at the rate of 10,000 hectares per year and it is estimated that if current trends continue, "the forest resource will be exhausted in a generation" (USAID 1990, 3).

Melons and Shrimp. In the late 1980s, capitalist investors in southern Honduras began investing in two new nontraditional export crops—cantaloupe and shrimp. During the 1980s, cantaloupe production expanded at a rate of 23 percent per year and shrimp production at a rate of 22 percent (USAID Honduras 1990, 2). Shrimp aquaculture has catapulted shrimp to third position in terms of Honduran exports (behind bananas and coffee). The Central Bank of Honduras reported that in 1992 shrimp farms in the south sold over 4 million kilos of shrimp worth $40.2 million. Approximately 11,900 people were directly employed by the 25 farms, six shrimp packing plants, and six ice-making operations (see DeWalt, Vergne, and Hardin 1996). As with the earlier booms in cotton and cattle, these earnings have been offset by both environmental and social costs.

On the positive side, cantaloupe production provides a substantial number of jobs in production and in packing for export. Accompanying the boom in production, however, have been escalating levels of soil degradation, aphid-borne viruses, and insect pests like leaf miners and white fly. Even with two to three applications *per week* of pesticides, crop losses in 1989–90 were 56 percent of harvest projections (Meckenstock et al. 1991, 5). Runoff of pesticides poses a threat to community water supplies in the region as well as to the estuaries in the Gulf of Fonseca where shrimp farming has become big business.

Despite beginning only in the early 1980s, by 1993 a total of 11,515 hectares were in shrimp farms. The expanding shrimp farms have already displaced over 4,300 hectares that were once covered by some type of mangrove. Although this level of environmental destruction is already substantial, it pales in comparison with what could occur. The Honduran government has already granted an estimated 31,000 hectares of concessions for possible shrimp farm development, of which only about a third has been developed. A significant portion of the remaining concessions are located in areas with higher vegetation cover. This means that the amount of mangrove that could be destroyed by shrimp farm construction, if the remaining concessions are developed, will be significantly higher than what has taken place thus far (DeWalt, Vergne, and Hardin 1996). There may be a repetition in Honduras of the extensive mangrove destruction that occurred along the coast of Ecuador in connection with development of shrimp farming in that country (LACR 1989). There are indications that habitat destruction has exacerbated the problem of acquiring naturally occurring postlarval and juvenile shrimp that are used to stock the ponds, thereby raising costs and reducing profits (Leonard 1987, 144).

Parallels in the social processes associated with the recent boom in shrimp mariculture and the earlier expansions of export commodities (cotton, sugar, and livestock) in the region are striking. Past "enclosure movements" in which small farmers were removed from relatively good agricultural land often by force and with the compliance of local authorities are being repeated on the intertidal lands. Intertidal land once open to public use for fishing, shellfish collecting, salt production, and the cutting of firewood and tanbark is now being converted to private use (see DeWalt, Vergne, and Hardin 1996). The situation was neatly summarized by a poor farmer and artisanal fisherman who told us in 1988, "First we were evicted from our land . . . now they are throwing us out of the sea. Where will we go?"[5]

A Micro/Macrolevel Perspective on Land Access

During the last forty years, the political-economic conditions restructuring agriculture in southern Honduras have led to substantial inequalities in access to land. These trends have led to the region mirroring the inequalities in land access in the nation as a whole. Table 1 compares the distribution of land in the municipality of Pespire (the county in which the highland communities we studied were located), in southern Honduras, and in the country as a whole.[6] Landholding patterns are remarkably consistent across local, regional, and national levels. Approximately two-thirds of producers have access to less than 5 hectares of land; this multitude share only 9 to 10 percent of the total land area. In contrast, the 10 to 12 percent of the population with access to over 50 hectares control more than 50 percent of the land area. These commercial producers are those who have invested in cattle, melons, and other export commodities.

The increased concentration of land has impoverished both the landscape and an increasing percentage of the population.[7] The general trend has been toward resource oligopoly, patterns of exploitation and production that jeopardize future systemic sustainability in exchange for quick profits, wanton destruction of natural resources, and underemployment. The question remains, what are the small producers, the majority of the population, doing as large commercial concerns expand?

Adaptive Strategies in Smallholder Agriculture

Except for a few communities that benefited from the relatively modest land reform carried out in Honduras in the 1970s, most small producers in the south are concentrated on the steep mountain slopes that are marginal for agriculture. Although large landholdings are relatively rare in these communities (the mean size of landholdings is less than 6 hectares), there is still considerable inequality in access to land (see table 2). A large percentage of people in communities studied by us and other anthropologists (Durham 1979; Boyer 1983) are landless or have access to less than one hectare of land. The result is that many people depend on renting, borrowing, or sharecropping relatively small amounts of land.[8]

In these communities, agriculture is based on a system of shifting cultivation[9] that involves interplanting maize and sorghum (see DeWalt and DeWalt 1982 or DeWalt 1985 for a description of this system). In the past, two or three years of cultivation were followed by a period of fallow, during which the soil was allowed to recover its fertility. Now, however, an increasing proportion of the land is being converted to pasture for livestock.

TABLE 1. Comparison of Inequality of Landholdings in Pespire, in Southern Honduras, and in Honduras

Size of Holdings (hectares)	Percentage of Farms			Percentage of Area		
	Pespire	South[a]	Honduras	Pespire	South	Honduras
<5	63.4	68.4	63.9	10.1	10.3	9.1
5–9.9	15.9	13.6	14.5	9.9	8.1	7.7
10–19.9	9.8	8.8	9.8	12.2	10.4	10.2
20–49	7.4	6.0	7.8	19.6	14.8	17.5
50–99	2.2	1.7	2.3	12.8	9.5	11.5
>100	1.3	1.6	1.7	35.3	46.8	44.0
Total	1,714 farms	25,412 farms	195,341 farms	19,383 ha.	304,462 ha.	2,629,859 ha.

[a]The south includes the two provinces of Choluteca and Valle.

TABLE 2. Comparison of Land Tenure Characteristics in the Highland Communities Studied

	Research Communities[a]				
	1	2	3	4	5
Mean size of holdings (hectares)	2.3	3.7	5.9	4.6	3.1
Maximum size of holdings	14	69	39	47	214
% of landowners in community	63	27	46	72	—
% with holdings less than 1 hectare	10	24	49	29	40
% that purchased land	41	19	44	31	—

[a]Community 1 = San Antonio (Stonich 1986)
  Community 2 = Esquimay (Stonich 1986)
  Community 3 = Cacautare/El Naranjito (DeWalt and DeWalt 1982)
  Community 4 = Mean of villages in Langue (Durham 1979)
  Community 5 = Mean of 7 communities (Boyer 1983)

The conversion of land to pasture involves decisions by both the landowners and the land-poor; the conjunction of their decisions has created a short-term symbiotic relationship. Poor people in Cacautare, for example, had relatively little difficulty renting land from larger landowners (see DeWalt 1985). The rental cost of one *manzana* (.69 hectares) in 1981 was only about eight dollars per year and an agreement by the renter to leave the crop residue in the field for cattle to eat. Landowners are willing to rent their land cheaply because the most expensive and labor-intensive aspect of hillside agriculture is clearing secondary-growth forest. Rather than paying laborers to cut brush and trees, landowners rent out their land in forest for a year or two. Part of the rental agreement is that pasture grasses will be sown in the field between rows of subsistence crops so that the landowner will be left with a new pasture. We have estimated that this arrangement saves the landowner at least one hundred dollars in labor costs for each hectare of new pasture (see B. DeWalt and K. DeWalt 1982). The result is that the percentage of land in pasture in the south of Honduras expanded by about 50 percent in only twenty years, at the expense of forest and fallow land.

Landowners are interested in growing pasture to feed livestock because the potential returns are much greater than they are in growing basic grains or export crops (DeWalt 1985, 177–8; Parsons 1976, 126). Several of the relatively well-off smallholders with whom we spoke in Cacautare in 1982 reported that they had little interest in planting sorghum and maize because market prices were too low, labor costs had climbed, laborers no longer worked as hard as they did in the past, and the weather, insects, and other natural forces made grain harvests too unpredictable. Our calculations indicate that their average profit from selling one steer exceeded the total profit from several manzanas of grain.

In spite of the short-term symbiotic relationship between larger landowners and those who have to rent land, for the land-poor the expansion of pasture implies a serious problem in the long term. Their dilemma was succinctly expressed by one of our informants who said:

Right now we have land available to rent, but each year you can see the forested land disappearing. In a few years, it will all be pasture and there will be no land available to rent. How are we to produce for our families then? We see what is happening, but we have no choice because our families have to eat now.

During this period of commercialization in which wealthy farmers and large corporations have displaced the poor from productive agricultural lands (and more recently from even the mangrove swamps), and during which those with a little bit of land in the highlands have used the landless and land-poor to convert land to pastures, the population of the region has continued to increase rapidly. Population density increased from 29.8 persons per square kilometer in 1950 to 63.9 in 1985 (Stonich 1986, 145).

The concentration of landholdings in southern Honduras combined with continuing population increase is leading to a more intensive use of land resources, especially by small landholders. Farmers in Cacautare, for example, reported that fields *should* be cultivated for only 3 years in a row (mean = 2.93; range 1 to 5 years) and *should* lie fallow for at least 6 years (mean = 6.22; range 1 to 15 years). There is a direct relationship between the size of landholdings and the amount of time fields lie fallow (Stonich 1986; Stonich 1993; Durham 1979). Table 3 shows this relationship for the highland villages around Esquimay. Farmers with over 20 hectares allow their land to lie in fallow for 5 to 6 years. Those with less land resume cultivation of their land after only 2 or 3 years of fallow (Durham 1979, 144–45). Boyer (1983) reports that in other communities in the south, a fallow period is no longer part of the agricultural system.

Boserup (1965) and others (see Pingali, Bigot, and Binswanger 1987)

TABLE 3.   Agricultural Practices by Land-Tenure and Farm Size in Southern Highland Villages, 1983

Type of Tenancy	N	Percent of Land in Food Crops[a]	Percentage of Land in Pasture	Mean Number of Cattle Owned (range)	Length of Fallow (years)
Renters[b]	74	95	—	0.17 (0–4)	2.7
Owners					
<1 ha[c]	23	80	—	0.22 (0–3)	2.7
1–5 ha	87	51	4	0.22 (0–3)	3.2
5–20 ha	15	23	21	2.5 (0–13)	3.8
20–50 ha	5	6	48	8.0 (7–9)	5.0
>50 ha	1	6	20[d]	50.0 (50)	6.0

Source: Stonich 1989, 287
[a]Maize, sorghum, and beans
[b]Mean area of rented land, 1.4 ha.
[c]51 percent of owners also rent land.
[d]Largest landowner rents additional grazing land in lowlands.

have argued that increased population leads to the more intensive utilization of land through adoption of practices to add fertilizers and conserve soil (see DeWalt and Stonich 1992). The problem, however, is that although farmers in the south are utilizing the land more frequently, they are not *intensifying* their operations.

Contained in table 4 are data on a variety of technologies that can be used in southern Honduras to improve the productivity and sustainability of land use. These are techniques that are being advocated and promoted by development projects in southern Honduras. What is striking in these data is that those individuals with the smallest amounts of land are *least likely* to engage in land-conserving practices. The few farmers who are intensifying their operations are those who own relatively larger tracts of land. Without time to recover fertility, soil fertility is being depleted, yields are declining and soil erosion is a substantial problem. The deforestation of the hillsides has led to frequent landslides when torrential rains hit the region, exacerbating problems of soil erosion.

TABLE 4. Intensification of Agriculture in Two Highland Communities of Southern Honduras (percentages using various practices)[a]

| Practice/Technique | Total Access to Land (Rented, Owned, Sharecropped) | | | | |
	<1 ha. (n = 23)	1–5 ha. (n = 87)	5–20 ha. (n = 15)	>20 ha. (n = 3)	Total (n = 128)
Trees left in field before planting	13	44	100	100	46
Do not burn fields	39	37	80	67	43
Use check dams	9	40	87	67	41
Sow across slopes	17	46	20	67	38
>50 percent of field crops sown on flat land	0	11	93	100	20
Employ terraces	0	2	87	33	13
Utilize live barriers	0	1	27	100	6
Utilize ditches	0	5	13	0	5
Utilize manure	0	0	27	67	5
Utilize trash barriers	0	2	20	0	4
Mean number of conservation practices employed	.8	1.7	6.3	6.0	2.2
Percent of land in each tenure category[b]	1	25	49	24	100

Source: Stonich 1993

[a]Computed from household survey data

[b]Computed from analysis of digitized cadastral maps of research areas

Nutritional and Demographic Consequences
of These Strategies

The effects of these political-economic processes on the biological populations of these communities are quite profound. Regional level data indicate that 41 percent of all southern families did not meet minimum subsistence levels (SAPLAN 1981). Average nutritional levels were lower in the
late 1980s than in 1970 and the average energy deficit in rural areas was
approximately 20 percent (USAID 1989a). Families living in "semi-urban
communities" consumed even fewer calories than rural families (Stonich
1986, 152–4).

Our work in nine communities showed that 65 percent of children
under five years of age were less than 95 percent of standard height for age
(that is, stunted); 14 percent of children were under 90 percent of standard
weight for their height (wasted).[10] Figures are similar for the highland and
lowland samples. These data indicate that two-thirds of children in these
communities experienced undernutrition at some time in their first five
years of life, but that acute undernutrition, as measured by low weight for
current height, is less of a problem at any one time. The children of tenant
farmers and households headed by single women were at greater nutritional risk than the children of landowners (see K. DeWalt and B. DeWalt
1987).

An analysis of dietary adequacy for all families showed that, on the
average, families met 110 percent of their energy needs and 200 percent of
their protein needs.[11] This masks considerable variation because 49 percent of the families did not meet their estimated energy requirement. Only
1 percent of families failed to meet their need for protein indicating that
calories are a much more significant limitation than protein. In a region in
which cattle production is so pervasive, however, only 3 percent of all the
protein consumed by these villagers comes from meat (DeWalt and
DeWalt 1987, 39).

Health problems abound in these communities. Infant mortality in the
nine communities we surveyed averaged 99/1,000, well above the national
rate of 64/1,000 (World Bank 1992, 272). Furthermore, an average of 16
percent of all children born in the nine communities did not survive
beyond the age of five.

Despite the health and nutritional problems in the region, the natality
rate in southern Honduras is higher than the national average. This is dramatically manifested in the communities we studied. Our surveys in nine

communities recorded an average of 6.3 live births per woman, and many women had yet to complete their families. In spite of a dwindling resource base and severe nutritional and health problems, families in southern Honduras continue to have high fertility rates. The explanation for this, I believe, relates to the adaptive strategies of people attempting to cope with bleak natural and social environmental circumstances.

Despite the very high natality rates, population growth rates in southern Honduras have been slower than in the rest of the nation. Partially this results from the high infant mortality rate. Far more important in reducing the population growth rate, however, has been regional outmigration. When families cannot survive on the land, they seek opportunities elsewhere (Durham 1979). Many people recognize that their future and that of their families lies in leaving the south and migrating to other areas of the country. Thus, the problems plaguing the south are being exported to other regions of Honduras.

Since 1974, outmigration from the southern region has averaged 1.3 percent annually. Approximately half as many people leave the region permanently every year as are added to the population by both its high birth rate and in-migration. To give some sense of this, in villages around Esquimay, 39 percent of all children over 13 years of age from households studied were no longer living in the community. In terms of temporary migration, 70 percent of male household heads and 20 percent of female household heads in Cacautare had migrated at least once to work outside the community.

Many of these permanent or temporary migrants end up in the cities of Honduras. The urban population growth rate in Honduras was 5.8 percent between 1974 and 1980, and 5.4 percent between 1980 and 1987, a rate much higher than the population growth rate of about 3.5 percent (USAID 1989a). Migrants from environmentally degraded areas in the south are also settling in Olancho and the vast, relatively unpopulated areas of the Mosquitia in northeastern Honduras. The colonization of tropical forest areas has even extended into the Rio Platano Biosphere Reserve.[12] Approximately 6,500 colonists from degraded land in southern and western Honduras are now occupying lands in this reserve and 9,000 more colonists occupied the area immediately outside the reserve (Poole 1989). Thus, the destruction of the dry tropical forest and the mangroves in the south is now having direct effects on deforestation of the humid tropical forest in other regions of Honduras.

Because the poor have increasingly come to depend on the remittances from those members of their family who engage in temporary or permanent migration, they are unwilling to invest time and resources in attempting to intensify their agricultural operations in the south. Ultimately, this is what accounts for their lack of interest in adopting the techniques listed in table 4.

Evolution, Adaptation, and Political Economy

The political ecology perspective complements the use of evolutionary theory and the concept of adaptation as a means to understand the processes occurring in southern Honduras and in development more generally (see DeWalt 1991). In the context of the data presented, in this final section I would like to outline my thoughts concerning how cultural and biological anthropology should use these two perspectives to better understand human behavior.

Among the basic propositions of evolutionary theory, three are quite important in the present context. Evolutionary theory posits that *variation* is a ubiquitous feature of all living things. *Selection* acts on these variations and is the force that gives rise to and alters the categories of living things. The interaction between variation and selection results in adaptation and extinction; *adaptation* is always relative to particular organisms and specific environments and is never permanent (see Greenwood 1984, 66).[13]

It is important for us to avoid the simplistic notion that evolution is a process of natural selection of variant traits, in which human beings are passive beneficiaries or victims (Smith and Reeves 1989, 10). Instead, humans "engage and transform the environment through decisions and actions; they actively and selectively create and organize their niches, and in the process affect those of other species, communities and individuals" (Wiley 1992, 220). There are three important implications of this active human modification of their environs. One is that the physical environment is not a fixed entity but instead is constructed by social processes; the natural and social environment are indistinguishable. Second is that human decisions have substantial effects on other humans as well as the constructed environment that is continually being modified and reshaped by those decisions. Third is that the constructed environment differentially affects individuals, more severely constraining some, providing greater opportunities and advantages for others, and is constantly being manipulated and modified by the actions of those individuals. The activities of the organism, in this case humans, "sets the stage for its own selection"

(Levins and Lewontin 1985, 58). The selective forces at work also substantially involve human agency in the form of social, political, economic, and cultural factors.

The way in which I have tried to tap into the variability of human activities is by looking at adaptive strategies. I have used the ideas of Bennett for whom adaptive strategies are "the patterns formed by the many separate adjustments that people devise in order to obtain and use resources and to solve the immediate problems confronting them" (1969, 14). By understanding the constraints on their decisions and by knowing their goals, it is possible to appreciate the reasons for *variability* within and among communities with regard to why people utilize the adaptive strategies they do (see DeWalt 1979).

The adaptive strategies of people in southern Honduras are quite clearly constrained by the political-economic circumstances within which they live. Decisions of poor people to (1) abandon the fallow periods that were an essential part of the agricultural system; (2) rent land from larger landholders and convert this land to pasture; (3) have large numbers of children; and/or (4) migrate to cities or other regions of the country are quite understandable. Renting land or more intensively using the small amounts of land they control are short-term necessities for producing enough food on which to live. Having large numbers of children is a means of trying to insure longer-term survival; some children can migrate to cities or colonize other areas of the country and perhaps provide some resources to their parents and siblings. Temporary or permanent migration are means to augment the resources from which a living can be derived.

At the same time, for rational reasons these poorer members of the population are less interested in investing time and resources into intensifying their agricultural operations. They have determined that, with the small amounts of land they have available, their long-range futures depend on gaining access to resources in other regions or in the cities. Thus, development efforts in the region that are attempting to arrest the processes of resource degradation are unlikely to be successful with the poorest farmers.

As we have seen, those individuals in the highlands who do have access to land resources will be most successful, given current economic policies, by investing their time and resources in cattle and pastures. While many of these individuals are engaging in practices to try to conserve the soil and land resources, they are also contributing to deforestation in the region. Thus, although their adaptive strategies may be more successful in the long term if they are able to discover sustainable means of livestock raising, at least in the short term, their practices are also contributing to resource degradation.

The wealthy landowners and corporations who have large livestock operations, are producing melons or cotton, or are investing in shrimp production on the coastal plain and in the mangrove-lined estuaries, are also responsible for a considerable amount of resource degradation in the region. Their concern with achieving short-term profits means that they provide few opportunities for wage labor, engage in the abusive use of pesticides, and are engaged in *mining* the soil and water resources of the region. What is adaptive, at least in the short-term economic sense, for this small group creates substantial problems to which the majority of the population has to adapt as best they can, in many cases being forced into choices that cause further environmental destruction.

Thus, the main trends of the past four decades of "development" in southern Honduras have been to create adaptive strategies that threaten the long-term viability of the region. The main effects have been:

1. Increasing inequality in access to physical resources like land, swamps, and water
2. A decline in wage labor opportunities for those displaced from access to the physical resources
3. Resource destruction—of the tropical dry forest, of mangroves, pesticide contamination, etc.—on a grand scale by commercial producers
4. Resource destruction—because of intensification of agriculture on steep slopes—on a grand scale by land-poor and landless agriculturalists
5. An increase in the "diseases of poverty"—hunger, malnutrition, infant mortality, and very high birth rates—among the poorest segments of the population

The political-ecological perspective has great utility in analyzing what is occurring in southern Honduras. This research demonstrates how the local-level biological processes of nutrition, demography, and resource destruction must be articulated with and contextualized within political-economic processes of the region and the nation. It is important to view the adaptive strategies of people in southern Honduras as attempts to cope with the immediate problems with which they have to deal and to understand these adaptive strategies in longer term perspective. We need to understand the historical political-economic forces that have created the current conditions within which decisions—of the poor, of small farmers, and of wealthy landowners and transnational corporations—are being made.

In conclusion, the development efforts of the World Bank, USAID, and the Honduran government that have promoted commercialization and export agriculture have been prejudicial to the majority of the population of the southern region. Current development projects that are attempting to arrest the resource destruction occurring in the region are unlikely to address the root causes of this destruction and are thus likely to fail. Although the future evolution of this system cannot be predicted with certainty, it is apparent that without a change in the underlying political economy of the region and the nation, the natural resource base will continue to deteriorate as will the quality of life of a substantial part of the population.

NOTES

1. The top 20 percent of the population held 68 percent of the wealth in the 1970s. The comparable figure for the top 20 percent in Mexico was 58 percent and, for Argentina, it was 50 percent (Sheahan 1987).

2. In addition to sorghum and millet, other projects focus on such commodities as peanuts, beans and cowpeas, and small ruminants. Other collaborative efforts focus on tropical soils, pond dynamics, integrated pest management, and sustainable agriculture and natural resource management. McCorkle (1989) is a compilation of the social science work done as part of these collaborative research programs.

3. Sorghum is widely grown in the United States, Mexico, Argentina, and other Western Hemisphere countries. In these countries, it is used only as a feed crop for livestock (see Barkin, Batt, and DeWalt 1990).

4. In 1969, the government of Honduras expelled several thousand Salvadoran immigrants, many of whom had lived in Honduras for over a generation. El Salvador retaliated by invading Honduras. This so-called Soccer War (because it occurred shortly after the soccer teams representing the countries competed in World Cup qualifying matches) was widely attributed to "population pressure"— the competition of poor Hondurans and Salvadorans for increasingly scarce arable land. Many analysts concluded that a Malthusian scenario was being played out in which the population had exceeded the carrying capacity of the land. Durham's classic analysis of this situation demonstrated that it was the use and distribution of land, rather than its carrying capacity, that resulted in the problems of food production and the inability of families to meet subsistence needs (1979).

5. Moreover, although development documents written in the mid-1980s stressed the importance of incorporating resource-poor households in the shrimp development process primarily through the formation and support of cooperatives, more recent reports conclude that only the larger, more intensive operations are profitable (USAID Honduras 1989b). These large operations generate very few employment opportunities, typically employing fewer than one person per hectare (González et al. 1987; cited in SECPLAN/DESFIL 1989, 179).

6. This inequality of land distribution is also found in the other Central American countries (see DeWalt and Bidegaray 1991, 24).

7. A recent report by agricultural scientists reported: "Since the 1950s, the agricultural economy of southern Honduras has been dominated by a series of boom and bust cycles of export commodities. Cattle, cotton and sugar have each reached their zenith only to dissipate in the face of declining productivity and adverse world markets. Much of this instability has been self-inflicted through degradation of the natural resource base which has reduced productivity and profitability. At present, non-traditional export crops like melon and shrimp are experiencing the great expectations and up-swing of this cycle; however, signs of limitations and stress on production are becoming apparent" (Meckenstock et al. 1991, 2).

8. For example, 54 percent of the sample in villages around Cacautare were renters, sharecroppers, or borrowers. The comparable figure for villages around Esquimay was 55 percent (Stonich 1986, 202). Durham reported that 39.4 percent of people in Langue were renters; he did not report any borrowing or sharecropping of land (1979, 144).

9. Although the type of cultivation that is practiced by small farmers in southern Honduras is usually described as slash-and-burn agriculture, the way that a field enters the cultivation cycle is more accurately described as a slash-and-mulch system. Here, the secondary forest growth is cut down, but rather than being burned it is left lying on the ground to serve as a mulch for the grain crops that are planted.

10. Estimates of nutritional status of households were based on anthropometric measurements of children 60 months of age and under. Length was measured in centimeters using an infantometer for children unable to stand unaided. Height was measured for children able to stand using a measuring board in which a metal meter tape had been imbedded. A sliding headboard was used to read the height. Weight was measured to the nearest 100 gms. using a spring-type scale for children under 10 kilograms. Children over 10 kgs were weighed using a dial face spring scale (both Salter scales). Children's weight for age, height for age, and weight for height were calculated as a percentage of standard using the World Health Organization's standards (WHO 1979).

11. Calculations were based on estimates of family food intake from 24-hour recalls of family meals and a food-use interview that focused on the week before the interview date. Amounts of energy and protein available to the household were calculated and expressed as a percentage of household needs. Protein and energy needs were calculated using WHO (1973) estimates of protein and energy requirements for individuals of the same age and sex as household members. These were summed for the household.

12. The Rio Platano Biosphere Reserve located within the region referred to as la Mosquitia was established in 1979 and became a world heritage site in 1980. It covers almost the entire watershed of the Rio Platano, approximately 525,000 hectares on the Caribbean coast of Honduras. At the time it was created there were approximately 4,450 inhabitants, mostly Miskito Indians and a few Pech and ladino villages within the boundaries. At that time the reserve was inaccessible by road. By 1990 there still were no conventional roads into the reserve, however, illegal access was facilitated by widespread logging and gold-mining roads. By then several hundred Nicaraguan Miskito Indians had settled within the reserve.

13. Evolutionary theory provides a macro framework within which to view human processes. It does not necessarily provide *explanations* or predictions concerning the best possibilities for the future (see also Wiley 1992, 232). Indeed, many people would agree that even in the biological area evolutionary theory is primarily useful for post hoc explanation rather than prediction. Thus, we need to use other theories that can help us to better account for human behavior.

REFERENCES

Barkin, David, Rosemary L. Batt, and Billie R. DeWalt. 1990. *Food Crops vs. Feed Crops: Global Substitution of Grains in Production.* Boulder, CO: Lynne Rienner.

Barkin, David, and Billie R. DeWalt. 1988. Sorghum and the Mexican Food Crisis. *Latin American Research Review* 23:30–59.

Bennett, John. 1969. *Northern Plainsmen.* Chicago: Aldine.

Bennett, John. 1976. *The Ecological Transition: Cultural Anthropology and Human Adaptation.* New York: Pergamon Press.

Boserup, Ester. 1965. *The Conditions of Agricultural Growth.* Chicago: Aldine.

Boyer, Jefferson. 1983. *Agrarian Capitalism and Peasant Praxis in Southern Honduras.* Ann Arbor, MI: University Microfilms (Ph.D. diss.).

Daly, Martin, and Margo Wilson. 1983. *Sex, Evolution, and Behavior.* Boston: Willard Grant Press.

DeWalt, Billie R. 1979. *Modernization in a Mexican Ejido: A Study in Economic Adaptation.* New York and Cambridge: Cambridge University Press.

DeWalt, Billie R. 1985. Microcosmic and Macrocosmic Processes of Agrarian Change in Southern Honduras: The Cattle are Eating the Forest. In *Micro and Macro Levels of Analysis in Anthropology: Issues in Theory and Research,* ed. Billie R. DeWalt and Pertti J. Pelto, 165–86. Boulder, CO: Westview.

DeWalt, Billie R. 1989. Halfway There: Social Science in Agricultural Development and the Social Science of Agricultural Development. In *Social Sciences in International Agricultural Research: Lessons from the CRSPs,* ed. Constance McCorkle, 39–61. Boulder, CO: Lynne Rienner.

DeWalt, Billie R. 1991. Anthropology, Evolution, and Agricultural Development. In *Social Science Agricultural Agendas and Strategies,* ed. Glenn C. Johnson and James T. Bonnen, with Darrell Fienup, C. Leroy Quance, and Neill Schaller, 60–68. East Lansing: Michigan State University Press.

DeWalt, Billie, and Pedro Bidegaray. 1991. The Agrarian Bases of Conflict in Central America. In *Understanding the Central American Crisis: Sources of Conflict, U.S. Policy and Options for Peace*, ed. Kenneth Coleman and George Herring. Wilmington, DE: SR Books.

DeWalt, Billie R., and Kathleen M. DeWalt. 1982. *Cropping Systems in Pespire, Southern Honduras*. Farming Systems Research in Southern Honduras Report #1. Lexington: University of Kentucky Department of Anthropology.

DeWalt, Billie R., and Pertti J. Pelto, eds. 1985. *Micro and Macro Levels of Analysis in Anthropology: Issues in Theory and Research*. Boulder, CO: Westview.

DeWalt, Billie R., and Susan C. Stonich. 1992. Inequality, Population and Forest Destruction in Honduras. Paper presented in the IUSSP Seminar on Population and Deforestation in the Humid Tropics, Campinas, S.P. Brazil.

DeWalt, Billie R., Susan C. Stonich, and Sarah Hamilton. 1993. Honduras: Population, Inequality and Resource Destruction. In *Population and Land Use in Developing Countries*, ed. Carole L. Jolly and Barbara Boyle Torrey, 106–23. Washington, DC: National Academy Press.

DeWalt, Billie R., Jorge Uquillas, Kathleen M. DeWalt, William Leonard, and James Stansbury. 1990. *Dairy Based Production and Food Systems in Mejia and Salcedo*. Report # 1 on the Research, Extension and Education Project Baseline Surveys. Lexington, KY: Nutrition and Agriculture Cooperative Agreement and Fundación para Desarrollo Agropecuario.

DeWalt, Billie R., Philippe Vergne, and Mark Hardin. 1996. Shrimp Aquaculture Development and the Environment: People, Mangroves and Fisheries on the Gulf of Fonseca, Honduras. *World Development* 24 (7): 1193–1208.

DeWalt, Kathleen Musante. 1993. *Nutritional Strategies and Agricultural Change in a Mexican Community*. Ann Arbor, MI: UMI Research Press.

DeWalt, Kathleen M., and Billie R. DeWalt. 1987. Nutrition and Agricultural Change in Southern Honduras. *Food and Nutrition Bulletin* 9 (3): 36–45.

DGECH (Dirección General de Estadística y Censos). 1976. *Censo Nacional Agropecuario 1974*. Tegucigalpa, Honduras: Dirección General de Estadística y Censos.

Durham, William. 1979. *Scarcity and Survival in Central America: Ecological Origins of the Soccer War*. Stanford: Stanford University Press.

Gilpin, Robert. 1987. *The Political Economy of International Relations*. Princeton, NJ: Princeton University Press.

González, J. R., et al. 1987. *Situación de la Carcinocultura en la Costa Sur de Honduras*. Tegucigalpa, Honduras: RENARE (cited in SECPLAN/DESFIL 1989).

Greenwood, Davydd. 1984. *The Taming of Evolution: The Persistence of Nonevolutionary Views in the Study of Humans*. Ithaca, NY: Cornell University Press.

Jarvis, Lovell S. 1986. *Livestock Development in Latin America*. Washington, DC: World Bank.

LACR (Latin American Commodities Report) Shrimp / Ecuador. 1989. *Latin American Commodities Report*, CR-89–09 (Sept. 15): 8. London: Latin American Newsletters, Ltd.

Leonard, H. Jeffrey. 1987. *Natural Resources and Economic Development in Latin America*. New Brunswick, NJ: Transaction Books.

Leonard, William R., Kathleen M. DeWalt, Jorge E. Uquillas, and Billie R.

DeWalt. 1993. Ecological Correlates of Dietary Consumption and Nutritional Status in Highland and Coastal Ecuador. *Ecology of Food and Nutrition* 31:67–85.

Leonard, William R., Kathleen M. DeWalt, Jorge E. Uquillas, and Billie R. DeWalt. 1994. Diet and Nutritional Status Among Cassava Producing Agriculturalists of Coastal Ecuador. *Ecology of Food and Nutrition* 32:113–27.

Levins, Richard, and Richard Lewontin. 1985. *The Dialectical Biologist.* Cambridge, MA: Harvard University Press.

McCorkle, Constance, ed. 1989. *Social Sciences in International Agricultural Research: Lessons from the CRSPs.* Boulder, CO: Lynne Rienner.

Meckenstock, Dan, David Coddington, Juan Rosas, Harold van Es, Manjeet Chinman, and Manuel Murillo. 1991. Honduras Concept Paper: Towards a Sustainable Agriculture in Southern Honduras. Paper presented at the International Sorghum/Millet Collaborative Research Support Conference, July 8–12, Corpus Christi, TX.

Parsons, J. J. 1976. Forest to Pasture: Development or Destruction? *Revista de Biologia Tropical* 24 (Supp. 1): 121–38.

Pingali, Prabhu, Yves Bigot, and Hans Binswanger. 1987. *Agricultural Mechanization and the Evolution of Farming Systems in Sub-Saharan Africa.* Baltimore: Published for the World Bank, Johns Hopkins University Press.

Poole, Peter. 1989. Developing a Partnership of Indigenous Peoples, Conservationists, and Land Use Planners in Latin America. Latin America and Caribbean Technical Department Working Paper #WPS 245. Washington, DC: World Bank.

Redclift, Michael. 1984. *Development and Environmental Crisis.* New York: Methuen.

Redclift, Michael. 1987. *Sustainable Development: Exploring the Contradictions.* New York: Methuen.

Reeves, Edward C., Billie R. DeWalt, and Kathleen M. DeWalt. 1987. The International Sorghum/Millet Research Project. In *Anthropological Praxis: Translating Knowledge into Action,* ed. Robert M. Wulff and Shirley J. Fiske, 72–83. Boulder, CO: Westview Press.

SAPLAN (Sistema de Análisis y Planificación de Alimentación y Nutrición). 1981. *Análisis de la Situación Nutricional durante el Periodo 1972–1979.* Tegucigalpa, Honduras: Consejo Superior de Planificación Económico (mimeographed).

SECPLAN (Secretaria de Planificación, Coordinación, y Presupuesto) and DESFIL (Development Strategies for Fragile Lands). 1989. *Perfil Ambiental de Honduras 1989.* Tegucigalpa, Honduras: SECPLAN.

Sheahan, John. 1987. *Patterns of Development in Latin America.* Princeton, NJ: Princeton University Press.

Smith, Sheldon, and Edward Reeves. 1989. Introduction. In *Human Systems Ecology,* ed. Sheldon Smith and Edward Reeves. Boulder, CO: Westview.

Stares, R. C. 1972. *La Economia Campesina en la Zona Sur de Honduras, 1950–1970: su Desarrollo y Perspectivas para el Futuro.* Informe Presentado a la Prefectura de Choluteca, Honduras.

Stonich, Susan C. 1986. *Development and Destruction: Interrelated Ecological,*

Socioeconomic, and Nutritional Change in Southern Honduras. Ann Arbor, MI: University Microfilms (Ph.D. diss., University of Kentucky).

Stonich, Susan C. 1989. The Dynamics of Social Processes and Environmental Destruction: A Central American Case Study. *Population and Development Review* 15:269–96.

Stonich, Susan C. 1991. Rural Families and Income from Migration: Honduran Households in the World Economy. *Journal of Latin American Studies* 15 (2): 131–61.

Stonich, Susan C. 1993. *Enduring Crises: The Political Ecology of Poverty and Environmental Destruction in Honduras.* Boulder, CO: Westview.

Stonich, Susan C., and Billie R. DeWalt. 1989. The Political Economy of Agricultural Growth and Rural Transformations in Honduras and Mexico. In *Human Systems Ecology: Studies in the Integration of Political Economy, Adaptation, and Socionatural Regions* ed. Sheldon Smith and Edward Reeves, 202–30. Boulder, CO: Westview.

Stonich, Susan C., and Billie R. DeWalt. 1996. The Political Ecology of Deforestation in Honduras. In *Tropical Deforestation: The Human Dimension,* ed. Leslie Sponsel, Thomas Headland, and Robert Bailey, 187–215. New York: Columbia University Press.

USAID (United States Agency for International Development). 1982. *Country Environmental Profile.* McLean, VA: JRB Associates.

USAID (United States Agency for International Development). 1989a. *Strategic Considerations for the Agricultural Sector in Honduras.* Office of Agriculture and Rural Development, USAID/Honduras, draft copy.

USAID (United States Agency for International Development). 1989b. *Plan de Desarrollo del Camarón en Honduras.* Tegucigalpa, Honduras: USAID.

USAID (United States Agency for International Development). 1990. *Agricultural Sector Strategy Paper.* Tegucigalpa, Honduras: USAID Office of Agriculture and Rural Development.

White, Robert A. 1977. *Structural Factors in Rural Development: The Church and the Peasant in Honduras.* Ph.D. diss., Cornell University.

Wiley, Andrea. 1992. Adaptation and the Biocultural Paradigm in Medical Anthropology: A Critical Review. *Medical Anthropology Quarterly* 6:216–36.

Williams, Robert G. 1986. *Export Agriculture and the Crisis in Central America.* Chapel Hill: University of North Carolina Press.

World Bank. 1992. *World Development Report, 1992.* New York: Oxford University Press.

World Health Organization. 1973. *Protein and Energy Requirements.* Geneva: WHO.

World Health Organization. 1979. *Measurement of Nutritional Impact.* Geneva: WHO/FAO.

Chapter 13

The Biocultural Impact of Tourism on Mayan Communities

Magalí Daltabuit and Thomas L. Leatherman

focus on how tourism affects gender relations & health

Throughout Latin America and much of the developing world, nations are turning to tourism as a path of economic development for generating much needed foreign exchange. Mexico is the leader of this trend in Latin America, and a primary destination is Quintana Roo on what is called the Mexican Caribbean. In the last two and a half decades, the recently formed state of Quintana Roo on the eastern portion of the Yucatán peninsula has experienced a massive penetration of tourism, transforming it from one of the most isolated areas of Mexico into a tourist bonanza. This development has been an unqualified success for the Mexican government and international investors, but less certain is how this change has affected the Maya: their environment, diet and health, and culture. It is clear, however, that rapid tourism development in this region has economic and sociocultural costs for local populations (Pi-Sunyer and Thomas 1997). As environmental resources and labor become increasingly commoditized and symbols of prestige become increasingly Western, substantial disruptions to local patterns of life are inevitable. Among the areas most vulnerable to disruption are subsistence strategies, modes of household and community organization, gender and social roles, and the nature and meaning of cultural identity. These social disruptions have counterparts in human biological costs as Mayan populations become assimilated into a tourist economy. Yet, there has been little consideration of how social and economic changes in the contexts of tourism development might be linked to biological changes in nutrition and health.

This paper presents a short history of tourism development in the Yucatán and examines its potential role in affecting transformations in the local society, economy, and patterns of health in the Mayan community of Yalcoba. It addresses the pervasive problem of tourism's impact on

317

indigenous societies and documents the way macro political-economic processes (in this case tourism) interconnect with local histories to affect the biology of individuals. Specifically it examines patterns of diet, nutrition, and health in Mayan households and explores how gender differences in illness might be related to shifting gender roles and women's work in household reproduction.

Tourism and Development

Third World countries have climates, cultures, and landscapes that are attractive to the people of industrialized nations: sun and sand, "rustic" ways of life, exotic landscapes. The interest of third world countries to promote tourism is based on the fact that it generates jobs and profits for foreign exchange. Yet, tourism also intensifies migration patterns, increases the peripheralization and marginalization of local communities, and displaces existing economic activities such as farming or fishing that are basic for the survival of local populations (Jud 1975; Manning 1982; Pi-Sunyer 1977; Smith 1982).

Massive tourism emerged after World War II and is an international industry that transports and entertains millions of individuals that travel between developed countries or between developed countries and the Third World (Pi-Sunyer 1981, 1982). This industry is made up of the airlines, the large hotel consortiums, travel agencies, car rental agencies, construction companies, and so on. While tourism is clearly one of the most important elements in the economic development of the third world countries, it is a remarkably capital-intensive industry. It requires large expenditures for building infrastructure and purchasing sophisticated technologies—expenditures most developing countries can not afford without foreign investment. As a result, most of the hotels, travel agencies, and airlines are owned by foreign companies, which means that a large portion of profits from the tourist economy flow to the home nations of the multinational corporations that dominate the tourism industry worldwide (Smith 1982; Callimanopulos 1982). This has led Smith (1982) to characterize tourism as a phenomenon sponsored by the government, regulated by international agencies, and supported by multinational enterprises.

In virtually all instances, massive tourism is a form of development initiated and controlled by external agencies and institutions. Participation of local groups in planning and management is absent or minimal, and little concern is given to the long-term consequences of tourism for the local inhabitants or the environment upon which they depend. More recent developments in eco-tourism and archeo-tourism are based in a concern over environmental preservation and sustainability. But while they may entail more direct contact between tourists and rural indigenous populations, local populations are still largely left out of the planning process.

Tourism in Mexico and Quintana Roo

Mexico, like other developing countries, has been attracted by the myth of tourism as a miracle industry able to transform its failing economy. During the last fifteen years tourism has contributed to the balance of payments by generating foreign exchange second only to the oil industry. Mexico has the largest tourist sector in Latin America and the sixth highest number of visitors in the global tourist market (De la Torre 1985). Since the beginning of tourism development in Mexico during the 1950s, a relationship between local investment and multinational corporations was established. In the 1960s national tourism programs centered upon regional development, infrastructure construction, and modernization to capture a larger number of visitors, and on credit concessions to reinforce private investment. In 1974 FONATUR (Fondo Nacional de Fomento al Turismo) was created to sponsor tourism programs and to orient investment to areas of official interest for regional development such as Cancún in Quintana Roo, Ixtapa in Guerrero, Los Cabos and Loreto in Baja California and more recently Huatulco in Oaxaca (Cesar and Arnaiz 1985).

A generation ago, Quintana Roo in the eastern part of the Yucatán peninsula remained one of the most inaccessible locations in Mexico, an economic and political frontier where the institutions of the state were minimally represented. Today, the Maya of this region find themselves part of a totalizing experience driven by the exigencies of modern tourism. Quintana Roo was selected by the government as an area with strong tourist potential for several reasons. It was one of the most underdeveloped areas in Mexico, characterized by geographical and political marginality, and by an indigenous rural population with a high level of poverty. In many ways it was the last frontier of economic expansion in a process of national integration and development. Other reasons were that it has an abundance of resources needed for tourism such as 200 annual days of sunshine, beautiful beaches, archaeological sites, cheap labor, and political stability. Its proximity to Miami and the Caribbean Sea allows Quintana Roo to compete for the Caribbean tourist trade (Lee 1978).

Early development of the tourism industry in Quintana Roo took place on the islands of Cozumel and Isla Mujeres. At this stage of development, capital investment remained in local hands, allowing for controlled development, more profits for local economies, and a more direct and accommodating relationship between tourists and local inhabitants of these islands. Tourism on a massive scale, planned and controlled by the state, started in 1974 with the development of Cancún by multinational corporations. In the early 1970s Cancún was an isolated fishing village with 426 inhabitants, but now it has become the state's most important city with a population of approximately 400,000 people and an alarming annual growth rate of 20 percent. It has come to dominate the economy of the whole Yucatán peninsula, overshadowing Mérida, the capital of the state of Yucatán and the former center of the peninsula.

The main objectives of this massive tourism project were to promote regional economic development, to create employment for the local population, and to obtain a profit. In the Cancún project, the Mexican government assumed responsibility for the construction of roads, an airport, and hotels, as well as providing public services. Credit was received from the World Bank, the Bank of International Development, and private national banks (Crick 1989). The main companies that invested in the first stage of tourist development were the Downtowner Motor Inn, Western International, Club Mediterranean, and more recently the International Telegraph and Sheraton Hotels, among others (Cesar and Arnaiz 1985). The period of greatest growth in hotel construction occurred between 1976 and 1978. In 1982 a national economic crisis slowed development, but since 1986 it has increased again with the construction of more than 30 new hotels. The development of smaller resorts southward along the Cancún–Tulum coastal corridor has increased in the past five years to the point where a hotel or resort complex stands on every available beach. Several new communities composed of service personnel have grown up around resorts, primarily comprised of migrants from elsewhere in the Yucatán.

The dominant influence in Quintana Roo tourism remains Cancún, a huge resort city with over 137 hotels and approximately two million visitors a year, of which a million and a half are foreigners. Cancún serves as the port of entry for the majority of foreign tourists arriving in the area, of which 91 percent are American. The average foreign visitor is less than forty years old and has an annual income of over $50,000 (FONATUR 1993, 12). National tourists come mainly from Mexico City (43 percent) and the state of Yucatán (20 percent), and the vast majority are also under forty years of age (FONATUR 1987). The employment generated by the tourist industry within Cancún is of two types: (1) direct employment related to hotels, restaurants, travel agencies, tourist transportation, marinas, and so on, and (2) indirect employment that includes commerce, public workers, construction, and taxi and bus drivers. Twenty-five percent of the inhabitants of Cancún are involved in direct employment, while more than 50 percent are involved in indirect employment. The construction business generates most of the indirect employment (Cesar and Arnaiz 1985).

Tourism development in the Yucatán and Quintana Roo has had a profound impact on the Mayan landscape. Today, an infrastructure of roads crisscrosses the state, facilitating a growing degree of economic and political penetration. Tourism, government services, and commercial activity directly or indirectly touch all Mayan communities, although the extent and specific nature of these influences, as well as local responses to them, vary considerably. Mayan communities of the Yucatán peninsula have exhibited both resistance and resilience to their marginal situation within the national Mexican economy. Though profoundly influenced over the centuries by capitalist penetration, their success in remaining largely self-sufficient has depended upon access to sufficient land and labor to support slash-and-burn agriculture. In recent decades, however, processes of economic development have begun to exacerbate a set of environmental problems such as decreased land availability and productivity, and they have drawn labor away from rural communities into the tourist sectors. As a result, agricultural production has declined, and Mayan communities are going through a process of transformation from self-production to a market economy.

The highly capital-intensive development of Cancún and the coast created a labor market based largely in construction and in service industries to tourists. At present the employment offered in construction attracts many Mayan peasants from the Yucatán peninsula who need to sell their labor to support their families. The Mayan migrants constitute a reserve of cheap labor that is necessary for the development of the tourism industry. The migrations to the tourist centers have altered the demographic profile and economic strategies of the surrounding rural areas from which these workers are drawn. Even in communities in the interior that tourists rarely see, large numbers of men as well as adolescent males and females migrate for work to Cancún and the coast, returning home on weekends or once a month. For established families, this places an added burden on women, who must maintain home and family in their husbands' absence. It has also led to a shift in desires and expectations among younger generation Maya who are less interested in making milpa (slash-and-burn horticulture) and tending kitchen gardens. For those remaining in the community, the time and labor are now often unavailable to make milpa and harvest forest resources as in the past. Important shifts in ethnic and cultural identity, household and community relations, and the loss of indigenous knowledge are additional costs of the economic transformation that has taken place in Quintana Roo and the Yucatán over the past two decades.

In many ways, the sort of social, economic, and cultural changes noted here have been replicated to differing degrees in other regions of the Third World as a result of capitalist economic development. The situation in Quintana Roo is remarkable because the penetration of a modern tourist industry has not only been fast and recent, but massive in scale. The speed and totalizing nature of this shift, and the fact that it carries a strong ideological component in the images of wealth and prestige presented to the Maya in the form of foreign tourists, make these social impacts even more dramatic and critical to document. Our concern, however, is the understudied aspects of dietary, nutritional, and health costs that may accompany these changes. We turn now to a case study of one community located in the hinterland of the peninsula, but which is nevertheless strongly affected by the tourism-led economic development throughout the Yucatán. The discussion combines the results of research carried out over a period from 1986 through 1996 by the authors and their students.

The Case of Yalcoba

Social and Economic Transformations

Yalcoba is a Mayan village of about 1,450 inhabitants located in a Maize Production Zone in the interior of the Yucatán peninsula approximately 140 kilometers (or 85 miles) from Cancún. It is a community of contrasts. A typical house of *bajareque* construction (pole and thatch) has a television in a prominent place. There is no good source of clean water, waste disposal, or sanitation in the village—but there is cable TV. The majority of the inhabitants (±75 percent) practice slash-and-burn agriculture, but wage work outside the community is the major source of household income. The regional tourist economy in which they work is seen both as a source of economic salvation and as a negative force influencing the attitudes of a younger generation and disrupting the social and cultural fabric of village life.

Until recently the main economic activity was slash-and-burn agriculture that produces crops such as maize, beans, squash, and tubers. Agriculture was supplemented by raising cattle, pigs, chickens, and bees, as well as by home gardens, hunting, and collecting wild plants. The transformation of self-production into a cash economy with wage labor as the main activity is reinforced by increasingly limited access to *ejido* (communal) lands, which makes traditional subsistence strategies less viable. Increased consumption norms and the commoditization of basic needs, including food, makes a steady source of cash income essential to daily household reproduction. In 1986, 43 percent of the families had at least one member that migrated to Cancún on a weekly basis. Estimates from 1991 suggest that between 60 and 75 percent of households have migrating members. In 1986, 76 percent of male heads of household reported that agriculture was a main source of household income, supplemented with temporal wage labor. Only 9 percent of heads of household mentioned wage labor as their primary occupation. In 1993, 59 percent of household heads reported agriculture as a primary occupation, and 23 percent reported wage work in construction as the primary source of household income. In 53 percent of households surveyed ($n = 108$), male heads were employed outside the village, mainly in Cancún, even if they did not list wage work as their primary occupation (Miller 1994).

Some younger unmarried women, and a few divorced or widowed women, work in Cancún as maids in hotels or in other service industry jobs. However, migrants are predominantly males, 15 to 45 years old, who migrate weekly to work in the construction industry. This is hard work under difficult and dangerous conditions and with very low salaries (U.S. $3.50 per day). Most do not receive any benefits such as medical care or insurance. Many report that they become alienated and face discrimination even from other workers who come from elsewhere in Mexico.

As men migrate into Cancún, women are left in the village to attend to local production and household reproduction activities. Men who work in Cancún return to Yalcoba on the weekends, and some return only every two weeks. Women often anxiously wait for them to return and bring their earnings, which provide the vast majority of funds to meet all basic family needs. Their situation is often exacerbated by the fact that their husbands may not find work in Cancún for several weeks, or may spend the majority of their earnings before returning home for the weekend. Women have few local income-generating activities and engage in a range of activities such as making hammocks, keeping chickens, and sewing and embroidering *huipils* (traditional dresses), none of which provide a sizable or steady income. Thus, in the context of tourism-led economic development, these women are increasingly operating in spheres of production and household reproduction, and with relatively little control over household budgets (Daltabuit 1989). These multiple roles are recognized in the "double day" of work that many women must perform. In addition to multiple roles, women marry and begin having children early, usually by age 19 but as early as age 15. Mean completed fertility is between 7 and 8 births, and women spend much of their adult life pregnant, lactating, or caring for a small child. For those women living in marginal socioeconomic conditions, high fertility in conjunction with high work levels presents a biological and psychosocial stress that may well result in more illness (Harrington 1983).

Within the social sphere, greater involvement in the tourism-based cash economy can diminish family networks and promote the abandonment of traditional cultural and social activities. Traditional agricultural ceremonies such as the *chac chac,* a rain ceremony carried out in the summer, are in decline. Young couples still reside next to the husband's parents, but some decline to pool resources, opting instead to prepare meals and manage their household independently. This is seen by many older residents as a threat to the very structure of the Mayan family. The most dramatic change is seen in young men who openly express their disdain for the drudgery of milpa work, and who prefer to seek their future in Cancún. They return each week with clothing, language, and a value system reflecting the urban environment of Cancún and the Mexican national culture.

These symbols of First World penetration are supported, valorized, and reproduced within the community through the televised media (Miller 1994). In 1993, 74 percent of households in Yalcoba owned televisions which received two channels carrying programs from Mexico City and occasionally the United States. The most frequently viewed programs were *telenovelas* (soap operas) that depict the lives of upper-class urban dwellers and occasionally an *indio* maid or gardener. Interspersed within these soaps is a barrage of advertisements for food, toys, clothing, and other commodities, and for sun and sand tourism. Advertisements for Coca-Cola and Pepsi appeared with increased frequency amid a cola war, whereby Pepsi was seeking a greater share of the huge soft drink market in Mexico.

Thus, the effects of tourism-based development on Mayan communities such as Yalcoba can range from transformations in household economies and a growing commoditization of basic needs, to a loss of indigenous knowledge and control over local resources, to changing ethnic identities (Pi-Sunyer and Thomas 1997). It can also have implications for the health and nutrition of Mayan households. As food systems become increasingly commoditized, diets shift from a reliance on local products to consumption of more purchased products from outside the community and region (dietary delocalization). As gender roles and the division of labor shift in a wage economy, differences in gender-based patterns of illness can emerge (Leatherman 1996). In the following section, we explore these potential impacts of social and economic change on nutrition and health among households in Yalcoba. Specifically, we address three aspects of nutrition and health: dietary delocalization and the penetration of junk foods, household health and gender differences in illness, and the potential impact of women's work and reproductive stress on their health.

Dietary Delocalization and the Penetration of Junk Foods

One of the most visible effects in many rural communities experiencing economic change and increased monetization is a dietary delocalization (Pelto and Pelto 1983), in which there is an increase in foods from outside a region in the local diet. Food commoditization and dietary delocalization are associated with improved levels of nutrition in industrialized nations, but often with negative nutritional effects in developing nations (Pelto and Pelto 1983, 507). Growth in markets and commoditization of foodstuffs can result in increased food availability (i.e., diversity in the market), but decreased access and hence reduced dietary diversity for the many rural populations that cannot afford market prices. Dewey (1989), for example, reviewed the effects of food commoditization on diet and nutrition in three areas in Latin America, including Mexico, and concluded that communities and households reliant on nonlocal commercialized foods showed reduced dietary diversity and impaired nutritional status compared to those with a greater reliance on subsistence production of local crops to meet basic food needs.

In order to evaluate changes in dietary patterns and dietary delocalization in Yalcoba, Daltabuit compared the frequency of consumption of locally produced and commercial foods among Yalcoba households (1989, table 1). The foods that were eaten almost daily by the majority of families included tortillas, lard, beans, bread, eggs, other wheat products, sugar, and soft drinks. Several foods that were in the past very important in the local diet had a low frequency of consumption, including honey, tubers, squash seeds, posoles, and wild meats. Commercial foodstuffs were consumed with about the same frequency as locally produced foods. It is particularly telling that sugar, soft drinks, and snack foods were among the five most frequently consumed items in 1986.

Particularly dramatic is the consumption of soft drinks, especially the ubiquitous Coca- Cola and other sodas. Soft drink industry analysts estimate that each year the 90 million plus population of Mexico consume 560 eight ounce servings of soft drinks per capita, accounting for 20 percent of Pepsi's and 15 percent of Coke's international sales (Jabbonsky 1993). Pendergrast (1993, 413) estimated that the consumption of Coke alone in Mexico reached 273 servings (i.e., cans or bottles) per capita per annum by the early 1990s, second only to the U.S. estimate of 296 servings. More recent reports suggest that Mexico has now surpassed the U.S. in per capita consumption of Coke (Coca-Cola Company 1993) . Local distributors of soft drinks in Yalcoba in 1994 reported weekly sales that suggested a per capita consumption of one Coke per day. In 1996, 75 school-aged children between the ages of 6 and 13 were asked about consumption rates of soft drinks and other snack foods. They reported average weekly intakes of 7.4 soft drinks (mostly Coke or Pepsi), 10.2 snack foods (e.g., chips or cookies), and 11.8 candies (e.g., suckers). Maximum daily consumption rates reported were about 4 to 5 sodas, 7 snack foods, and 6 candies. During a morning school break in Yalcoba it is typical for children to buy a Coke and a snack, which contributes about 350 calories, about one-quarter of an elementary school child's daily requirement (Daltabuit 1989; McGarty 1995).

The average daily intake of calories and protein were estimated for individuals in 40 households in 1986 (Daltabuit 1989, table 2). The general tendency was for children and adolescents to be below standard for daily allowances of calories and protein (at 70 to 75 percent of the standard) based on Mexican standards, and for adults to be at or above standards for calories and at about 85 percent of the protein RDA. Younger females in particular had very low intakes of calories and protein, while older women were above standard. Such a pattern when accentuated can reflect the characterization by Dickinson et al. that a large part of the Yucatecan population "spends most of its life under nutritional stress: when they are young, malnutrition is highly prevalent (i.e., stunting), when they are older, obesity is quite common" (1993, 315).

While calorie deficits and protein calorie malnutrition were common in the Yucatán in the 1960s and are clearly problems for portions of the present population, recent studies have cited the importance of micronutrient deficiencies (Gurri and Balam 1992). A restudy on a small household sample ($N = 13$) in 1994 found calories and protein to be adequate, but nutrient density for vitamin A and zinc to be potentially compromised. While these more recent results are still preliminary, they gain importance in high maize diets and when considering the shifts in dietary diversity toward the consumption of more soft drinks. Allen and co-workers (1992) in the Mexican highlands showed that iron, zinc, and vitamin A deficiencies are almost unavoidable when maize intakes are over 60 percent of the diet. In addition, the high levels of phosphoric acid in Coke can compromise the bioavailability of calcium and other positively charged elements such as zinc and iron (Calloway 1993). Thus, when the remaining "non-maize" calories come from sugar, soft drinks, and snack foods it is almost a certainty that marginal nutrition will become worse (Calloway 1993).

TABLE 1.   Frequency of Consumption of Traditional versus Commercialized Foods in Yalcoba Households, 1986 (in percentages)

Food Items	3–7 Times/Week	1–2 Times/Week	1–3 Times/Month	0–3 Times/Year
Traditional				
Tortillas	100	0	0	0
Lard	98	2	0	0
Eggs	80	20	0	0
Citric fruits	51	16	6	27
Beans	50	45	5	0
Honey	12	15	27	45
Pumpkin seeds	10	37	40	12
Meat	7	41	19	33
Tubers	7	16	34	43
Wild meats	2	3	12	83
Commercialized				
Sugar	98	2	0	0
Soft drinks	83	17	0	0
Junk food	58	12	7	23
Instant coffee	55	15	0	30
Wheat products	49	30	6	14
Powdered milk	35	10	7	36
Chocomilk	32	25	7	36
Oil	2	0	0	98
Chocolate	47	33	13	7

While delocalization of diets often has negative nutritional effects in developing nations, the added penetration of soft drinks and "snack foods" in local diets may well exacerbate the effects on nutritional status.

In order to evaluate the nutritional status in Yalcoba, anthropometric data on Yalcoba school children were collected in 1986 and 1996 and classified for stunting and wasting based on the classification system of Waterlow (1984) and using reference standards for Mexican (Ramos Galvan 1975) and U.S. populations (NCHS standard, Frisancho 1990; see table 3). Stunting, or low height for age, was common in 1986; 49 percent of the boys and 55.8 percent of the girls were stunted. The vast majority of children (98 percent) had normal weights for height; 1 percent were wasted and 1.4 percent were overweight. The recent anthropometric survey carried out in 1996 confirmed earlier results that many of the children were stunted but with normal weight for heights. Based on NCHS reference standards (which overestimate stunting compared with the Ramos Galvan reference standard), 61 percent of the children were stunted and none were wasted, although 4.5 percent were overweight. Also, Daltabuit (1989) reported that all adults were at or above standards of weight for height,

TABLE 2.   Calorie and Protein Intakes in Yalcoba Households

Age Groups	N	Calories		Protein	
		Kcal	%RDA[a]	Grams	%RDA[a]
A. Daily Intake by Females					
1–3	(2)	745	87%	20	70%
4–6	(4)	1,145	78%	34	85%
7–10	(5)	1,357	68%	40	77%
11–18	(4)	1,562	68%	51	76%
19–34	(8)	2,112	106%	60	85%
35–54	(7)	1,848	100%	61	86%
B. Daily Intake by Males					
1–3	(6)	835	73%	23	79%
4–6	(4)	1,208	80%	33	82%
7–10	(5)	1,528	76%	43	83%
11–18	(10)	1,504	56%	47	72%
19–34	(2)	2,141	78%	73	88%
35–54	(3)	3,112	125%	82	99%
55+	(5)	2,040	91%	64	77%

Source: Bourges, H., A. Chavez, and P. Arroyo 1970. *Recommendaciones de Nutrimentos para la Poblacion Mexicana.* Pub L-17, Instituto Nacional de la Nutricion, Mexico.
[a]Recommended daily allowances for the Mexican population

and that 19 percent of men and 75 percent of women were overweight. In table 4, mid-arm muscle area (a rough indicator of protein status), mid-arm fat, and the sum of triceps and subscapular skinfolds were classified into five categories based on percentile cutoffs used by Frisancho (1990): low, below average, average, above average, and high levels of muscle or fat. Fifty percent of the children measured in 1996 are below reference standards for muscle status, and 25.5 percent have low muscle. Yet, only 8.6 percent of the children are below standard for fat status and an equal number have above standard fat status. These results indicate the prevalence of chronic moderate malnutrition in Yalcoba children and can be interpreted as an indicator of social deprivation in the population. Similarly they can reflect chronically low protein and/or micronutrient status but perhaps more adequate caloric intakes. In a limited number of cases, especially where adult women are overweight or obese, we are beginning to see signs of what Dickinson et al. (1990) have noted elsewhere in the Yucatán (especially in the urban periphery): the double-edged problem of childhood malnutrition and adult obesity. It should be noted that the tendency toward obesity is often a first stage in health problems associated with diabetes and hypertension that appear to plague a number of indigenous populations experiencing rapid changes in diet and life-style (McGarvey et al. 1989). *diseases of affluence.*

Patterns of Illness

Data on medical case records collected from the local clinic for 1981 through 1986 and 1989 through 1990 found that respiratory and gastrointestinal complaints accounted for over 70 percent of illness consultations at the clinic. Skin diseases, parasites, and chronic skeletal-muscular ailments (e.g., arthritis, rheumatism) accounted for many of the remaining complaints. Severe nutritional deficiencies (e.g., anemia, pellagra, severe malnutrition) represented a small but important number of cases, and a variety of reproductive problems (e.g., miscarriages, dysmenorrhea, postpartum infections) were reported by women. Also illness symptomatological surveys of 124 women in 1986 and of 30 women in 1989 also found that respiratory and gastrointestinal illness were leading health problems. The predominance of respiratory and gastrointestinal diseases follows a general morbidity pattern for Mexican rural communities, and information from earlier studies confirms that the health problems in Mayan rural communities have remained basically the same since the early 1930s (Saunders and Connell 1933).

Health surveys were carried out in 30 households in 1989 and 1991 (table 5) to examine economic and gender-based variation in health status. In both years, at least 50 percent of the households reported an illness in one to two family members in the preceding month, and about half reported illness events serious enough to disrupt their work. The most prevalent illness categories reported in these health surveys were respiratory, gastrointestinal, skeletal muscular, and dermatological, very similar to the clinic records. Households of lower economic status reported about 8 percent more illness cases but these differences were not statistically significant. More moderate income households ranked their family health as above average (50 percent vs. 33 percent in lower income households), and more felt that they could obtain help from outside the family in times of illness (25 percent vs. only 6 percent of the low income households).

Between 30 and 40 percent of adult women from the two health surveys reported an illness in the previous month, while only between 4 and 7 percent of adult males were reported to have been ill. Low levels of illness (7 to 9 percent) were also reported for children. These estimates may be

TABLE 3. Nutritional Status in Children: Prevalence of Stunting (Low Height-for-Age) and Wasting (Low Weight-for-Height) in 1986 and 1996

Nutritional Status[a]	N in 1986	($N = 288$) (%)	N in 1996	($N = 154$) (%)
Stunted	150	(52.1)	94	(61)
Wasted	3	(1.0)	0	(0)
Normal	281	(97.6)	147	(95.5)
Overweight	4	(1.4)	7	(4.5)

Source: Reference standards used to calculate Z-scores for 1986 are from Ramos-Galvan (1985), and for 1996 are NCHS standards published in Frisancho 1990.

[a]Based on Waterlow (1984) classification using –2.0 Z-score cutoffs for stunting and wasting

TABLE 4. Muscle and Fat Status Among Children in Yalcoba (ages 6–12 years: 1996)

Nutritional Status	Mid-Arm Muscle N	%	Mid-Arm Fat N	%	Sum of Fat Folds N	%
Low	39	25.5	3	1.96	1	0.7
Below average	37	24.2	36	23.5	12	7.9
Average	73	47.7	107	69.9	125	82.8
Above average	4	2.6	3	1.96	7	4.6
High	0	0	4	2.6	6	4.0

biased by the fact that so many adult males were away during the week, and because a portion received on-the-job health care. Thus potential health problems might be overlooked or minimized in reports by the adult females who most often provided the information on household health. Nevertheless, the magnitude of differences indicated here suggests a real gender bias in health status. Reasons for these differences might lie in the interaction of high work loads, marginal diets, and the biological costs of reproduction (Daltabuit 1989; Browner 1989; Larme 1993). In the present contexts of tourism, this interaction may be exacerbated by the increased work loads and the added work and psychosocial stress of being effectively a single head of household for much of the time.

Women's Work, Reproduction, and Health

Earlier research in 1986 (Daltabuit 1989) found that women in Yalcoba performed heavy work loads and experienced heavy reproductive stress. Our subsequent work in 1989 attempted to connect these factors more directly to the health status of women. Time allocation information on household work was collected along with reproductive histories and illness symptomatologies of 30 women. We calculated a "reproductive stress index" for each woman and enumerated the number and type of symptoms reported by women at different levels of reproductive stress. The stress index is a measure of the percentage of a woman's reproductive life spent pregnant and lactating.

The time allocation data illustrated that women worked longer hours and with fewer rests than men, confirming an earlier and more extensive survey by Daltabuit in 1986. They are in charge of virtually all domestic work and increasingly spend their limited free time in small-scale income-generating activities such as making hammocks, embroidering huipils, and

TABLE 5. Household Health and Gender Differences in Illness in Yalcoba Households, 1989 and 1991 (*N* = 30)

	1989	1991
Households with illness	63.3%	50.0%
Sick persons/household	1.0	1.7
Adult females sick	30.0%	40.0%
Adult males sick	7.0%	4.0%
Children sick	7.0%	9.0%

taking in laundry. Both men and women reported that women were resilient in the face of illness and kept working through most problems, in part because their efforts were essential to the daily operation of the household. In particular, women with little social support may have no choice but to work in spite of illness (Daltabuit 1989). Interestingly, there is also an ideology that women are inherently weaker (e.g., have *sangre debil*, "weaker blood") and thus are more prone to illness. Birth and post-partum periods are times of particular weakness when various sanctions against certain work must be followed to prevent illness. Women should rest for one week following birth and avoid heavy work for one to two months. They should avoid exposure to "winds" for about forty days, and this means staying close to home.

Reproductive histories confirmed earlier findings (Daltabuit 1989) that women in Yalcoba reproduce early and frequently until age thirty-five, and rarely past age forty. Average age at first pregnancy is nineteen, but 40 percent of the women were pregnant by age seventeen, and 12 percent by age fifteen. Over their reproductive life, women average between seven and eight pregnancies, one miscarriage, and five to six living children. They breast-feed their babies to between one and a half and two years and introduce weaning foods at around six months. Following Daltabuit (1989) and earlier work of Harrington (1983), a "reproductive stress index" was calculated for each of the thirty women. About one-half the women had a medium to light stress index—where less than 60 percent of their reproductive life was spent pregnant or lactating; and one-half had a heavy stress index of greater than 60 percent. These convenient cutoffs were then used to classify the women into high and low stress categories for reproductive stress.

Almost 20 percent more of the women in the high stress category reported a health problem in the previous two-week period, and 25 percent more ranked their own health as poor. The high stress women also reported about 6 percent more symptoms than low stress women (table 6). Of primary interest is that the largest differences are seen in symptoms related to skeletal muscular problems, nerves, and weakness. These are the types of chronic symptom groupings found by Oths (1991), Finerman (1983), Larme (1993), and Browner (1989) to be associated with reproduction-related illness elsewhere in Mexico and Latin America. Oths (1991), for example, found that women in northern Peru reported symptoms of chronic malaise labeled as *debilidad,* which she related to reproductive stress. Finerman (1983) related the prevalence of *nervios,* a folk illness with symptoms related to chronic weakness and nervous feelings, to high fertility levels among Ecuadorian women. In two Andean communities, Larme (1993) has identified *sobreparto* as a reproductive illness associated with symptoms of chronic skeletal-muscular complaints, weakness, fatigue, and general malaise. Finally, Carole Browner (1989) found that Mexican women with four or more pregnancies reported significantly more minor complaints like headaches, backaches and other body aches, weakness, and fatigue.

If women's health problems are due to the combined effects of heavy work loads and high reproductive stress, then high stress women in poor households whose spouses have migrated in search of work should be under greater stress. Figure 1 examines these associations by comparing the prevalence of all symptoms and chronic symptoms in women of low vs. high reproductive stress, in those with high reproductive stress who are poor, and in those poor women who have spouses that migrate from the community on a regular basis. Total symptom prevalence increases moderately in these categories (from about 28 to 42 percent), but chronic symptoms show a more marked increase from about 18 percent prevalence in low stress women to a 47 percent prevalence in high stress, poor women with migrant husbands (several of whom are in charge of effectively female-headed households). Small sample sizes limit the analysis, but the data suggest that as work and reproductive loads become increasingly high, health status becomes worse, particularly in terms of chronic fatigue, weakness, and pain. In the present contexts of tourism, increased work loads and the added stress of being effectively a single head of household for much of the time may exacerbate this interaction.

TABLE 6.   Reproductive Stress and Symptom Prevalence Among Mayan Women in Yalcoba

Symptom Category	Low Stress ($N = 12$)	High Stress ($N = 18$)
All symptoms	27.5	33.3
Respiratory	27.5	33.8
GI-urinary	18.6	25.0
Heart-circulatory	20.0	22.5
Skeletal-muscular	15.0	25.0
Weakness	25.0	42.0
Nerves	12.0	24.0

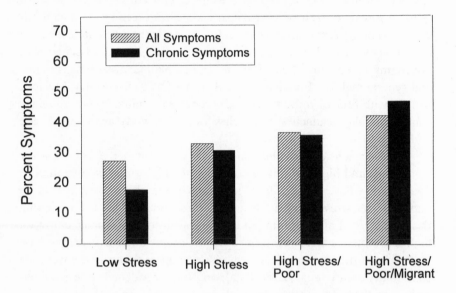

Fig. 1.   Symptom prevalence and levels of reproductive stress among women in Yalcoba

West fucking [rest the rest]
metaphor.

Conclusion

In the last two and a half decades, the massive penetration of tourism in Quintana Roo and the rest of the Yucatán has begun a transformation of Mayan environments, economy, society, and culture that we can only begin to envision. This penetration has been met by resistance and accommodation, by outrage and resignation. Local populations recognize the potential damage that tourism brings to all aspects of their lives, but also recognize the present necessity of the jobs it creates to meet the basic needs of their families. The older generation wonders what the world is coming to, while the younger generation hopes it comes to them. Tourism is a relatively recent force in the Yucatecan landscape, but we can already see its real and potential impacts on the lives and health of Mayan populations.

One observation we can make is that the unprecedented economic growth in the past two decades in the Yucatán has not brought newfound prosperity for the laborers who work in construction or service industry jobs. Rather it has served to create a large underclass of wage workers with low pay, few benefits, and poor job security. Nor has prosperity found its way into the hinterland communities such as Yalcoba from which these workers come. Rather, the standard of living and quality of life remain low for rural populations. Throughout the Yucatán peninsula, malnutrition, disease, and lack of access to basic services such as clean water, electricity, and even medical facilities are common to most Mayan communities.

There are some indications that tourism is making matters worse for rural households in the Yucatán. Milpa production has declined, and diets are shifting away from a base in local produce to commercialized foodstuffs. The increased proportion of caloric intake that is met through sodas and snack foods cannot improve nutrition and may prove to be particularly detrimental. Health status remains poor and relatively unchanged over past decades. Health status among women may be worsening due to the combined effects of heavy work loads, high fertility, and marginal nutriture. It is unclear exactly what effects the tourist economy specifically has on women's health, but it is suggested that the disruptive effects to family relations and household economies may make women particularly vulnerable.

Thus, for Mayan peoples, the social and biological costs of assimilation into the Mexican modern capitalist economy may be high. To date, the Maya have been granted little input in the planning of a development process, in which they are seen primarily as sources of cheap labor and ethnic backdrop at tourist sites. Individually or communally, they are absent in regulatory bodies and middle management strata. It is not too extreme to say that economic penetration is transforming them into a peripheral element in their own homeland, a situation that has powerful political and social implications, particularly in light of the long Maya history of cultural resistance.

REFERENCES

Allen, L., J. R. Backstrand, and E. J. Stanek. 1992. The Interactive Effects of Dietary Quality on the Growth of Young Mexican Children. *Am. J. Clin. Nutr.* 56:353–64.

Browner, Carole. 1989. Women, Household and Health in Latin America. *Social Science and Medicine* 28:461–73.

Callimanopulos, Dominique. 1982. Introduction. In *The Tourist Trap. Cultural Survival Quarterly* 6 (3): 3–6.

Calloway, D., S. P. Murphy, G. H. Beaton, and D. Lein. 1993. Estimated Vitamin Intakes of Toddlers: Predicted Prevalence of Inadequacy in Village Populations in Egypt, Kenya, and Mexico. *Am. J. Clin. Nutr.* 58:376–84.

Cesar Dachary, A., and S. Arnaiz Burne. 1985. *Estudios Socioeconomicos Preliminares de Quintana Roo: Sector Tourismo.* Centro de Investigaciones de Quintana Roo. Puerto Morelos, Mexico.

Coca-Cola Company. 1993. *Annual Report of the Coca-Cola Company for 1993.*

Crick, Malcolm. 1989. Representation of International Tourism in the Social Sciences: Sun, Sex, Sighs, Savings, and Servility. *Ann. Rev. Anthrop.* 18:307–44.

Daltabuit, Magalí. 1989. *Mayan Women: Work, Nutrition and Child Care.* Ph.D. diss. University of Massachusetts, Amherst.

Daltabuit, M., and Oriol Pi-Sunyer. 1990. Tourism Development in Quintana Roo, Mexico. *Cultural Survival Quarterly* 14 (1): 9–13.

De la Torre, Oscar. 1985. *El Turismo. Fenomeno Social.* Fondo de Cultura Economica. Mexico.

Dewey, K. 1989. Nutrition and the Commoditization of Food Systems in Latin America. *Social Science and Medicine* 28:415–24.

Dickinson, F., M. T. Castillo, L. Vales, and L. Uc. 1993. Obesity and Women's Health in Two Socioeconomic Areas of Yucatan, Mexico. *Coll. Antropol.* 2:309–17.

Finerman, R. 1983. Experience and Expectation: Conflict and Change in Traditional Family Health Care among the Quichua of Saraguro. *Social Science and Medicine* 17:1291–98.

FONATUR. 1987. Panel Aeropuerto: Estudio Continuo entre Visitantes por Via Aerea 1987. Subdireccion General de Mercadotecnia. Gerencia General de Estudtios de Mercado. Cancun, Quintana Roo.

FONATUR. 1993. Panel Aeropuerto: Estudio continuo de Visitantes por Via Aerea. Subdireccion General de Comercializacion. Mexico, D.F.: Fonatur.

Frisancho, A. R. 1990. *Anthropometric Standards for the Assessment of Growth and Nutritional Status.* Ann Arbor: University of Michigan Press.

Gurri, F. D., and G. Balam. 1992. Regional Integration and Changes in Nutritional Status in the Central Region of Yucatan, Mexico: A Study of Dental Enamel Hypoplasia and Anthropometry. *Journal of Human Ecology* 3 (2): 417–32.

Harrington, A. J. 1983. Nutritional Stress and Economic Responsibility: A Study of Nigerian Women. In *Women and Poverty in the Third World,* ed. M. Buvinic, M. Lycette, and A. McGreevey. Baltimore: Johns Hopkins University Press.

Jabbonsky, L. 1993. The Mexican Resurrection. *Beverage World* 112 (1547): 38–40.

Jud, D. 1975. Tourism and Crime in Mexico. *Social Sciences Quarterly* 56:324–30.

Larme, A. 1993. Work, Reproduction and Health in Two Andean Communities. Working paper no. 5, from Production, Storage and Exchange in a Terraced Environment on the Eastern Andean Escarpment, Bruce Winterhalder, series editor. Chapel Hill: University of North Carolina.

Leatherman, Thomas. 1996. A Biocultural Perspective on Health and Household Economy in Southern Peru. *Medical Anthropology Quarterly* 10 (4): 476–95.

Lee, L. Rosemary. 1978. Who Owns Roadways: The Structure of Control in the Tourist Industry of Yucatan. *Studies in Third World Societies,* pub. 6, Tourism and Economic Change. Williamsburg, VA.

Manning E. F. 1982. The Caribbean Experience. *Cultural Survival Quarterly* 6 (3).

McGarty, Catherine A. 1995. *Dietary Delocalization in a Yucatecan Resort Community in Qintana Roo, Mexico: Junk Food in Paradise.* Honors Thesis, School of Nursing, University of Massachusetts, Amherst.

McGarvey, S. T., J. Bindon, D. Crews, and D. Schendel. 1989. Modernization and Adiposity: Causes and Consequences. In *Human Population Biology,* 263–79. New York: Oxford University Press.

Miller, Cynthia. 1994. The Social Impacts of Televised Media Among the Yucatec Maya. M.A. thesis, University of South Carolina.

Nash, D. 1978. An Anthropological Approach to Tourism. *Studies in Third World Societies,* pub. 6, Tourism and Economic Change. Williamsburg, VA.

Oths, K. 1991. *Medical Treatment Choice and Health Outcomes in the Northern Peruvian Andes.* Ph.D. diss. Case Western Reserve University.

Pelto, G. H., and P. J. Pelto. 1983. Diet and Delocalization: Dietary Changes since 1750. *Journal of Interdisciplinary History* 14:507–28.

Pendergrast, M. 1993. *For God, Country and Coca-Cola: The Unauthorized History of the Great American Soft Drink and the Company that Makes It.* New York: Charles Scribner's Sons.

Pi-Sunyer, O. 1977. Through Native Eyes: Tourists and Tourism in a Catalan Maritime Community. In *Hosts and Guests: The Anthropology of Tourism,* ed. V. Smith, 149–55. Philadelphia: University of Pennsylvania Press.

Pi-Sunyer, O. 1981. Tourism and Anthropology. *Annals of Tourism Research VIII* no. 2: 271–84.

Pi-Sunyer O. 1982. The Cultural Costs of Tourism: The Tourist Trap. *Cultural Survival Quarterly* 6 (3): 7–10.

Pi-Sunyer, Oriol, and Brooke Thomas. 1997. Tourism, Environmentalism and Cultural Survival in Quintana Roo, Mexico. In *Life and Death Matters: Human Rights and the Environment at the End of the Millennium,* ed. Barbara Johnston, 187–212. Walnut Creek, CA: Altamira Press.

Ramos Galvan, R. 1975. Somatometria Pediatrica. *Archivos de Investigacion Medica,* vol. 6. Instituto Mexicano del Seguro Social. Mexico.

Saunders M. G., and H. F. Connell. 1933. *The Peninsula of Yucatan. Medical, Biological, Meteorological and Sociological Studies,* 431–500. Carnegie Institution of Washington.

SECTUR. 1987. Informe de Labores 1986–87. Secretaria de Turismo. Mexico.

Smith L. V., ed. 1982. *Hosts and Guests: The Anthropology of Tourism.* Philadelphia: University of Pennsylvania Press.

Waterlow, J. C. 1984. Current Issues in Nutritional Assessment by Anthropometry. In *Malnutrition and Behavior: Critical Assesment of Key Issues,* ed. J. Brozek and R. Scherch. Lausanne: Nestle Foundation.

Chapter 14

Poverty and Nutrition in Eastern Kentucky: The Political Economy of Childhood Growth

Deborah L. Crooks

This chapter discusses child poverty in the United States and the role of biological anthropologists in poverty research. Biological anthropologists have made important contributions to research on poverty in the developing world via a focus on child growth and development. Child growth is an accepted marker of the quality of a child's environmental circumstances because of its well-documented sensitivity to those circumstances (Huss-Ashmore and Johnston 1985; Schell 1986). In developing countries, child growth has been an effective monitor of economic and social conditions that limit resources and erode adaptive strategies of those living on the margins. Where political and economic agendas and policies combine to prevent access to adequate nutrition, housing, sanitation, and health-related resources, child growth often suffers.

With few exceptions biological anthropologists have paid less attention to this issue in the developed world. But given that childhood growth reflects the quality of a child's environment, research in this area could raise critical flags, calling attention to geographical areas and populations within the United States where more resources could improve children's lives. Thus by bringing their expertise to bear on these issues in the United States, biological anthropologists could bring much to the understanding of the relationship between poverty and childhood well-being.

Already, limited research in the United States has documented a relationship between poverty or socioeconomic status (SES) and child growth, indicating deficits in stature and weight, and, conversely, excesses in weight among some poor children in the United States, although some research indicates little/no effect on growth (reviewed by Crooks 1995).

Clearly there is variation in the research outcomes. However, it is not clear whether this variation results from methodology, for example, how poverty is defined and how it is used in the research, or whether it represents true variation based on the circumstances and experience of poverty for different groups in the United States.

What is clear is the need for more research to sort out the complex relationship between poverty and malnutrition in the United States, because the consequences of malnutrition may be devastating and lifelong. In the developing world, undernutrition, measured by low stature, weight, and body composition may have long-term consequences for adult productivity and success via cognitive deficits, compromised school performance, and even reduced work capacity (e.g., Grantham-McGregor 1984; Spurr 1983; Johnston and Low 1995). Similar consequences may hold for U.S. children, as well, especially as they relate to school achievement (Wilson et al 1986; Karp et al. 1992; Sewell, Price, and Karp 1993).

Another form of malnutrition, overnutrition, which is measured by high weight, body mass index, and/or skinfold thickness, may also have consequences for adult productivity. Although this remains to be documented, we can hypothesize a connection from childhood behaviors to adulthood behaviors that produce obesity, which is associated with chronic diseases, e.g., cancer, heart disease, and high blood pressure (Bandini and Dietz 1992; Dietz 1994; Greenwood et al. 1993; Webber et al. 1995). Where these diseases result in disability and where there is discrimination against overweight individuals, social and economic success may be compromised (Gortmaker et al. 1993).

Finally, a third form of malnutrition found among children in the United States is micronutrient deficiency. Not as easily recognizable as under- or overnutrition, micronutrient deficiencies result from inadequate diets in terms of quantity, quality, or both. Various micronutrient deficiencies are reported to be associated with negative child function (Buzina et al. 1989; Allen 1990; Kanarek and Marks-Kaufman 1991). Where these affect school achievement or health, adult productivity may be compromised.

These three forms of malnutrition occur in the context of poverty in the United States and may result from lack of resources for appropriate and adequate nutrition. However, the path from poverty to malnutrition in the United States is complex, with linkages that are multiple and often indirect (Crooks 1995). *Hypothesized* linkages include the ability of parents to secure a job that enables them to adequately provide for their children (education, job availability, transportation, and child care are all indirect links here), the ability of families to secure and/or produce quality food for their children (education, employment, land productivity/availability, and food prices/availability are all indirect links here), and parents' understanding of what constitutes quality nutrition and the importance of nutrition for their children's well-being (education, child-rearing practices, and the ability to allocate limited resources are all indirect links here).

Malnutrition in the Midst of Plenty

Why malnutrition should occur in the midst of affluence may be made more clear by an examination of the history of this issue. Malnutrition in the United States is a recurring phenomenon. In 1967, hungry and malnourished children were "discovered" in the Mississippi Delta, which prompted a major effort to document the nutritional status of poor children (Brenner et al. 1967; U.S. Department of Health, Education and Welfare 1972). Advanced and moderate malnutrition, hunger, and micronutrient deficiencies were documented for children in Appalachia and the South, in major cities of the North and West, and on Native American reservations. As research proliferated, poverty was identified as a key factor in poor nutritional status for many U.S. children and it became a critical focus in studies of U.S. child growth (Crooks 1993).

In terms of policy at this time, child growth became an important measure of the social and political will of Americans to deal successfully and respectfully with the problems of poor people, especially their basic right to food (Poppendieck 1995). Prompted by an aggressive network of activists, the public responded, and the U.S. Congress instituted and expanded numerous programs dealing with hunger and access to food, particularly the food stamp program, school lunch and breakfast programs, and the Special Supplemental Food Program for Women, Infants and Children (WIC) (Brown and Allen 1988; Poppendieck 1995). These programs were eminently successful (Brown and Allen, 1988), and concerns for hunger and child nutrition virtually disappeared from U.S. public discourse.

Then, in the 1980s, the specter of hungry and malnourished children rose again in the United States as increasing numbers of people, including children, appeared at urban soup kitchens, food pantries, and homeless shelters (Poppendieck 1995). The U.S. Conference of Mayors demanded federal assistance to deal with the situation, but this time met with little success (Brown and Gershoff 1989). Numerous agencies, both governmental (e.g., the U.S. Department of Agriculture, the Presidential Task Force on Food Assistance), and nongovernmental (e.g., the Center on Budget and Policy Priorities, Second Harvest, the Food Research and Action Center, and the Physicians' Task Force on Hunger), continued to document growing numbers of hungry and malnourished Americans (Brown and Allen 1988).

Today hunger and malnutrition among America's children continue to be problematic because poverty continues to be problematic. At the most recent rate of 22.7 percent, that is, 12.6 million children (table 1), U.S. child poverty rates are among the highest in the industrialized world. Canada, Australia, the United Kingdom, France, Sweden, the Netherlands, and Germany all have lower, single-digit rates, resulting from policies that have far greater success in lifting children out of poverty and providing for their welfare than do those of the United States (Smeeding and Torrey 1988; Garbarino 1992; Smeeding 1992).

But why do we find these increasing rates of child poverty in the United States and the disparity between the rates in the United States and elsewhere? Many suggest this is the direct result of the 1980s reversal of social policies, which reduced levels of federal spending for many social programs and shifted responsibility for programs to state governments, many of which were already economically strapped (Kelly and Ramsey 1991). Added to this, the economic restructuring of the 1980s resulted in high rates of under- and unemployment, a disproportionate creation of low-wage jobs and jobs without benefits (Segal 1991; Schorr 1992), and a redistribution of wealth upward resulting in increasing disparities (Schorr 1992). Differentially low wages and/or lack of equity in pay and fringe benefits for women, who head the majority of poor families,[1] compounded the problem, acting as barriers to movement out of poverty for many poor children (Schorr 1992; Gaventa, Smith, and Willingham 1993a). Therefore, as more families struggled at below-poverty wages and states shouldered more of the child welfare burden with fewer resources, rates of child poverty escalated. While children bear the brunt of poverty, the long-term costs of child poverty can be measured in terms of human capital, that is, large segments of the population who are unable to give their full potential to society, compromising the quality of the labor force, international competitiveness, and leadership (Smeeding and Torrey 1988; Dorsey 1991; Segal 1991).

Poverty: The Case of Appalachia

The children of Appalachia have been particularly affected by these macropolitical and macroeconomic circumstances. Appalachia is one of the areas originally identified in the 1960s as having unexpectedly high rates of hungry and malnourished children. Traditionally, many would blame Appalachians themselves, seeing Appalachia as different from the rest of the country, as existing outside mainstream America (for a critique, see Gaventa, Smith, and Willingham 1993b). Appalachian people have been called backward, victimized, fatalistic, "yesterday's people" (Caudill 1962; Weller 1965); mired in a "culture of poverty"[2] of their own making, and from which they cannot escape.

But others argue that this is little more than a victim-blaming stereotype and point out that Appalachian poverty is situational, not cultural (e.g., Billings 1974; Fisher 1993a, 1993b; Gaventa, Smith, and Willingham 1993a, 1993b; Couto 1994; Billings, Pudup, and Waller 1995). In the past, Appalachian people and resources fueled the Industrial Revolution, and Appalachian textiles, clothing, wood, and agricultural products played a major role in the U.S. economy (Couto 1994). Appalachian people have not "backwardly" resisted development, but actively sought it on their own terms, just as actively resisting exploitative practices that sought to undermine traditional cultural values (Fisher 1993b). Appalachia is not

TABLE 1. Poverty Rates in the United States, 1960–93

Year	All	Child	Adult	Elderly	White	African-American	Hispanic
1993	15.1	22.7	12.4	12.2	12.2	33.1	30.6
1990	13.5	20.6	10.7	12.2	10.7	31.9	28.1
1985	14.0	20.7	11.3	12.6	11.4	31.3	29.0
1980	13.0	18.3	10.1	15.7	10.2	32.5	25.7
1975	12.3	17.1	9.2	15.3	9.7	31.3	26.9
1970	12.6	15.1	9.0	24.6	9.9	33.5	NA
1965	17.3	21.0	NA	NA	NA	NA	NA
1960	22.2	26.9	NA	NA	NA	NA	NA

Source: Data from U.S. Bureau of the Census Current Population Reports, Series P60-188.

Note: Definition of poverty is based on income cut-offs or thresholds adjusted by various factors such as family size, head of household, number of children, and farm/non-farm residence. The threshold is based on the "Economy Food Plan," a plan of adequate nutrition designed by the Department of Agriculture. The Poverty Index was developed by Mollie Orshansky of the Social Security Administration and adopted in 1969 and thus pertains to those figures quoted above after 1969.

outside the mainstream, but has played a central role in the political economy of the United States.

Today, Appalachia continues to play a role in the mainstream economy, but an uneven one. In parts of Appalachia, we find economic prosperity, particularly in the Sun Belt or areas adjacent to large manufacturing cities of the North and South. In other areas, especially in rural central and southern Appalachia, we find rates of poverty equaled only by the inner cities of the North. Paradoxically, we find these high poverty rates existing in the midst of a national economic recovery.

Case Study: Poverty and Child Growth in Bridges County, Kentucky

Research currently under way in the eastern Kentucky region of central Appalachia utilizes a biocultural approach in an attempt to understand the consequences of poverty for childhood growth. Bridges County[3] is located in a persistently poor region of central Appalachia. It is currently designated by the Appalachian Regional Commission (ARC) as a "severely distressed" county,[4] but it has a long history of economic viability, going back to its location along a number of prominent Native American paths or trails that connected major villages in the north and south. European settlers moved into the area in the very late 1700s and farmed the rich bottomlands of a major river and numerous tributaries in the region; many mountain farms were successful as well. An abundance of natural resources also provided an economy of iron and manufactured iron products. By the time of its establishment as a county in the mid-1850s, Bridges County had a lively economy based on resource extraction (clay, limestone, timber, coal, oil, and iron ore), milling and forging, and agriculture.

Over time, however, the economy of various central Appalachian counties was subject to the exigencies of changing national and international conditions, mediated through local ones. Single-industry economies dominated by absentee owners, political corruption, and a highly stratified local class system created oppressive conditions for many people in the area (Fisher 1993b). Compounding this, Appalachia's "mature" industries[5] in mining, manufacturing, and agriculture were particularly sensitive to changes brought about by the economic restructuring of the 1980s. As economic restructuring took hold and the U.S. economy deindustrialized

and downsized, as technology replaced human labor, as the service and
financial sectors increased and the majority of newly created jobs were
low-wage and without benefits, poverty in Appalachia became more and
more entrenched (Fisher 1993a; Gaventa, Smith, and Willingham 1993a,
1993b; Couto 1994).

Bridges County was not exceptional in this process of economic deterioration. Today, most farmers cannot make a living solely by farming.
Instead Bridges County's economy rests on light industry, government,
and service jobs, many of which are seasonal. The average weekly wage
provides less than $300, the official unemployment rate is 10 to 11 percent
and the unofficial rate is 15 to 16 percent, high compared to the U.S. rate
of 5.8 percent. Nevertheless, I am told that residents of Bridges County are
"lucky" compared to others in that they are connected by a highway to
nearby counties that provide job opportunities. As long as one has transportation, that is, a vehicle and money for gas, a job may be only an hour's
distance away. But in a recent countywide needs assessment survey, lack of
transportation was indicated as a major impediment to employment.

With this level of under- and unemployment, the poverty rate in
Bridges County is also high, between 25 and 30 percent, compared to that
of the United States as a whole at 15.1 percent (1993 statistics) (Eller 1994;
U.S. Bureau of the Census 1995). The child poverty rate in Bridges County
at 30 to 35 percent also exceeds the U.S. child poverty rate of 22.7 percent
(Eller 1994; U.S. Bureau of the Census 1995). Other data indicate the
extent of poverty in the portion of the county served by Bridges Elementary School. Of the sample reported here, 78.4 percent of the children are
on free or reduced-priced lunch.[6]

To investigate the impact of poverty on children, I used the aforementioned convention of growth as a marker of child well-being and
employed standard techniques of anthropometry to measure height,
weight, and triceps skinfolds (Frisancho 1990). Body mass index was calculated from height and weight.[7] Z-scores[8] for height and weight were calculated against NCHS references using the computer software Anthro
Version 1.01 (Centers for Disease Control 1990); and Z-scores for triceps
skinfold and body mass index were calculated using the NHANES data in
Frisancho (1990).

As seen in table 2, boys generally exhibit adequate growth in height
(HAZ) (except for seven-year-old boys), with mean Z-scores very close to
0, indicating no detectable problem with chronic long-term undernutri-

tion. On the other hand, mean Z-scores for weight-for-age (WAZ), body mass index (BMIZ), and triceps skinfold (TRICZ) indicate a problem with overweight and fatness.

Girls' growth appears much more variable than boys'. HAZ, in particular, is below the mean for ages seven to nine, suggesting chronic undernutrition may be a problem for some of these girls. Weight (WAZ) is closer to the mean, except for ten-year-old girls, who also exhibit height, triceps skinfolds and body mass indices well above the mean. Whether or not this is sample bias, catch-up growth, or some other phenomenon, including early maturity for some girls, cannot be determined since these are cross-sectional data.

Since both overnutrition and undernutrition are suggested by mean Z-score data, the percentage of children falling below the 15th and 5th percentiles[9] of height (low height and very low height or stunting), and above

TABLE 2.   Z-scores for Height-For-Age (HAZ), Weight-For-Age (WAZ), Triceps (TRICZ) Skinfold and Body-Mass Index (BMIZ)

Age	N	HAZ	WAZ	TRICZ	BMIZ
			Boys		
7	5	−0.89	−0.09	1.05	0.58
		(1.18)	(1.38)	(1.24)	(1.50)
8	5	−0.02	0.58[a]	0.85	0.72
		(1.19)	(0.74)	(0.65)	(0.94)
9	11	0.17	0.84[a]	1.15[a]	0.96
		(0.97)	(1.49)	(1.30)	(1.56)
10	9	0.04[b]	0.66	0.65	0.67
		(1.27)	(1.27)	(1.04)	(1.27)
11	11	0.01	0.69	0.73	0.64
		(0.88)	(1.42)	(1.56)	(1.20)
			Girls		
7	3	−0.64	−0.16	0.13	0.23
		(1.34)	(1.00)	(1.12)	(1.25)
8	10	−0.88	−0.39[a]	0.12	0.07
		(1.03)	(0.99)	(0.85)	(0.87)
9	12	−0.47	−0.12[a]	0.23[a]	0.09
		(1.05)	(0.98)	(1.17)	(0.97)
10	15	0.92[b]	1.10	1.26	0.89
		(0.77)	(1.22)	(0.97)	(1.29)
11	6	0.67	0.35	0.24	−0.13
		(0.73)	(0.38)	(0.38)	(0.43)

[a]Significant difference between boys and girls at $p \leq .10$
[b]Significant difference between boys and girls at $p \leq .05$

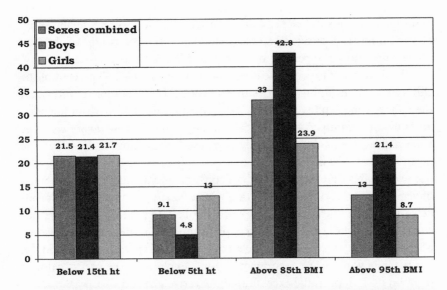

Fig. 1. Percentage of children who are undernourished (based on height-for-age) and overnourished (based on body mass index) percentiles

the 85th and 95th percentiles of BMI (overweight and very overweight or obesity) were calculated (fig. 1). Again, we find contrasting patterns. There is an excess of low-height children with 21.4 percent of boys and 21.7 percent of girls below the 15th percentile; but stunting, or height below the 5th percentile, appears to be problematic only for girls at 13 percent compared to boys at 4.8 percent.

On the other hand, overnutrition is quite prevalent among these children and is more apparent for boys than girls; 42.8 percent of boys and 23.9 percent of girls are at or above the 85th percentile of BMI, with 21.4 percent of boys but only 8.7 percent of girls at or above the 95th. This figure indicates very high levels of overnutrition in these children. Why this should be so in the context of poverty requires explanation.

Searching for that explanation, I evaluated the diets of these children. Dietary data were gathered over the course of a year in four 24-hour recalls, allowing for seasonality and day-of-week variation.[10] Data were analyzed with Nutritionist IV software (N-Square Computing 1993). Mean levels of many nutrients as percentages of RDAs (Recommended Daily Allowances established by the Food and Nutrition Board of the

National Academy of Sciences) are reported in table 3. Again, means often obscure important variation so I also calculated the percentage of children above and below 100 percent recommended RDA for the nutrients.

While mean caloric intake is not much above RDAs, 50 percent of the children are consuming calories in excess of RDA recommendations. At the same time, many children are consuming below recommended amounts of vitamins A and B-6, calcium, and zinc. But *we do not consume nutrients, we consume food.* Analysis of food consumption data (i.e., the mean number of daily food exchanges compared to USDA recommendations) indicates that Bridges children consume highly insufficient amounts of vegetables and fruit and moderately insufficient amounts of dairy products. These insufficiencies, along with the fact that most grains are not consumed as whole grains, could explain the dietary deficiencies of some micronutrients. Also, children are consuming servings of meat and fat foods far beyond RDA recommendations, explaining the excess calories from fat and, in part, the excess rates of overweight and obesity.[11]

Thus far, we have seen that children in this high poverty area of eastern Kentucky exhibit malnutrition. The excess stunting among girls cannot be explained by these data, since stunting is a long-term problem, beginning much earlier in life than can be accounted for here. What is intriguing, however, is a lower level of dietary intake of zinc in girls than boys (mean for girls is 82.3 compared to 93.3 for boys, and 72.4 percent of girls have zinc intake less than 100 percent RDA compared to 66.7 percent of boys). If this dietary deficiency is a long-term problem, it may help explain the greater prevalence of low height in girls (see, for example, Walravens, Krebs, and Hambidge 1983).

Malnutrition in terms of overnutrition is better explained by these data and may be a consequence of dietary quality, at least in part. In another paper (Crooks 1996), I presented data on variation within the population with respect to diet and socioeconomic status. Data in that paper indicate that poor children exhibit lower levels of most nutrients compared to nonpoor children, and that poor children exhibit dietary intake of micronutrients below RDA recommendations for vitamins A and B-6, calcium, and zinc. Taken together, those data plus the data presented here speak to the complexity of the effects of poverty on the growth and nutritional status of school-age children. Within a single, generally poor community, we have evidence of both stunting and overweight. We also have evidence of poor dietary quality that is probably related to socioeconomic status and poverty level.

Discussion

Although, as this and other studies indicate, the consequences of poverty for child growth are varied, child growth is a proven protocol for assessing child well-being. It is consistently used by U.S. anthropologists in the developing world, but has been less often used in the United States. The reason for this has not been adequately addressed, but it may be that anthropologists, who tend to employ the technique, are more likely to work outside the United States than within its borders. Or, since the majority of poor children in the United States are not suffering the kind of acute undernutrition that often prompts action and research in other countries, most Americans simply do not recognize that nutrition and health problems in the United States are severe enough to warrant their attention (Huston, McLoyd, and Coll 1994).

But our attention is warranted. Many poor children in the United States suffer consequences to growth and nutrition. The data presented here indicate malnutrition in various forms—undernutrition, overnutrition, and micronutrient deficiencies. These may be related to the quantity of food and the pattern of foods consumed. But we know little about why children are consuming the foods they consume, and this is where a political-economic perspective is so very important. Macro-level processes are linked to local-level circumstances that may constrain the ability of house-

TABLE 3. Mean Values for Daily Intake of Various Nutrients as Percentage of RDAs

	Boys			Girls		
	Mean	% Below RDA	% Above RDA	Mean	% Below RDA	% Above RDA
Calories	107.6	32.0	68.0	101.8	65.6	34.5
Protein	302.5	8.0	92.0	251.8	3.4	96.6
Vitamin A	125.4	52.0	48.0	132.7	34.5	65.5
Vitamin B-1	136.4	16.0	84.0	127.3	37.9	62.1
Vitamin B-2	168.7	16.0	84.0	157.1	20.7	79.3
Vitamin B-3	190.9	20.0	80.0	149.3	31.0	69.0
Vitamin B-6	113.4	56.0	44.0	102.8	58.6	41.4
Vitamin B-12	327.9	4.0	96.0	266.2	6.9	93.1
Vitamin C	186.2	28.0	72.0	188.2	24.1	75.9
Iron	132.9	20.0	80.0	108.3	44.8	55.2
Calcium	97.3	52.0	48.0	111.3	62.1	37.9
Zinc	93.3	66.7	33.3	82.3	72.4	27.6

holds to provide adequately for their children's well-being. A number of recent publications document the difficulties poor families experience in providing adequate nutrition for their children (Damio and Cohen 1990; Curtis and McClellan 1995; North Carolina Childhood Hunger Project 1995). For example, Curtis and McLellan (1995) argue that this is due to increased costs relative to wages and benefits and reductions in amount and eligibility for food assistance. The safety-net programs established in the late 1960s during the War on Poverty have worn thin, and a serious erosion of benefits to families and children occurred during the 1980s. Many children are falling through holes in the net.

Added to this, "supermarket flight" (i.e., to the suburbs) during the late 1970s and early 1980s left many poor inner-city and rural people no choice but to shop at smaller grocery stores where prices may be higher and food quality lower (Public Voice 1988; Curtis and McLellan 1995). Therefore, even with AFDC, Food Stamps, School Meals, and other food-related programs, and despite complex strategies for managing housing, medical, food, and other costs of everyday living, many American families must rely on lower-cost, poorer-quality foods to get by. Many run out of food well before the end of the month. This could produce both undernutrition and overnutrition as seen among Bridges children.

The research continues at Bridges Elementary School. The linkages between poverty and child growth await exploration, but for this, we need to move beyond the school to individual households and then to the community at large. Future research hopes to look at how families make decisions concerning allocation of resources for food versus rent, utilities, medical expenses, and so on; where families purchase food and why; what foods are available at the most-frequented places of purchase; what other resources for food are available to families; and which are being used and why.

I recognize that the research presented here is primarily descriptive, but it is only the first step in understanding the biocultural consequences of poverty for child growth. While it may lack methodological depth from a political-economic perspective, this is not from lack of realization of the importance of this perspective. Although Stack (1974), Leacock (1971), and others showed us over twenty years ago that understanding the complexity of poverty requires attention to individual and household strategies devised to deal with the varied and changing circumstances of poverty in everyday life, biological anthropologists are just coming to that realization. The challenge now is to find ways to combine quantitative and qualitative techniques with statistical and ethnographic methodologies to better understand the paths by which upstream processes affect local and household-level behaviors and the consequences thereof. Williams (1992) argues that a true understanding of poverty, its causes and consequences, requires contextualization of large-scale quantitative data with cultural-historical research, "looking at actual, rather than hypothetical neighbor-hoods" (168). Biological anthropologists can take this as a challenge to present a historically constituted and situationally specific "biology of poverty."[12] While, as a discipline, we are not there yet, we are beginning to formulate research strategies that may answer the challenge.

NOTES

Many people contributed to this research in various ways. I want to thank the children, parents, teachers, and staff of Bridges Elementary School for participating in the research. Thanks especially to the principal and director of the Family Resource Center, two individuals who are strongly committed to improving the lives of the children of Bridges Elementary School. This research was accomplished with the help of a grant from the National Institute of Child Health and Human Development, National Institutes of Health, #F32 HD07620. Thank you to Alan Goodman and Tom Leatherman for including my work in this volume and to Mary K. Anglin and Alan Goodman for thoughtful comments and editorial assistance on the manuscript.

1. In 1992, the poverty rate for families with children was 17 percent, while the rate for families headed by single mothers was 46 percent. This is not to suggest that single mothers are incompetent providers for their families, nor that single mother–headed families are a cause of child poverty. Rather, changes in "traditional" family structure may be a consequence of poverty, not a cause (see, for example, Zinn 1989).

2. This comes from the anthropological writings of Oscar Lewis, e.g., in Lewis (1966).

3. Bridges County is a pseudonym used to protect confidentiality. In addition, statistics quoted for Bridges County will be approximations and citations may not be provided where doing so would breach confidentiality.

4. ARC's ranking (as severely distressed, distressed, middle, strong, and very strong) is based on measures of unemployment, per capita income, and poverty rate, each compared to the national rate (Couto 1994).

5. Couto (1994, 44) defines "mature" economies as those "with little prospect for [the] growth in domestic demand . . . those that are resource-based and labor-intensive . . . sensitive to product substitution, e.g., oil for coal or plastic for wood."

6. To be eligible for the free lunch, children must come from families whose income does not exceed 130 percent of the federal poverty guidelines; for a reduced-price lunch, income is not to exceed 185 percent.

7. Height is a cumulative measure of growth. Thus, height deficit, compared to a population reference (usually the National Center for Health Statistics or NCHS), is an accepted marker of long-term, chronic undernutrition. Weight, although cumulative as well, is much more labile, being subject to short-term fluctuations in diet and health. It is an easy measure to collect, but its interpretation is dependent on its relationship to height. Therefore, body mass index (ht/wt^2) is often used as a measure of body composition and proportion. Triceps skinfold is a measure of body fat stores.

8. Z-scores provide a standardized measure allowing for the examination of growth measurements on a population basis. For example, growth scores for height can be aggregated across age and gender groups to determine the population group mean. Z-scores can also allow examination of the research sample's growth compared to that of another population. Thus, the standard practice is to compute the research sample's Z-scores using the means and standard deviations provided by the National Center for Health Statistics (NCHS) and the National Health Examination Survey (NHANES). In this way, the sample's growth can be readily compared to that of the overall U.S. population.

9. Again, these percentiles are those of the reference population, as calculated from NCHS and NHANES data.

10. People may eat differently on weekends compared to weekdays, and many foods are seasonal in availability or consumption patterns. Therefore, the standard practice is to collect daily dietary intake data from both weekends and weekdays and at various times during the year to capture this variation.

11. Overweight and obesity cannot be fully accounted for by diet; activity plays a large part. However, I do not have activity data at this time.

12. I am indebted to R. Brooke Thomas for introducing me to this concept, one in which he urges biological anthropologists to move beyond our standard research protocols, to "broaden the scope of data collection into a richer array of social variables, and to interpret these data with regard to the biological and social consequences of inequities" (Thomas, this vol., chap. 2).

REFERENCES

Allen, L. H. 1990. Functional Indicators and Outcomes of Undernutrition. *J. Nutr.* 120:924–32.

Bandini, L. G., and W. H. Dietz. 1992. Myths about Childhood Obesity. *Pediatric Annals* 21:647–52.

Billings, D. 1974. Culture and Poverty in Appalachia: A Theoretical Discussion and Empirical Analysis. *Social Forces* 53:315–23.

Billings, D. B., M. B. Pudup, and A. L. Waller. 1995. Taking Exception with Exceptionalism: The Emergence and Transformation of Historical Studies of Appalachia. In *Appalachia in the Making: The Mountain South in the Nineteenth Century,* ed. M. B. Pudup, D. B. Billings, and A. L. Walker, 1–49. Chapel Hill: University of North Carolina Press.

Brenner, J., R. Coles, A. Mermann, M. J. E. Senn, C. Walwyn, and R. Wheeler. 1967. *Children in Mississippi: A Report to the Field Foundation.* New York: Field Foundation.

Brown, J. L., and D. Allen. 1988. Hunger in America. *Ann. Rev. Public Health* 9:503–26.

Brown, J. L., and S. N. Gershoff. 1989. The Paradox of Hunger and Economic Prosperity in America. *J. Public Health Policy* 10:425–43.

Buzina, R., C. J. Bates, J. van der Beek, G. Brubacher, R. K. Chandra, L. Hallberg, J. Heseker, W. Mertz, K. Pietrzik, E. Pollitt, A. Pradilla, K. Suboticanec, H. H. Sandstead, W. Schalch, G. B. Spurr, and J. Westenhofer. 1989. Workshop on Functional Significance of Mild-to-Moderate Malnutrition. *Am. J. Clin. Nutr.* 50:172–76.

Caudill, H. 1962. *Night Comes to the Cumberlands: A Biography of a Depressed Area.* Boston: Little, Brown.

Centers for Disease Control. 1990. Anthro Software for Calculating Pediatric Anthropometry, Version 1.01. Atlanta: U.S. Department of Health and Human Services, Public Health Service, Centers for Disease Control.

Couto, R. A. 1994. *An American Challenge: A Report on Economic Trends and Social Issues in Appalachia.* Dubuque: Kendall/Hunt.

Crooks, D. L. 1993. Nutritional Status of U.S. Children. Poster presented at the annual meetings of the American Anthropological Association, Washington, DC.

Crooks, D. L. 1995. American Children at Risk: Poverty and Its Consequences for Children's Health, Growth and School Achievement. *Yrbk. Phys. Anthropol.* 38:57–86.

Crooks, D. L. 1996. Dietary Quality among Poor Appalachian School Children: A Question of Food Security? *Communicator* 19:5–8.

Curtis, K. A., and S. McClellan. 1995. Falling through the Safety Net: Poverty, Food Assistance and Shopping Constraints in an American City. *Urban Anthropology* 24:93–135.

Damio, G., and L. Cohen. 1990. *Policy Report of the Hartford Community Childhood Hunger Identification Project.* Hartford, CT: Hispanic Health Council.

Dietz, W. H. 1994. Critical Periods in Childhood for the Development of Obesity. *Am. J. Clin. Nutr.* 59:955–59.

Dorsey, L. C. 1991. The Rural Child. *J. Health Care for Poor and Underserved* 2:76–84.

Eller, R. D. 1994. *Kentucky's Distressed Communities: A Report on Poverty in Appalachian Kentucky.* Lexington: Appalachian Center, University of Kentucky.

Fisher, S. 1993a. National Economic Renewal Programs and Their Implications for Appalachia and the South. In *Communities in Economic Crisis: Appalachia and the South,* ed. J. Gaventa, B. E. Smith, and A. Willingham, 263–78. Philadelphia: Temple University Press.

Fisher, S. L. 1993b. *Fighting Back in Appalachia: Traditions of Resistance and Change.* Philadelphia: Temple University Press.

Frisancho, A. R. 1990. *Anthropometric Standards for the Assessment of Growth and Nutritional Status.* Ann Arbor: The University of Michigan Press.

Garbarino, J. 1992. The Meaning of Poverty in the World of Children. *Am. Behav. Sci.* 35:220–37.

Gaventa, J., B. E. Smith, and A. Willingham. 1993a. Toward a New Debate: Development, Democracy, and Dignity. In *Communities in Economic Crisis: Appalachia and the South,* ed. J. Gaventa, B. E. Smith, and A. Willingham, 279–91. Philadelphia: Temple University Press.

Gaventa, J., B. E. Smith, and A. Willingham, eds. 1993b. *Communities in Economic Crisis: Appalachia and the South.* Philadelphia: Temple University Press.

Gortmaker, S. L., A. Must, J. M. Perrin, A. M. Sobol, and W. H. Dietz. 1993. Social and Economic Consequences of Overweight in Adolescence and Young Adulthood. *N. Engl. J. Med.* 329:1008–12.

Grantham-McGregor, S. 1984. Chronic Undernutrition and Cognitive Abilities. *Hum. Nutr.: Clin. Nutr.* 38C:83–94.

Greenwood, M. R. C., P. R. Johnson, R. J. Karp, P. G. Wolman, J. Hurley, and E. Snyder. 1993. Obesity in Disadvantaged Children. In *Malnourished Children in the United States: Caught in the Cycle of Poverty,* ed. R. J. Karp, 115–29. New York: Springer.

Huss-Ashmore, R., and F. E. Johnston. 1985. Bioanthropological Research in Developing Countries. *Ann. Rev. Anthropol.* 14:475–528.

Huston, A. C., V. C. McLoyd, and C. G. Coll. 1994. Children and Poverty: Issues in Contemporary Research. *Child Dev.* 65:275–82.

Johnston, F. E., and S. M. Low. 1995. *Children of the Urban Poor: The Sociocultural Environment of Growth, Development, and Malnutrition in Guatemala City.* Boulder: Westview.

Kanarek, R. B., and R. Marks-Kaufman. 1991. *Nutrition and Behavior: New Perspectives.* New York: Van Nostrand Reinhold.

Karp, R., R. Martin, R. Sewell, J. Manni, and A. Heller. 1992. Growth and Academic Achievement in Inner-City Kindergarten Children. *Clin. Pediatrics* 31:336–40.

Kelly, R. F., and S. H. Ramsey. 1991. Poverty, Children and Public Policies: The Need for Diversity in Programs and Research. *J. Fam. Issues* 12:388–403.

Leacock, E. B. 1971. *The Culture of Poverty: A Critique.* New York: Simon and Schuster.

Lewis, O. 1966. The Culture of Poverty. *Scientific American* 215:19–25.

Martorell, R. 1995. Results and Implications of the INCAP Follow-up Study. *J. Nutr.* 125:1127S–38S.

N-Square Computing. 1993. *Nutritionist IV: Diet Analysis and Nutritional Evaluation,* Version 3.0. Salem, Oregon: N-Square Computing.

North Carolina Childhood Hunger Project. 1995. *Hidden Hunger: The Face of Hunger among Families and Children in North Carolina.* Chapel Hill: Department of Nutrition, School of Public Health, University of North Carolina.

Poppendieck, J. 1995. Hunger in America: Typification and Response. In *Eating*

Agendas: Food and Nutrition as Social Problems, ed. D. Maurer and J. Sobol, 11–34. New York: Aldine de Gruyter.

Public Voice. 1988. *Patterns of Risk: The Nutritional Status of the Rural Poor.* Washington DC: Public Voice.

Schell, L. M. 1986. Community Health Assessment through Physical Anthropology: Auxological Epidemiology. *Human Organization* 45:321–27.

Schorr, A. L. 1992. Ending Poverty: The Children's Hour. *Am. Behav. Sci.* 35:332–39.

Segal, E. A. 1991. The Juvenilization of Poverty in the 1980s. *Social Work* 36:454–57.

Sewell, T. E., V. D. Price, and R. J. Karp. 1993. The Ecology of Poverty, Undernutrition, and Learning Failure. In *Malnourished Children in the United States: Caught in the Cycle of Poverty,* ed. R. J. Karp, 24–30. New York: Springer.

Smeeding, T. M. 1992. Why the U.S. Antipoverty System Doesn't Work Very Well. *Challenge* (Jan./Feb.): 30–35.

Smeeding, T. M., and B. B. Torrey. 1988. Poor Children in Rich Countries. *Science* 242:873–77.

Spurr, G. B. 1983. Nutritional Status and Physical Work Capacity. *Yrbk. Phys. Anthropol.* 26:1–35.

Stack, C. B. 1974. *All Our Kin: Strategies for Survival in a Black Community.* New York: Harper and Row.

U.S. Bureau of the Census. (various dates). *Current Population Reports.* Washington, DC: U.S. Government Printing Office.

U.S. Department of Health, Education, and Welfare. 1972. *Ten-State Nutrition Survey 1968–1970.* DHEW Publication No. (HSM)72–8134. Atlanta: Centers for Disease Control.

Walravens, P. A., N. F. Krebs, and K. M. Hambidge. 1983. Linear Growth of Low Income Preschool Children Receiving a Zinc Supplement. *Am. J. Clin. Nutr.* 38:195–201.

Webber, L. S., V. Osganian, R. V. Luepker, H. A. Feldman, E. J. Stone, J. P. Elder, C. L. Perry, P. R. Nader, G. S. Parcel, S. L. Broyles, and S. M. McKinlay. 1995. Cardiovascular Risk Factors among Third Grade Children in Four Regions of the United States: The Catch Study. *Am. J. Epidemiol.* 141:428–39.

Weller, J. 1965. *Yesterday's People.* Lexington: University of Kentucky Press.

Williams, B. 1992. Poverty among African Americans in the Urban United States. *Human Organization* 51:164–74.

Wilson, D. M., L. D. Hammer, P. M. Duncan, S. M. Dornbusch, P. L. Ritter, R. L. Hintz, R. T. Gross, and R. G. Rosenfeld. 1986. Growth and Intellectual Development. *Pediatrics* 78:646–50.

Zinn, M. B. 1989. Family, Race and Poverty in the Eighties. *Signs* 14:856–74.

PART 4

*Steps toward a Critical
Biological Anthropology*

Chapter 15

Race, Racism, and Anthropology

George J. Armelagos and Alan H. Goodman

Race, a core concept in anthropology since its inception, has managed to resist any agreed-upon and repeatable definition (Brace 1982a; Molnar 1975). Rather, this most chameleon-like concept manages to blend into changing social and intellectual environments. With remarkable resilience, race, which originated as a typological and nonevolutionary folk taxonomy, became a scientifically recognized unit of evolutionary change. Yet, questions about race remain. Despite efforts to fit race into evolutionary thinking, is race still no more than a pre-Darwinian typological concept? Whatever we think of race, is it an effective pedagogic tool for teaching human variation? Is it the best unit of analysis for sampling and explaining variation in human populations? Does the scientific use of race reinforce its pseudoscientific misuse, fostering racism? What alternatives exist for describing and analyzing human variation?

These are some of the questions we wish to explore in the following chapter. We first examine the history of the race concept, and challenges that have emerged, both political and scientific, against the continuity of this chameleon-like concept. This simple task raises fundamental questions about the biological utility of race and the social, political, and economic factors that influence conceptions of human difference and similarity. We next outline how the concept of race is currently used in teaching and research. Race, we conclude, has failed to work as a core anthropological concept; it fails to describe and explain variation. What race does do, and does well, is type individuals, and this typing supports the existing structures of power. The last goal is to consider the history of abandoning the race concept, and, as a consequence, the avoidance of concern for the biological and social cost of racism.

This chapter is part of a book on political-economic perspectives in biological anthropology because the history of race so clearly and centrally illustrates the role of sociopolitical forces in the origin, adoption, and persistence of ideas. We suggest that a new biocultural anthropology should include sophisticated understanding of the history of concepts. Furthermore, a new area of biocultural collaboration involves the determination of the social and biological costs of racism.

Race: A Brief History of the Idea

Two basic assumptions limited how human variation was viewed before Darwinism. The biological world was assumed to be the result of special creation, and all life was static and immutable. Since race was divinely ordained, human variability was easily explained. Furthermore, races, as with all animate and inanimate objects, were ranked. Since the time of Aristotle, the *scala naturae* was a generally accepted concept in which all natural objects were arranged in an upward progression, and the *scala naturae* became temporalized in the concept of the "Great Chain of Being" (Lovejoy 1936). The distinctness of racial types was self-evident, as was the fact that races varied in organic complexity and their position relative to God (Eiseley 1968).

Carolus Linnaeus was one of the first scientists to develop a systematic classification of all living things. His racial classification reflected contemporary European folk ideas of the time, as seen in his inclusion of feral and monstrous races, which were then widely believed to exist, and his combining of social and biological characteristics to classify races. While Linnaeus felt that his classification reflected divine creation, in retrospect it reified and lent scientific weight to popular and politically useful ideas about human differences.[1]

In 1749 George Buffon began the process of formalizing the race concept and placing it on a more objective basis (Greene 1959, 181). Writing in a period during which the central question was whether the races had a monogenic or polygenic origin (Greene 1959; Harris 1968), Buffon was more concerned with racial origins than mere classification. Polygenists, who included the French intellectual F. M. A. de Voltaire, and American physical anthropologists, such as S. G. Morton, J. C. Nott, and G. R. Gliddon, believed in the multiple origins of races, thus supporting the notion that the races were actually separate species and providing a justification for slavery. Monogenists derived all races from a single origin (Adam and Eve). Not unexpectedly, the inequality of the races was accepted by both groups, but for different reasons. Polygenists explained racial difference by divine intent, while the monogenists claimed it resulted from degeneration from the original creation.

Later in the eighteenth century Blumenbach developed a fivefold classification (Black [Negro], Brown [Malayan], White [Caucasian], Yellow [Asian], and Red [American Indian]). Whereas his classification was based on biological characteristics alone, this did not prevent him from using racial differences to explain differences in cultural development. For example, as the original Caucasian race expanded into new regions, it was exposed to environmental and cultural factors that caused a degeneration eventually leading to the formation of new races. Degeneration explained the development of racial differences, and racial differences explained cultural development (Greene 1959, 223). Skin color, facial form, and head shape were measured to assess the degree of degeneration. This interpretation conformed to the ranking of races in the "Great Chain of Being."

Two key intellectual events, the development of the theory of natural selection (Darwin 1859) and the development of the synthetic theory of genetic evolution (Fisher 1930; Haldane 1932), should have challenged the continued use of race by providing an explanation for variation as due to evolutionary forces. However, without substantial change, race was incorporated into post-Darwinist, evolutionary paradigms. While some argued that race became thoroughly reinvented from a folk taxonomy to an evolutionary concept (for example, see Brues 1993), we have argued that the typological concept remained typological and incompatible with evolutionary and adaptive theory (Goodman and Hammonds, ms.). Lewin echoes this point: "inequality of races—with blacks on the bottom and whites on the top—was explained away as the natural order of things: before 1859 as the product of God's creation, and after 1859 as the product of natural selection" (1989, 3). Moreover, the rapidity with which scientists in such diverse fields as medicine, anthropology, education, sociology, and paleontology lent support to "proven" racial inferiority shows that racism was an integral part of the intellectual climate (Haller 1971, x–xi).

Two trends followed the development of evolutionary theory. First, there was an intensive search for racial traits that could be measured and quantified. Boas, as early as 1904, states that the major efforts of biological anthropologists were directed toward racial classification and searching for traits, such as the cephalic index, that could define them.[2] As the synthetic theory of genetic evolution developed, the search for racial traits switched from morphology to genetic polymorphisms. One of the strategies for dealing with race in light of natural selection was a search for nonadaptive traits. If the genetic traits were nonadaptive and linked to a specific racial group, their frequency would remain stable except for admixture with other racial groups. Theoretically, nonadaptive traits could be used to establish the racial history of a group (Hooton 1926, 1946).

Earnest Hooton trained many of the anthropologists that played a role in the development of modern physical anthropology. Hooton (1946) and Coon (1962, 1965) perpetuated the polygenetic view that dominated the work of Morton (1839, 1844, 1847) and Nott and Gliddon (1854) a century earlier (see Brace 1982a, 1982b; Harris 1968). Hooton's and Coon's concept of polygenesis was incarnated in a polyphyletic model of raciation that rejected the origin of race from separate species, but recognized a differential transformation of various races as they evolved from *Homo erectus* to *Homo sapiens* in various regions of the world (Brace 1982a, 1982b).

Aleš Hrdlička, as the founder and first editor of the *American Journal of Physical Anthropology,* a leading force in the founding of the American Association of Physical Anthropologists, and curator of physical anthropology at the Smithsonian Institution, was America's preeminent physical anthropologist of his generation (Blakey 1987). As such, he was frequently called upon to interpret the significance of issues related to human variability and race. Blakey (1987) shows that by 1918, Hrdlička expressed concern about the rudimentary state of racial studies. Eventually, Hrdlička would support the premise that social differences between human groups were the result of racial characteristics that reflect the limits of their evolution (Blakey 1987, 10). Blakey quotes Hrdlička (1927, 208–9) who says, "The real problem of the American Negro lies in his brain, and it would seem, therefore, that this organ above all others would have received scientific attention." In commenting on this period, Marshall (1968, 160) surmises that: "Historically, both scientific and lay concepts of race have served to support the economic and political privileges of ruling groups who regard themselves as superior by virtue of phylogenetic heritage rather than because of accidents of culture history."

Among influential anthropologists, only Franz Boas seemed to swim against the tide of racism (Boas 1940; also see Williams 1996).[3] First, he criticized the most basic aspect of the typology of race and attacked the assumption that the average represented the ideal. He believed these averages were abstractions that obscured reality and the extensive variability that existed in racial groups. Second, he argued against the fixity of races and demonstrated that one of the most cherished racial traits, the cephalic index, was influenced by the environment; individuals born in the United States had a significantly different cephalic index than their siblings born in Europe (Boas 1911). Since the cephalic index was a key racial trait, Boas's results were a severe blow to the belief in the immutability of race. Third, Boas criticized studies that linked race to character. Boas developed a strong antievolutionary stance that was a response to the established view that cultural development (evolution) was due to race (Harris 1968; Blakey 1987). Parenthetically, this antievolutionism grew to become one of the most influential forces in anthropology and is also a factor in the current biocultural split. By the 1940s, as a reaction to the rise of Nazism and racism in Germany, the scientific community began to support Boas's criticisms of linking character to race (Blakey 1987). Barkan (1992) and Littlefield and co-workers (1982) argue that the declining use of race in anthropology after World War II was prompted by political and social factors. Barkan suggests that the inclusion of outsiders (i.e., Jewish intellectuals and liberals) in anthropology was important in leading to a greater concern for egalitarianism. Whatever the motivation, scientific racism was questioned, but the race concept sailed on.

In William C. Boyd's influential *Genetics and the Races of Man* (1950) he argued that racial classification should be based on traits of known inheritance. He believed the reliance on morphological features of living and skeletal populations was misguided since they were subject to environmental influence. The blood types were mathematically manipulable, objective, and insulated from environmental influence. Boyd's genetic approach became the preferred method of racial classification. Blood types became the primary tool for describing race, even when they failed to comply with expectations and even when the blood types were suspected of undergoing selective change (Kelso and Armelagos 1963; Otten 1967).

Interestingly, in 1950 Coon, Garn, and Birdsell also published *Races: A Study of the Problem of Racial Formation in Man* and in this short book they tried to explain races as separate products of evolution and adaptation to different environments. Thus, at the same time, race was reinvented as both a result of nonadaptive genetic change and conversely as a result of selection to continental environments. This tension remains below the surface today, secondary to the greater problem that race does not fit either reformulation. In the following section we address why race does not work as an evolutionary unit and some of the political-economic factors that appear to support its persistence despite its scientific flaws.

Criticisms of Racial Analysis

Since the 1960s there has been a continued stream of challenges to the scientific validity and utility of the race concept (see, for example, Armelagos 1968; Brace 1964a, 1964b, 1982a; Goodman 1995; Gould 1977; Livingstone 1962; Marks 1995; Reynolds and Lieberman 1996; Wolf 1994). Critics raise a variety of objections. One of the earliest was race's contribution to racism. As Crick (1996) has said, if race is not a sufficient cause of racism, it is a necessary cause. In addition to scientific critique of the idea of race, particularly the notion of fixed and hierarchically arranged types, Boas (1911, 1940) suggested that the idea of race contributed to racism.

A related criticism is that racial data are often misapplied by racists. Many who accept the concept of race do not accept this as a sufficient reason for rejecting the scientific study of race; to do so would politicize the scientific process. Carleton Coon, for example, maintained that he had no responsibilities to the misapplication of his ideas on the separate evolution of races. Pat Shipman (1994) maintains this line of thinking and extends it to current debates over the "biology of violence." For Shipman there is a clear distinction between doing science (seeking truth) and its application, which scientists cannot control. However, the history of race is a prime example of the fact that politics is embedded in science; there is no science before politics. In the following chapter Blakey makes the radical suggestion for a type of science that acknowledges from the outset its ethical and political obligations (this vol., chap. 16).

But the "case against race" is not for sociopolitical reasons alone, contra Brues (1993); it is not just a politically correct stance. As Begley (1995) aptly writes in *Newsweek* on criticisms of race: scientists got there first. A fundamental scientific critique centers on the subjective nature of the classifications. If race is a valid scientific concept, any individual using acceptable procedures should be able to construct a racial classification that could be replicated by another individual using the same criteria. In a highly reflective statement Boas (1940, 173) suggests what is key to racial classification depends largely on the previous experience of the observer, not upon the morphological value of the observed traits. This explains the diversities of opinions in taxonomic classification. Following this reasoning, an argument can be made that racial classifications are social constructs that use biological traits in their classifications. While the use of biological traits provides an impression that race is a natural unit, it remains a cultural construct using biological descriptors. Classifications inform us more about society that they do about groups being classified.

Indeed, a number of examples exist of how racial classifications have been socially manipulated. Anderson (1962) describes how the Lapps, a European population, were classified as Mongoloids, following Blumenbach, even though there is little evidence of a direct biological relationship between the groups. Solomon (1965) describes how New Englanders, who are now classified as belonging to the same racial group, were initially separated into distinct races for political purposes (Marshall 1968). Irish immigrants were initially classified as Celts and thus separated from the Yankees, who dominated the economic and political power of the region and were classified as Anglo-Saxons. After the Irish gained political power, they were incorporated into the dominant racial group, and the new immigrants from the southern Mediterranean region were classified as a separate race. By a somewhat similar process, Jews became white folks in the United States after World War II (Sacks 1994). Blakey (this vol., chap. 16; 1988) notes how genetically similar members of the Nanticoke-Moors self-identified as either African American or Native American.

Racial categorization in Brazil relies on biological traits such as skin color and hair form, but the classification is also influenced by markers of socioeconomic status (Harris 1964). Thus, two individuals who have the same phenotype can be placed in different racial groups if they belong to different socioeconomic classes. Economic success whitens. Márquez (this vol., chap. 9) reports on a similar process governing social divisions in Mexico City in the nineteenth century.

Harris (1964) describes the principle of hypodescent. In North America an individual who is of "mixed racial heritage" is always placed in the race that is considered lower socioeconomically, regardless of the extent of the racial admixture. In the vernacular of the time, one "drop of Negro blood" makes an individual a Negro. Obviously, these social rules have great consequence for the use of race as a biological unit.

Livingstone (1962) recognized a tautology: traits or genes used to define a population as a race become identified as racial markers. The occurrence of such racial markers in a population is considered sufficient evidence for characterizing the racial identity of the group. For example, sickle cell gene was initially defined as a "Negro trait." If the sickle cell gene was found in a population, it was evidence that there was Negroid admixture. The higher the frequency of sickle cell trait, the greater the degree of admixture. Sadly, the racial explanation obscured the relationship between sickle cell gene and its selective advantage in a malarial environment.

Early studies showed that sickle cell anemia was exclusively found in Blacks. The discovery of sickle cell anemia in whites, rather than challenging the established knowledge that sickling was a racial disease of the black body, sanctioned the questioning of the racial purity of whites (Tapper 1995). As late as 1943, Ogden (1943, 178) summarizes:

> The problem of whether this condition is confined to the Negro race or may occur in members of white and yellow races without admixture of Negro blood is not yet satisfactorily solved. However, . . . I have a right to my strong convictions that the sickling trait is a condition found in the Negro race only [and] that all cases in which members of white families have such a trait . . . [is evidence that] an admixture of Negro blood has taken place. . . . It can be concluded that all white persons with sickle cell anemia . . . have been persons of Mediterranean origin (Greeks, Italians, and Spaniards), with the exception of one American family. . . Every living person, if one goes back twenty-four generations, had in the early thirteenth century 16,713,216 ancestors. If one considers this fact, it becomes obvious that it is practically impossible to exclude with any degree of certainty the existence of an admixture of Negro blood in some members of the white race.

Skin color and the ABO blood groups were similarly treated as racial traits. Garn (1961), for example, describes the Diego blood group as "Asiatic" (45) and Tay-Sachs as a probable "Jewish disease" (82). Today the idea of racially distinct diseases has been somewhat superficially replaced by the notion of race as risk factor (Goodman and Hammonds, ms). The problem remains that the definition of the risk group is unrepeatable, and it is rarely known whether the risk is attributable to genetics or lived experiences.

Alternatives have emerged in response to problems with racial analysis that provide a more effective means of understanding variation. Brace (1964b) and Livingstone (1962) argued for a clinal approach that overcomes the limitation of the racial model. Clinal analysis considers variation of a trait in terms of its geographical distribution. It is a more effective means for describing and understanding human variation and does not assume clustering of traits. Returning to the example of sickle cell, Livingstone's (1958) clinal analysis revealed a relationship between sickle cell gene and the occurrence of malaria that was obscured by a racial approach. Race is not the proper unit of study for work on resistance to hypoxic stress any more than it is to a question about cognitive abilities. In the former one might look at such things as the extent of capillary beds and lung volume and in the later infant stimulation, prenatal drug exposure, and parental intelligence. In neither of these examples is race a variable that will do any more than be interpreted in confusing and subjective ways.

Is Race Useful?

> Don't look for the meaning, look for the use.
> —Wittgenstein's Aphorism

Paul Baker (1968, 94) has argued that the case for or against race ought to be based on the concept's utility: "Among human biologists the concept of race has two functions: first as a pedagogic device for teaching human variation and second as a research tool for investigating biological variation." Baker supports the use of race because racial groups are defined by certain traits that cluster, thus becoming templates for describing the variability that exists in their region. For example, a population can be described as having a skin color similar to Africans' and ABO blood frequencies similar to American Indians'. Unfortunately, one will often find descriptions that a population has the "blood of Berbers in the bodies of Bedouins" and the implication is that there is some relationship between the racial groups.

In forensic anthropology, race is still widely used in teaching and research. The reason given for this, even among those who do not hold to the underlying validity of the concept, is that this is what law enforcement agencies require (St. Hoyme and Iscan 1989). Unfortunately, qualification about race seems to infrequently enter into teaching. A quick perusal of France Casting's fall 1992 catalog provides a vivid illustration of this fact.[4]

One skull is labeled in bold capital letters "NEGROID MALE." The description of the skull states that it "illustrates racial traits very well. . . . this is a wonderful cast!" The skull below it is labelled "CAUCASOID FEMALE," and its description is similar: "illustrates racial traits very well. . . . This is in excellent condition!"

Essential information is how well each of these skulls fits the ideal racial type—Negroid and Caucasoid. The orientation of students is not to learning about the discontinuous and nonconcordant nature of human variation. They learn nothing of the complexities of biology. Rather they are sold a comfortingly simple story: there are old and static ideal types and with a minimum of training one can play the game of fitting the crania to the ideal type. In spite of contestations of belief in evolutionary theory, race really has not changed. This is solid typology. Plato would be proud.

It is the forensic anthropologist's goal to provide "bureaucratic race," that which is officially recognized (St. Hoyme and Iscan 1989). But bureaucratic races change, and they may have little to do with biology (Lee 1993). Brues (1993) apparently believes that "just providing race" is scientific and nonpolitical, whereas belief that there are no races is a political statement. However, Lee (1993) cogently makes the opposite argument in documenting the political pressures that go into becoming an "official race" in U.S. national statistics. The "I'm just doing my job" approach is a political statement and suggests strongly that the ideology is accepted from above.

The survey research of Lieberman and colleagues (1989) strongly suggested that belief in the salience of race declined in anthropology up until the mid-1980s. Ironically, this decline, without clear presentation of the dynamics of race and racism, may have left anthropologists unable to respond to potential problems. For example, Rushton (1994) uses race to explain differences in sexual behavior and intelligence. He argues from a model of r/K selection that Blacks are more r selected (read sexual) than whites and orientals (who are more intelligent). This scheme is an example of the amateur evolutionary idea that nature puts energies into either one characteristic or another (see Hoberman 1997). Although Rushton's work is both unscientific and racist, it is amazing that some highly respected physical anthropologists are fascinated by it (Harpending 1996).

Today race is also applied in the cause of a more balanced view of history. For example, race is used to counter a perspective in which civilization is seen to result from the influence of European genes and culture (Bernal 1987, 1991). A counter movement, Afrocentricity, has become such a force that the cover of the September 23, 1991, *Newsweek* poses the question "Was Cleopatra Black?" Unfortunately, while it is important to counter a Eurocentric interpretation of the historical rise of civilizations, resorting to an outmoded concept seems to do little to systematically solve the problem. It is not that we deny African influence, rather, what seems to be salient to us is cultural influence, not genes or race.

The use of race as a research tool is fraught with methodological difficulties. Adams and Covino's (1958) study is typical of a racialist human biology. They were interested in variation in physiological response to cold, and so they sampled seven Negroes, seven Caucasians, and six Eskimos. They concluded that there was a racial difference in response to cold. However, the results can be questioned on a number of points. Do the twenty individuals represent the variation that exists in the three racial groups? Can we generalize from the seven Caucasians to all Caucasians? If the differences are statistically significant, are they biologically meaningful? Are the physiological factors that cause the differences in the response to cold revealed by racial analysis, and are the differences racial?

Two fundamental problems, what we have previously referred to as the "double leap of faith" (Goodman, 1995), repeatedly arise when assuming that the measured racial differences in disease rates, size, physiological function, or other characteristics are biological and can be generalized to a racial propensity or predisposition. First, the environment is rarely controlled for, and thus a condition is assumed to be genetic before the alternatives have been adequately explored. Second, once assumed to be genetic, genetic is equated with pan-racial, that is, the genes are assumed to align with purported races.

Biological anthropologists have had difficulty agreeing on the utility of race, as evidenced in sending a statement on race back to committee (Goodman 1995). However, a report from the Centers for Disease Control and Prevention (CDC) is clearer (MMWR #42, 1993). Among its conclusions are that "because most associations between disease and race have no biological basis, race—as a biological concept—is not useful in public health surveillance" (MMWR 1993, 12). Furthermore, they conclude, racial categories are too broad to be meaningful, there is no clear definition of race, the OMB Directive 15 (which determines racial categories for federal agencies) has no scientific basis, distinctions between race and ethnicity are unclear, concepts of race change over time, and meanings differ among individuals. The CDC report goes further still in its conclusion that emphasis on race in public health reinforces stereotyping and racism and diverts attention from underlying socioeconomic factors (MMWR #42, 1993, 12–13). Somewhat conversely, it maintains that it may be useful to keep race as a social construct and as a means to monitor the health consequences of racism.

Hahn and co-workers (1992) likewise paint a picture of a misapplication of race and ethnicity in infant mortality data. They find that the racial designation of infants who die during their first year frequently changes from birth to death. Mothers who record the racial designation at birth may not be the source of racial determination of the infant at death, and consequently the racial and ethnic identity changes. As a consequence, the infant mortality rates for American Indians may be 46.8 percent higher than reported.

Finally, Navarro (1990) argues that the use of race obscures the reporting of health statistics in the United States. He suggests that the role of class is hidden by reporting health statistics by race (the United States is the only Western developed nation not to collect mortality data by class).[5] For example, in 1988, the difference in life expectancy at birth is 75.5 for Whites and 69.5 for Blacks, and the differential is increasing. Without reporting mortality by class, the cause of this increase is difficult to determine.

Konner (1990) comments that Black men from Harlem are now less likely to survive to their sixty-fifth birthday than men in Bangladesh. While one might assume that it is the homicide (15% excess deaths which is equal to cancer deaths) and drugs (7% excess) that increase mortality, most of the excess is explained by cardiovascular disease.

Where there is evidence of class difference in morbidity, the results are more informative in that one can begin to understand what it is (and isn't) about race that leads to excessive morbidity and mortality. For example, Navarro (1990) reports data on chronic disease by race and economic status and suggests that economic status is more important than race. This does not meant that race and racism are unimportant; rather, Navarro concludes: "If a prerequisite for finding the right answer is to ask the right question, then it is unlikely that by concentrating solely on race differentials we will ever be able to understand why our health indicators for minorities are getting worse" (1240).

Others will still argue that race is useful and often point to forensic research as one area of utility. However, we have shown that misidentifications are likely to be highly common, much more common than proposed (Goodman 1997). The use of race in forensic research has probably led to countless misidentifications. Similarly, the use of race in medical research has likely led to equal proportions of misdiagnoses. Race doesn't work as a research tool because it fails to reflect human variation, because it is ill defined and changing, and because it conflates biology (genes) with lived experience.

Does Anthropology Have an Obligation to Investigate the Cost of Racism?

Unfortunately, regardless of whether anthropologists discarded race as an inappropriate model for understanding human variation or resurrected it to aid in the interpretation of the origins of modern *Homo sapiens,* they seem relatively uninterested in examining the implications of their actions. The molecular biologists, paleontologists, and skeletal biologists who consider only the ease of analysis of race are solid in their lack of interest in the social conception and use of race. Similarly, those who have rejected race as a concept for understanding biological variation have failed to consider its continued use as a social category and the biological and social costs that result from the racism that it perpetuates (Chase 1977; Hacker 1992). While the scientific interest in race has declined because of a more adequate means for understanding human variation, the case can be made for an increased emphasis for teaching about race and racism. The concept of race has been a core concept in anthropology for a long time (Stocking 1968; Wolf 1994), and it will remain a core concept of private discourse for even longer. It is not time to abandon race, but rather to refocus on the dynamics of race and racism (see Mukhopadhyay and Moses 1997). Whereas much of this might seem to be outside of the purview of biological anthropologists, there are many biological consequences that may be explicated. Furthermore, such studies of race and racism that bring together ideological, historical, and political analyses with biological analyses offer a new direction for biocultural studies.

Conclusion

The continued use of race has clear scientific and political-economic implications. Moreover, contra Shipman (1994), the two sets of implications are not separable. As N. W. Pirie (1950) argues:

> Some people think that the philosophy a scientist accepts is not of very much importance; his job is to observe the phenomena. A sensible philosophy controlled by a relevant set of concepts saves so much research time . . . A scientist can have no more valuable skill than the ability to see whether . . . the concepts he is using are applicable.

C. L. Brace (1982a, 12) specifies the problem for physical anthropology:

> ... the assumption that contemporary human variation can be under-
> stood in terms of 'racial variation', despite pointed critiques (Brace
> 1964, Livingstone 1962), sails on without any substantial change from
> the time when Hrdlička and Hooton were shaping the field into its
> subsequently recognizable form. The factors that influenced their
> shaping, then, stem from an earlier era.

Race, according to R. C. Lewontin (1972), explains a bit less than 6
percent of human variation. Given the difficulties with a racial model in
explaining human variation, the time and energy spent during the last 250
years attempting to recast race to deal with these problems of racial analysis suggest that our initiatives should be directed in other areas. The rejection of the racial model should not, however, preclude our interest in
understanding biological and cultural variability. Anthropology was
founded on the core concepts of race, culture, and evolution. While anthropology has transcended race, it can reassert its authority to speak to the
issues related to culture, biology, and evolution. Anthropologists can and
should contribute their knowledge, experience, and skills concerning such
topics as adaptation and its impact on health and disease, as well as the biological and social costs of racism, sexism, ageism, and classism. All of these
should be essential parts of a new biocultural agenda for anthropology.

Anthropology has lost its voice in dealing with many of the issues that
are vital to us (Perry 1992; Weiner 1992). Speaking to this issue as it relates
to multiculturalism, Annette Weiner (1992, B2) maintains: "As multiculturalism controversy has gained increasing public attention, anthropologists have remained silent—perhaps discouraged by the simplistic assumptions about cultural identity promulgated by those on the right and the far
left." Anthropology—as a humanistic perspective and as a biocultural science—should refocus and be poised to meet the issues of the 1990s and the
next century. One old challenge—racism—remains. Will anthropology,
will we as anthropologists, finally respond?

NOTES

This chapter was developed from our prior writing on race and anthropology.
Michael Blakey has particularly influenced our thinking on race, although he is not

to be blamed for any of our limitations. Bryan Byrne and Lynn Sibley commented on a prior version of this chapter.

1. The typology classification included a feral and monstrous race. American Indians (*Homo americanus*) are reddish, choleric, erect, obstinate, merry, free, paints himself with fine red lines and is regulated by customs. Asians (*Homo asiaticus*) are sallow, melancholy, stiff, severe, haughty, and avaricious, have black hair and dark eyes, covered with loose garments and ruled by opinions. Africans (*Homo afer*) are black, phlegmatic, relaxed, crafty, indolent, negligent, have silky hair, flat noses anoints himself with grease and governed by caprice. Europeans (*Homo europaeus*) are white, sanguine, muscular, gentle, acute, inventive, have long flowing hair, blue eyes, are covered with close vestments and governed by law. (Linnaeus from Slotkin 1968, 177–78). Linnaeus was European.

2. To illustrate the racial climate of the period, we need only to refer to the "Anthropology Day" held during the Olympic Games that were part of the 1904 World's Fair in St. Louis. For two days, "wild tribes" were tested against Olympic standards to see how far civilization had come (Carlson 1989, 19). After the World's Fair, Ota Benga, a "pygmy," became a popular attraction at the Bronx Zoo where he was caged with an orangutan (Bradford and Blume 1992; Carlson 1989).

3. Note the use of the qualifier "influential." It is interesting too that Frederick Douglass in the mid-1800s had already developed a clear idea about the problems of race and racial analysis. Du Bois certainly did too. Both of these influential African Americans (and many others of whom we know less today) were essentially ignored by white physicians and scientists.

4. This discussion of France Casting is from Goodman (1995) and Goodman and Armelagos (1996). After a prior draft of this paper was circulated, racial terms were dropped from the catalog. Also see Goodman (1997) for comments on the accuracy of "racing" skeletons.

5. The reliance on race as a variable in health statistics may be a way to deemphasize the class structure of American society and make it appear that the differences are genetic (and pan-racial), and therefore not a function of social and economic inequality or racism.

REFERENCES

Adams T., and B. G. Covino. 1958. Racial Variation to a Standardized Cold Stress. *J. Appl. Physiol.* 12:9–12.

Anderson, Robert T. 1962. Lapp Racial Classification as Scientific Myths. *Anthropological Papers of the University of Alaska* XI:15–31.

Armelagos, George J. 1968. Review of *Readings in Race,* Stanley M. Garn, Springfield, IL: C. C. Thomas. *American Anthropologist* 71:1190–91.

Baker, Paul T. 1968. The Biological Race Concept as a Research Tool. In *Science and the Race Concept,* ed. M. Mead, T. Dobzhansky, E. Tobach, and R. E. Light. New York: Columbia University Press.

Barkan, Elazar. 1992. *The Retreat of Scientific Racism.* Cambridge: Cambridge University Press.

Begley, Sharon. 1995. Three Is Not Enough. *Newsweek,* February 13, 69–71.

Bernal, Martin. 1987. *Black Athena: The Afroasiatic Roots of Civilization,* vol. I. New Brunswick: Rutgers University Press.

Bernal, Martin. 1991. *Black Athena: The Afroasiatic Roots of Civilization,* vol. II. New Brunswick: Rutgers University Press.

Blakey, Michael. 1987. Skull Doctors: Intrinsic Social and Political Bias in the History of American Physical Anthropology with Special Reference to the Work of Aleš Hrdlička. *Critique of Anthropology* 2:7–35.

Blakey, Michael. 1988. Social Policy, Economics, and Demographic Change in Nanticoke-Moor Ethnohistory. *American Journal of Physical Anthropology* 75:493–502.

Blumenbach, J. F. 1969. *On the Natural Varieties of Mankind.* New York: Bergmann. (Translation by T. Bendyshe of the third edition originally in 1795 in Gottinberg.) This translation was originally published for the Anthropological Society of London in 1865.

Boas, Franz. 1911. *Changes in Bodily Form of Descendants of Immigrants.* Final Report. 61st Congress, 2d Session, Senate Document 208. Washington, DC: GPO.

Boas, Franz. 1940. *Race, Language and Culture.* New York: Free Press.

Boyd, W. C. 1950. *Genetics and the Races of Man.* Boston: Little Brown.

Brace, C. Loring. 1964a. On the Race Concept. *Current Anthropology* 4:313–14.

Brace, C. Loring. 1964b. A Nonracial Approach Towards the Understanding of Human Diversity. In *The Concept of Race,* ed. A. Montagu, 103–52. New York: Free Press.

Brace, C. Loring. 1982a. The Roots of the Race Concept in American Physical Anthropology. In *A History of American Physical Anthropology,* ed. Frank Spencer, 11–29. New York: Academic Press.

Brace, C. Loring. 1982b. Comments: Redefined Race: The Potential Demise of a Concept in Physical Anthropology, by A. Littlefield, L. Lieberman, and L. T. Reynolds. *Current Anthropology* 23: 641–47.

Bradford, Phillips Verner, and Harvey Blume. 1992. *Ota Benga: The Pygmy in the Zoo.* New York: St. Martin's Press.

Brues, Alice. 1993. The Objective View of Race. In *Race, Ethnicity, and Applied Bioanthropology,* ed. Claire Gordon, 74–78. NAPA Bulletin #13, American Anthropological Association.

Carlson, Lew. 1989. Giant Patagonians and Hairy Ainu: Anthropology Days at the 1904 St. Louis Olympics. *Journal of American Culture* (fall): 19–26.

Chase, A. 1977. *The Legacy of Malthus: The Social Costs of the New Scientific Racism.* New York: Alfred A. Knopf.

Coon, Carelton S. 1962. *The Origin of Races.* New York: Alfred A. Knopf.

Coon, Carelton S. 1965. *The Living Races of Man.* New York: Alfred A. Knopf.

Coon, Carelton, Stanley Garn, and J. B. Birdsell. 1950. *Races: A Study of the Problem of Race Formation in Man.* Springfield, IL: C. C. Thomas.

Crick, Bernard. 1996. Foreword. In *Race: The History of an Idea in the West,* Ivan Hannaford, xi–xvi. Washington, DC: Woodrow Wilson Center Press.

Darwin, Charles. 1859. *On the Origin of Species by Means of Natural Selection or the Preservation of Favored Races in the Struggle for Life.* London: John Murray.

Edmonson, Munro. 1965. A Measurement of Relative Racial Differences. *Current Anthropology* 6(2): 167–98.

Eiseley, Loren. 1968. Race: The Reflections of a Biological Historian. In *Science and the Concept of Race,* ed. M. Mead, T. Dobzhansky, E. Tobach, and R. E. Light, 80–87. New York: Columbia University Press.

Fisher, R. A. 1930. *The Genetical Theory of Natural Selection.* London: Oxford University Press.

France Casting. 1992. Fall Catalog. Fort Collins, CO: France Casting.

Garn, S. M. 1961. *Human Races.* Springfield, IL: C. C. Thomas.

Goodman, Alan H. 1995. The Problematics of "Race" in Contemporary Biological Anthropology. In *Biological Anthropology: The State of the Science,* ed. N. T. Boas and L. Wolfe, 215–39. Bend, OR: International Institute of Human Evolutionary Research.

Goodman, Alan H. 1997. Bred in the Bone? *Sciences* (March/April): 20–25.

Goodman, Alan H., and George J. Armelagos. 1996. The Resurrection of Race: The Concept of Race in Physical Anthropology in the 1990s. In *Race and Other Miscalculations, Misconceptions and Mismeasures: Papers in Honor of Ashley Montagu,* ed. L. T. Reynolds and L. Lieberman, 174–86. Dix Hill, NY: General Hall Publishers.

Goodman, Alan H., and Evelynn Hammonds. (ms.) Reconciling Race and Human Adaptability: Carleton Coon and the Persistence of Race in Scientific Discourse.

Gould, S. J. 1977. Why We Should Not Name Human Races: A Biological View. In *Ever Since Darwin,* ed. S. J. Gould, 231–36. New York: W. W. Norton.

Greene, John C. 1959. *The Death of Adam.* New York: Mentor.

Hacker, Andrew. 1992. *Two Nations: Black and White, Separate, Hostile, Unequal.* New York: Charles Scribner's Sons.

Hahn, Robert A., Joseph Mulinare, and Steven Teutch. 1992. Inconsistencies in Coding of Race and Ethnicity Between Birth and Death in US Infants. *JAMA* 267:259–63.

Haldane, J. B. S. 1932. *The Causes of Evolution.* London: Longmans, Green.

Haller, John S. 1971. *Outcasts from Evolution.* Urbana: University of Illinois Press.

Harpending, Henry. 1996. Human Biological Diversity. *Evolutionary Anthropology* 4 (3): 99–103.

Harris, Marvin. 1964. *Patterns of Race in the Americas.* New York: Walker.

Harris, Marvin. 1968. *The Rise of Anthropological Theory.* New York: Crowell.

Hoberman, John. 1997. *Darwin's Athletes: How Sports Has Damaged Black America and Preserved the Myth of Race.* New York: Houghton Mifflin.

Hooton, E. A. 1926. Significance of the Term Race. *Science* 63:75–81.

Hooton, E. A. 1946. *Up from the Apes.* New York: Macmillan.

Hrdlička, Aleš. 1927. Anthropology of the American Negro: Historical Notes. *American Journal of Physical Anthropology* 10:205–35.

Kelso, A. J., and George J. Armelagos. 1963. Nutritional Factors as Selective Agencies in the Determination of ABO Blood Group Frequencies. *Southwestern Lore* 29:44–48.

Konner, Melvin. 1990. Still Invisible, and Dying, in Harlem. *New York Times,* Feb. 24.

Lee, S. M. 1993. Racial Classifications in the US Census 1890–1990. *Ethnicity and Racial Studies* 16:75–94.

Lewin, Roger. 1989. *Human Evolution.* Boston: Blackwell Scientific Publications.

Lewontin, R. C. 1972. The Apportionment of Human Diversity. *Evolutionary Biology* 6:381–98.

Lieberman, L., B. W. Stevens, and L. T. Reynolds. 1989. Race and Anthropology: A Core Concept Without Consensus. *Anthropology and Education Quarterly* 2:67–73.

Littlefield, A., L. Lieberman, and L. T. Reynolds. 1982. Redefined Race: The Potential Demise of a Concept in Physical Anthropology. *Current Anthropology* 23: 641–47.

Livingstone, Frank B. 1958. Anthropological Implications of Sickle Cell Gene Distribution in West Africa. *American Anthropologist* 60:533–60.

Livingstone, Frank B. 1962. On the Non-existence of Human Races. *Current Anthropology* 3:279–81.

Lovejoy, A. O. 1936. *The Great Chain of Being.* Cambridge: Harvard University Press.

Marks, Jonathan. 1995. *Human Biodiversity.* Chicago: Aldine.

Marshall, Gloria. 1968. Racial Classifications: Popular and Scientific. In *Science and the Concept of Race,* ed. M. Mead, T. Dobzhansky, E. Tobach, and R. E. Light, 149–64. New York: Columbia University Press.

MMWR/Centers for Disease Control. 1993. The Use of Race and Ethnicity in Public Health Surveillance: Summary for the CDC/AT[SDR] Workshop 42:1–17.

Molnar, Stephen. 1975. *Race, Types and Ethnic Groups.* Engelwood Cliffs, NJ: Prentice Hall.

Morton, S. G. 1839. *Crania Americana.* Philadelphia: Dobson.

Morton, S. G. 1844. *Crania Aegyptica.* Philadelphia: Penington.

Morton, S. G. 1847. Hybridity in Animals, Considered in Reference to the Unity of the Human Species. *American Journal of Science* (series 2) 3:39–50, 203–12.

Mukhopadhyay, Carol, and Yolanda Moses. 1997. Reestablishing "Race" in Anthropological Discourse. *American Anthropologist* 99:517–33.

Navarro, Vicente. 1990. Race or Class Versus Race and Class. *Lancet* 17:1238–40.

Newman, Marshall T. 1963. Geographic and Microgeographic Races. *Current Anthropology* 4:189–92.

Nott, J. C., and G. R. Gliddon, eds. 1854. *Types of Mankind.* Philadelphia: Lippincott, Grambo.

Ogden, M. A. 1943. Sickle Cell Anemia in the White Race. *Arch. Int. Med.* 71(1): 164–82.

Otten, Charlotte. 1967. On Pestilence, Diet, Natural Selection, and the Distribution of Microbial and Human Blood Group Antigens and Antibodies. *Current Anthropology* 8:209–26.

Perry, Richard J. 1992. Why Do Multiculturalists Ignore Anthropologists? *Chronicle of Higher Education,* March 4, A52.

Pirie, N. W. 1950. Concept Out of Context: Pied Pipers of Science. *British Journal of Philosophical Sciences* 2:269–80.

Reynolds, Larry T., and Leonard Lieberman, eds. 1996. *Race and Other Miscalculations, Misconceptions and Mismeasures: Papers in Honor of Ashley Montagu.* Dix Hill, NY: General Hall Publishers.

Rushton, J. P. 1994. *Race, Evolution and Behavior: A Life History Perspective.* New Brunswick, NJ: Transactions.

Sacks, Karen. 1994. How Did Jews Became White Folks? In *Race,* ed. Steven Gregory and Roger Sanjek, 78–102. New Brunswick, NJ: Rutgers University Press.

St. Hoyme, L. E., and M. Y. Iscan. 1989. Determination of Sex and Race: Accuracy and Assumptions. In *Reconstruction of Life from the Skeleton,* ed. M. Y. Iscan and K. A. R. Kennedy, 53–93. New York: Alan R. Liss.

Shipman, Pat. 1994. *The Evolution of Racism.* New York: Simon and Schuster.

Slotkin, J. 1968. *Readings in Early Anthropology.* Chicago: University of Chicago Press.

Solomon, Barbara. 1956. *Ancestors and Immigrants.* Cambridge: Harvard University Press.

Stocking, George W., Jr. 1968. *Race, Culture and Evolution: Essays in the History of Anthropology.* New York: Free Press.

Tapper, Mel. 1995. Interrogating Bodies: Medico-Racial Knowledge, Politics and the Study of a Disease. *Comparative Study of Society and History* 1:76–93.

Weiner, Annette. 1992. Anthropology's Lesson for Cultural Diversity. *Chronicle of Higher Education,* July 22, B1–2.

Williams, Vernon J. 1996. *Rethinking Race: Franz Boas and His Contemporaries.* Lexington: University of Kentucky Press.

Wolf, Eric R. 1994. Perilous Ideas: Race, Culture, People. *Current Anthropology* 1:1–11.

Chapter 16

Beyond European Enlightenment: Toward a Critical and Humanistic Human Biology

Michael L. Blakey

With an examination of the history and ideological influences of physical anthropology, this chapter sets out to make four points: (1) studies of the biology of human populations have been consistently influenced by political ideologies; (2) the historical tendency toward the use of naturalistic explanations has often supported apologetic programs (while cultural and social determinism have been preferred explanations among societal critics); (3) a critical, social scientific approach to human population biology is advocated as one that best contributes to exposing the causes and biological effects of societal problems; and (4) publicly engaged and activist approaches to science further elevate the critical capacity and social significance of anthropological research, while promoting a qualitative transformation of our understanding of biology toward a more humanistic way of knowing. A critical and humanistic approach to biological anthropology is proposed. Examples are given of historical demographic, psychophysiological, and bioarchaeological studies that contain elements of the proposed program and show some of the intellectual and societal encounters that have informed my conclusions.

Epistemology

The fundamental premise of the perspective developed here is that science is inextricably cultural. If biological anthropology is understood and practiced as a component of a subjective cultural institution (science), then it might be transformed even further from the feudal religious epistemology from which the sciences have evolved since the Enlightenment. Biological

379

anthropology might become a more critical science that reveals and explores its social and political influences with one hand, while raising a critical mirror to the broader society with the other.

What we are now confronting is the prospect of a way of knowing that takes its "culturalness" seriously, and in so doing simultaneously recognizes both the limits of objectivity and the value of subjectivity. A science that does not ignore or deny its culturalness in order to reify its command of universal truth is freed to self-consciously apply subjective, yet realistic cultural lenses to the universe. Those interpretations may not be adequate for understanding all things at all times for all people. But with a critical science we would become more consciously aware of why that is so, and more aware of the subjective conditions that have guided interpretation.

There is a paradox of science and ideology that bothers and excites me, because it points to a fundamental inadequacy of positivism as resolved by critical science. It has been argued that science should be dislodged from ideology according to the notion of a strict dichotomy between science and ideology. Religious ideologies, from which science evolved, constitute prime examples. Ideological knowledge is characterized by faith in dogma (as dogmatic, closed, and capable of obscuring reality). Science, on the other hand, is characterized by self-critical approaches to objective knowledge (as self-critical, open-ended, and capable of producing real knowledge). This is not an uncommon characterization of differences between science and religion. The dichotomy has been adhered to even by some "critical theorists" (Leone et al. 1986). Yet, paradoxically, scientific knowledge is replete with unnoticed assumptions, closed to critique precisely when they appear most objectively and self-evidently real (the long-standing idea that craniometry could assess human "mentality" is an example of an untenable assumption of extensive international research that was seldom questioned for more than a century). In other words, the more objectively or consensually true a fact appears to be, the less one is likely to be critical of it. One could say that adherence to positivism itself is ideological, if nonetheless scientific, because there is no method for observing whether the facts accumulated today will remain true in the potentially boundless future. The pursuit of "real" knowledge (as objective truth) and self-criticism/open-endedness are partly contradictory.

Ideology and scientific knowledge do have commonalities. After all, they are historically intertwined. When the scientific facts conform to popular ideology (conventional wisdom) one's critical facilities are deeply impaired. Theories, biological and otherwise, that conform to dominant political ideologies compel methods for organizing data so that they will make sense in that theory's particular terms. By creating information consistent with the ideology in which the theory is embedded, research results can appear to be most real (objective) when they are most ideological (dogmatic).

Enlightenment natural historians showed, whether by their own intuition or the insistence of the church, a synthesis of Christian and scientific ideas (and a heritage of ancient Greek philosophy and political ideology). The tenacity of concepts of fixity and ranking (exemplified by Linnaeus, Lamarck, and Morton) during the emergence of natural history exemplifies just such retentions. These cosmologies competed under the impetus of social change, bringing about a current, vital institutionalization of a way of knowing based on the systematic *interpretation* of material evidence: science.

Christianity, of course, also has continued to evolve, and the questions it shares with anthropology continue to be important ones. I am suggesting here that the appeal of excessive naturalism in "Western science," although materialistic, is also partly rooted in prescientific European ideas regarding the preeminence of external agency in human affairs. Within that materialistic or scientific development, there has been (for the past 150 years) a struggle between nature and nurture approaches in anthropology and other social and biological sciences. Excessive naturalism is ideologically similar to the earlier feudal Christian view of life's phenomena as god-given.

This use of nature extends far beyond and precedes that of religion. Aristotle's *Politics* is a pre-Christian example in which he argues, tautologically, for a natural order of slavery and male domination; an argument which he explicitly uses to resolve the morally uncomfortable contradiction between inequitable practices and a belief in the "virtue" of elite Hellenic men. In every case, naturalism resolves contradictions between morality and practice.

"Naturalism," as it is used here, refers to any interpretation in which phenomena are attributed to natural causes as distinct from human decision making. This usage essentially expands upon the definition of biological determinism to encompass ecological and evolutionary explanations of human social life as well as sexual, racial, and genetic determinism. Previously, naturalism in the service of ideology has been referred to as the nature politic (Blakey 1991, 1996). The nurture view, emphasizing the sway of culture over biology, presents greater opportunities for a more derived, humanistic, and critical biology.

Naturalism as it informs empirical method shows the human element in data analysis as contaminating, deviating from ultimate truth. Culture, therefore, becomes a thing to be purged (or denied) in apprehension of legitimate truth. Natural science is viewed as objective, hard science. Social science is regarded as less objective and is popularly disregarded by many as not science at all. Thus, a natural science of humanity would appear to be the ideal anthropology (as Wilson 1975 and sociobiologists point out).

The proper order of human life according to this view is to be found outside human society. Whether the method is belief in gospel or systematic evidence, religion and natural science obtain an allure of being able to reveal knowledge derived from beyond human agency. The scientist, or holy man, hopes to be perceived as a vehicle rather than creator in conveying his knowledge of the influences of the extrahuman (spiritual or natural) universe of facts upon a human world.

The confounding of natural science theory with an objectified nature, so common in Western society, appears to neglect the observation that people modify nature in both theory and practice. (1) Natural science theory is as much a product of culture as is social science theory and religious philosophy. Each has a social history, and this is often intertwined (as with the interrelated influences of Malthus's political economy, Darwin's natural history, Spencer's sociology, and E. O. Wilson's zoology, in modern evolutionary theory). (2) Nature is constructed conceptually as it is explained. (3) Cultural evolution has brought about increasing modification of material nature by humans. Nature is being transformed into culture (as symbol, technology, energy, and food).

There are similarities in the ways we create nature through theory and the ways in which the supernatural has been created. Edward Tylor argued that humanity created God in its own image. In *Primitive Culture* (1871) Tylor wrote: "Among nation after nation it is still clear how, man being the type of deity, human society and government became the model on which divine society and government were shaped."

The same can be said of Morton's (Gould 1981) and Hrdlička's (Blakey 1987) craniometric ranking of race, Herbert Spencer's social Darwinist views, Thomas Hobbes's characterization of primitive people, Malthus's explanation of natural economy, and Aristotle's natural social order: each invokes a convenient view of a familiar, contemporary social order to explain the natural order. Thus, the social order is naturalized. Each explains human inequity as 'nature given.' (Of interest here is the observation that, while much of evolutionary theory was acceptable to them, Soviet scientists tended to reject the Malthusian aspect of natural selection both for reasons of the seeming limitlessness of the habitable land about them, and its contradiction to a socialistic way of life [Todes 1989].) In sum, scientific knowledge can be viewed as a branch of ideology.

The demystification of science may be as useful as the demystification of religion. If one does not question the unquestionable, one gains a sense of externalized control and command of objective, authoritative knowledge at the expense of our comprehension of the cultural assumptions and political agenda that create that knowledge.

A belief in materialism and reliance upon systematic evidence, minimally distinguishes science. But when these means are applied to apprehend objective facts, immutably true, they are apt to do so in the limited sense of asserting a fact beyond question—especially when these facts complement one's sociopolitical assumptions and experiences.

Fundamental questions that science has raised regarding religious dogma have not been equally applied to itself. Those who raise such questions, such as Feyerabend (1978) or Gould (1981), risk accusations equivalent to heresy. At the moment one believes oneself to have obtained an objective fact, immutable to the whims of time and place, that fact is relegated to the most powerful body of assumptions, which both lay beyond serious question and frame future knowledge. Reproducible results (such as was proposed by the old craniometry) can be false because of a form of mystification that claims objective knowledge.

The argument being made here, however, is that competition between scientists ascribing to diverse paradigms and theories, associated with varied sociocultural experiences and political camps, is often what brings about criticism that makes science change. Yet even Thomas Kuhn (1970) tellingly disregards broad social and political forces at work on science in examining paradigmatic competition as internal discussion among scholars. He severs its cultural innervations. The fact that the physical sciences constitute Kuhn's main frame of reference might make those connections less obvious than in the sciences of society (while the obviousness of links between physics and militarism should not be underestimated). Postmodernist critiques are often equally ahistorical, apolitical, and nonsociological. Even important critical theorists cling to the proposition that critical demystification will lead to real, unconditional, and objective knowledge. Perhaps it can. But the observed historical record of biological anthropology, among other sciences, shows us that we can expect only *differently* conditional knowledge. There is no method for observing otherwise. No one sits in the "Restaurant at the End of the Universe" to attest to evidence of a single fact that is immutable to change throughout all time and space. Social historians of science such as Allen (1975), Bernal (1987), Blakey (1987, 1996), Drake (1980), and Gould (1981), document a record of changing, ideologically loaded, scientific truths.

Emergence of a Dilemma

Biological anthropologists did not hesitate to study urban industrial populations during the first half of the twentieth century. Those using evolutionary and racial approaches such as Hrdlička, Hooton, and Coon were producers of apologetic explanations for the status quo of economic inequality, racial oppression, and imperialism. Eugenics was viewed as the comprehensive application of mainstream evolutionary and racial studies in the United States and Europe (Blakey 1987, 1991, 1996). These were not mad, renegade, or peripheral pseudoscientists. These were leading representatives of mainstream American anthropology practicing the scientific method with all its intrinsic subjectivity.

Franz Boas, in opposition to the mainstream, emphasized biological plasticity in immigrants and the biological and social influences of acculturation. He too was biased, despite his empiricism, by the integrationist politics of his youth in Germany and by his experience as a German and American Jew at a time when that community was oppressed, making the mainstream's racial hierarchies seem counterintuitive. His students and those he had influenced elaborated upon the Boasian antiracist tradition from the 1930s onward, when such liberal and antifascist views began to capture the imagination of the American public. The German Nazi application of eugenics made clearer the fallacies and implications of excessive naturalism (Blakey 1987; Drake 1980; Glick 1982; Herskovits 1953; Stocking 1976, 1–54).

Marginalized African-American antiracist scientists and critiques of biological determinism (from Frederick Douglass in the nineteenth century to W. Montague Cobb in the twentieth century) similarly stressed the influences of culture on biology. The specific aspects of culture on which these scholars focused, however, were social and economic differences, analyses that bolstered the application of their knowledge to the development of an ideology of human and civil rights struggle and a call for policy correctives (Rankin-Hill and Blakey 1994). Of course, members of every social group have taken up perspectives on virtually every side of most issues. But I argue that social and ethnic categories, nonetheless, are as relevant to scientific perspectives as they are to the political and other social tendencies with which such groups are closely associated in American life.

Racial determinism surrendered to the liberal environmentalists after World War II, albeit only conditionally. The condition in this case is the retention of an emphasis upon naturalism, in keeping with the continuing belief that making nature an ultimate cause made a research program more scientific. Yet in order to maintain the emphasis on nature, many major populations and applications were ignored. While racial hierarchy and determinism were rejected (and genetic determinism became greatly contested), the continuing adherence to dogmatic naturalism pressed the human ecologists of the 1960s and 1970s to seek out extreme environments (high altitude, deserts, etc.) and seemingly isolated, traditional cultures where natural science theories had the most explanatory power. Physical anthropology, which had initially included vital (though deeply troubled) research in the urban industrial world, stripped of racial evolutionary explanations and eugenic applications in the post–World War II era, fled the social conditions of the United States in order to study its naturalistic *theories.* There is little evidence that the most significant social and biological problems of the species were a research priority.

Since the 1960s, physical anthropological knowledge, while becoming no less apologetic, did become less relevant to human problem solving. While adhering to principles of naturalism, biological anthropology appears to have dealt directly with less and less of human society because the natural domain of human life was more narrowly defined during the postwar period. Viewed in this way, the solution to waning relevancy could either involve expanding again upon the range of natural dominion as has been occurring through sociobiology and other excesses of naturalism, or the development of a more humanistic and social theoretical approach to understanding human biology in which human agency and social structures derived from it become the causative foci. The following discussion addresses advantages of the latter alternative.

Critical Examination and Construction of Theory

A humanistic science is one in which scientists as people take responsibility for their explanations of a universe (biological or otherwise) in which humans influence their own affairs. Such a science assumes, therefore, that its practitioners and the rest of society share responsibility for the world they help create. This responsibility is for more than (but includes) professionalism and honesty. They also need to take responsibility for understanding the interpretive influences of their own cultural values and political motivations, influencing the results and applications of research. It should be considerate of the humane and humanitarian sensibilities. A humanistic biology is necessarily critical and reflective, rational and holistic. The observation that anthropology is fundamentally cultural and subjective, and that its knowledge results from human decision making rather than a reality external to human decision making, underscores the idea that we are responsible for our explanations whether or not this is acknowledged.

As pointed out earlier, excessive naturalism seems designed to disavow human responsibility for the production of knowledge in the name of objectivity. Simultaneously, excessively naturalistic explanations of human society abdicate societal responsibility for human problems. A *humanistic* science focusing on secular human agency stands, therefore, in opposition to naturalism. Taking its assumptions seriously, a humanistic biological anthropology should contend openly with its subjectivity, on the one hand, and should foster the development of theories that examine the accountability of society for its own biological variations, on the other. The application of systematic evidence in pursuit of explanation is no less required of such a science and, indeed, may be enhanced by the reduced mystification inherent in objectification and its paradoxical relationship to self-criticism.

A humanistic approach is a theory of theory. It provides assumptions for a more critically acute approach to developing and choosing the subjects, theories, methods, and interpretations of data. This approach should not be confused with other strains of critique and reflexivity. As mentioned earlier, the rubric of "critical theory" has been applied to epistemologically and politically diverse approaches. Humanistic science, the brand of critical theory for which I have argued, requires the following. With regard to any body of theory, one must, I think:

   a. Acknowledge and examine its social and institutional history.

   b. De-emphasize immutability of truth; all assumptions are operational and open to questioning.

   c. Seek cultural and institutional diversity of perspective. Balance or "democratic participation" of voices in an ever-developing discussion of facts partly substitutes for "objectivity." The participants in the discussion should include both scholars and representatives of public interests (not only governmental and elite funding organizations, as it exists today, but the people impacted by scientific research).

   d. Acknowledge and examine the sociopolitical vantage point of any approach. Such biases are not necessarily simplistically rightist or leftist, but are often composites of socially and politically loaded assumptions, meanings, and implications.

   e. Reconcile any approach with one's accepted cultural values, and explicate them. These values might, as examples, include a belief in human equality and social equity, self-determination and social responsibility, pluralism, individualism, progress, or their opposites. What one chooses to study and how one studies it are influenced by such values.

The "Statement to the Profession" of the Panel on Disorders of Industrial Societies organized by the American Anthropological Association and the Wenner-Gren Foundation (Forman 1994) proposes a similar program, which is meant to be applicable to all subdisciplines of anthropology. Social theories of human biological and health variation (prominently including political economy) appear to have the greatest potential for implementing all of the principles of a humanistic approach, in direct opposition to the principles on which naturalism rests. Yet, political-economic approaches vary greatly in theory and politic.

To take critical theory to its logical extension is to entertain the possibility of an epistemological species of science as different from modern science as modern science is different from theology. Nothing could be more exciting, or more predictable in view of the accelerating pace of cultural evolution. Perhaps what is needed is an emphatically social science of human biology, one that acknowledges its subjectivity and which is self-consciously critical. (Contrast this with the sociobiologist's natural science of human society.) Ultimately such a sociological approach (not to be confused with the discipline) should not be expected to stand alone, but will enhance the dialectical arena of knowledge that is currently so heavily skewed toward the tendencies of natural determinism and objectivism. Once liberating, relative to theology and the feudal order in which religion operated as hegemonic ideology (see Levins and Lewontin 1993), these tendencies of positivism now stand as an obstacle in the way of epistemological evolution and social change.

The biology I am espousing has a legacy in some of the ideas of Ashley Montagu, Montague Cobb, Franz Boas, W. E. B. Du Bois, and Frederick Douglass. In "Claims of the Negro Ethnologically Considered" (1854) Frederick Douglass speaks of the "effect of circumstances upon the physical man," stating that "a man is worked upon by what *he* works on. He may carve out his circumstances, but his circumstances will carve him out as well." He goes on: "I told a boot maker, in New Castle on Tyne, that I had been a plantation slave. He said I must pardon him; but he could not believe it; no plantation laborer ever had a instep. He said he had noticed, that the coal heavers and work people in low condition had, for the most part, flat feet, and that he could tell by the shape of the feet, whether a man's parents were in high or low condition." More poignantly, of occupation he writes, "The right arm of the blacksmith is said to be larger and stronger than his left." Douglass then proceeds to discuss similarities of the social behavior and physical appearance of impoverished Irish laborers and enslaved African Americans, and shows differences among Anglo-Americans occurring "even in one generation" depending on their "climate and habit" (304–5).

He also recognized the political embeddedness of American anthropology at its origin. His theory of a dialectical relationship between "circumstances" and "physical man" was used in the context of a nature–nurture debate on the works of Morton and Agassiz who, like Aristotle in the Hellenic twilight, proposed a natural legitimation of slavery on its last legs. Douglass recognized that both the craniometry and Egyptology of his time were for the legitimation of slavery. His alternative approach to scholarship sought not neutrality, but a human position for science. Douglass speaks of the "common nature" and "wants" of all humankind as a "common basis" of "human rights" (307). As a critical approach, he claimed that scholars, like other civic leaders, should take responsibility for their ideas; that claims of scientific neutrality were fatuous, "ignoble," and "cowardly" (1854, 289). Douglass is thus at the origins of the African-American tradition of scholar activism later seen in Du Bois's and Cobb's anthropology, presaging publicly engaged anthropology. Although Douglass acknowledges his limitations as a nonscientist, his treatise, by virtue of its date and clarity of thought, is ahead of Boas and Marx on these issues. It has nearly all of the elements from which to develop the scientific approach that I am seeking to advance.

Further, Douglass makes a practical decision about which aspects of causality (and by extension, application) to pursue. Writing about both social and natural ecological "circumstances," Douglass concludes, "If a cause, full and adequate, can be found here, *why seek further?*" (306). I take this to mean that if well-documented social causes of social and health problems have been identified, one should focus on their solution rather than search incessantly for genetic or racial influences which, even if found, are often unlikely to explain more than a tiny fraction of the variation being considered. Recent research on population differences in essential hypertension, IQ, and criminal behavior is a case in point. Heavy investment in a naturalistic agenda dulls acknowledgment of well-established data on social causes and impedes the creation of policies and programs meant to solve these social problems today as in the past.

An emphasis on social and economic causality might be preferred also, because social and economic variables are directly subject to human decision making and therefore may be altered comprehensively along with their biological effects by *social policy.* I have also considered that nature is increasingly being brought under human social control, for better and worse. A society is left with a responsibility for finding solutions to its biological problems. This brand of biology, therefore, becomes a source of systematic societal criticism, rather than apology. It seeks change, tests it applications, and invites criticism and revision more than (and differently from) positivism. By example, the following studies show important sociological influences on the formation of biocultural research on living, historical, and archaeological populations involving a variety of methods. Each case represents specific subject matter and methods that other researchers might gainfully extend and amplify. These cases also show epistemological problem solving or processes of thinking critically and humanistically about scientific research in general.

Examples

The following are examples of the relationship of my own research to the program I have described. Through these examples I hope to show ways in which a research program has evolved through influences of theory, data, public concerns, sociocultural perspectives, politics, and funding. I acknowledge that these studies have been brought under the framework of critical biology in only an embryonic sense.

The study of the social history and ideology of physical anthropology (Blakey 1987, 1996; Rankin-Hill and Blakey 1994), archaeology, and museology (Blakey 1983, 1990) has powerfully influenced the research I conducted between 1978 and the present. While science history and philosophy might seem a logical and affectively distanced means of assessing the potential implications of one's choice of research direction, political understandings were clearly brought to that critical historiography from the beginning.

My approach to these studies developed during the course of graduate study in physical anthropology at the University of Massachusetts, Amherst, when I urged classmates and faculty to think about them and was informed by those dialogues in constructive ways. The assumptions, problems, and ideas that started me on that path, however, were informed by the critical African-American intellectual tradition of vindicationist (see Drake 1980) and activist scholarship learned previously as a Howard University student. The societal problems (and optimism about their solutions) grappled with during the Civil Rights era, along with persistent encounters with academic racism, greatly impressed me at that juncture. I sought an approach to the study of humankind that would be as effective in correcting problems of social inequity as I knew anthropology had been in creating them. The three examples that follow include research in historical demography, social psychophysiology, and bioarchaeology.

Nanticoke-Moor Historical Demography: Political Economy, Critique, and Cultural Vantage.   The Nanticoke-Moors consist of currently segmented communities on the Delmarva Peninsula of the eastern United States, which had been a single community during the early nineteenth century. They are descended from refugee Africans, disaffected Western Europeans, and the refugee native Nanticoke whose community they integrated during the eighteenth century. Colonialism, genocide, and slavery initially brought refugees of diverse ethnic backgrounds together under the umbrella of the Nanticoke, who defined their ethnicity in cultural rather than biological terms.

What, I asked, had brought about subsequent segmentation of the community and what were the demographic effects of that segmentation? A departure from naturalism seemed justified, since "studies of the processes of biocultural change have tended to emphasize relationships between populations and the natural ecology, and the adaptive role of culture. Yet as culture and technology have evolved to create an increasingly elaborate and effective interface between humankind and the natural ecology, the sociocultural arrangements themselves have become increasingly independent of natural constraints and prominent among the conditions directly influencing human social and biological responses" (Blakey 1988, 493–94). The study would focus on community responses to historical political and economic changes, and their demographic effects.

Their local church was, as in many old rural communities, the central public institution. Each Nanticoke-Moor community had its own church, and a school (grades 1–8) and cemetery associated with the church. The study involved ethnohistorical research and a demographic analysis of cemetery headstone data from three Nanticoke-Moor communities. These had once been a single community, and nearly everyone in the three groups had familial or consanguineal ties to the other groups.

The Nanticoke-Moors of the original Indian River Community in Sussex County, Delaware, had begun to prosper during the mid–nineteenth century. They had accumulated large tracts of land and were profiting from agriculture and small retail and crab-packing businesses. At least two individuals were considered among the most wealthy landholders in the county (Porter 1978). These events precipitated envy and fear among local Euro-Americans who used the available legal means to redefine the group as "Negro" according to the rule of hypodescent (the "one drop" theory) (Fisher 1895). The Nanticoke-Moors also believed that their first church was burned by local whites during the 1860s to force them to integrate within mainstream African-American communities. During the period of Jim Crow segregation, the state school system and the national Methodist Conference attempted to squeeze the Nanticoke-Moors into the "colored" educational and religious institutions (Weslager 1943).

As a result, some Nanticoke-Moors incorporated as Indians, denied consanguineal relations with African ancestors, and rejected sharing churches with African Americans with whom they had worshiped since the period of slavery. They became prejudiced against African Americans and their own relatives who associated with African Americans. These were the means of preserving their autonomy and Indian identity under the racist climate and policies that extended from the mid–nineteenth until the mid–twentieth centuries. Their autonomy, however, would cost them access to state institutions and the growing agribusiness and industrial economy. A family farming economy (which did not require a post–eighth grade education in a segregated black school) persisted to the point of their economic underdevelopment. Infant mortality rose and life expectancy persistently declined for seventy years.

Other Nanticoke-Moors seemed less emphatic about protecting Indian identity at the expense of African-American associations. They continued to share a church (African Methodist Episcopal) and school with mainstream African Americans. Although initially a separate, endogamous group, they gradually increased intermarriage with blacks, often attended African-American high schools and colleges, and became incorporated into the growing wage labor agricultural and industrial economies. There was no evidence of growing infant mortality, and life expectancy increased consistently, even above that for Euro-Americans and African Americans. As low-pigmented, African-American acculturated Nanticoke-Moors, they had the advantage of becoming part of an advantaged caste of African Americans. Their employment opportunities in the white-controlled economy were greater than for many other black Delawareans. And they were viewed alternately with denigrating prejudice, envy, and elevated status among mainstream African Americans whose culture was deeply influenced by criteria of social status that were honed in the white supremacist society they had negotiated historically. This group's life expectancy increased throughout the late nineteenth and twentieth centuries.

Previous research (Porter 1978) attributed migration and economic problems in the Indian River community to adherence to traditional Nanticoke customs regarding hunting territory and to the natural limitations of the marginal land to which they had taken refuge during the colonial period. These factors should be considered, but Nanticoke-Moor history and demography cannot be adequately understood without considering their responses to the force of racist policies during a period of economic transformation.

This analysis departed significantly from most earlier research on the Nanticoke for reasons that could be tied directly to racial attitudes among anthropologists and Nanticoke-Moors, and to my own social background and political interests. Previous ethnographies by Babcock (1899), Weslager (1943), and Porter (1978) were biased due to the same racial problems that had brought about the community's segmentation in the first place. They each sought the advice and support of different generations of chiefs of the Indian River community. The chiefs denied the existing familial and historical connections between their community and the other communities that I have analyzed as Nanticoke-Moors. The chiefs were seeking to define themselves as Indian under the rule of hypodescent, and the anthropologists were interested in studying Indians (the study of African Americans was of little interest to cultural anthropologists) in accordance with the hypodescent rule. Indeed, Frank Speck (see Weslager 1943) introduced Western Native American craft production to the Nanticoke in an effort to help revitalize them as a traditional people (read "real Indians").

On the other hand, I had intimate knowledge of the extent of the community and some of its social divisions. These were my maternal kin. I knew, as my genealogical research would confirm, that a broad spectrum of communities were related to the Indian River group, and I expanded the unit of analysis to include them. The sociological and biological issues of my analysis are far less visible under the assumption that only one community constitutes the real unit of analysis. A general interest in the impact of racism and political economy constitutes a bias that opened some windows and closed others on my view of their history. Indeed, my analysis was intuitive and acceptable for some individuals among the various segments, but was rejected by the current chief, the third chief in his lineage and a person to whom I had familial ties. I had originally expected, given the strength of their motivation to be separate from blacks, that the Indian River community had achieved the highest physical quality of life by separating from their African-American affiliated kin. In the end I felt that I had exposed some of the reasons why their approach to ethnic maintenance has had negative demographic consequences instead.

The dearth of physical anthropological research on the Nanticoke-Moors and similar groups throughout the eastern seaboard United States had been explained to me by T. Dale Stewart, a senior physical anthropologist at the Smithsonian Institution (personal communication, 1979). Apparently, biological research concerning what were then called "trihybrid" populations had become associated with racism and eugenics, causing physical anthropologists to avoid them altogether. Obviously, I believed that studying them differently was a better solution. Clearly, racial politics and social backgrounds played important roles in all of these analyses or the lack thereof.

The London Stress Study: Political Economy, Critique, and Cultural Vantage. As previously discussed, biological anthropologists had turned away from studies of contemporary urban industrial populations because racism and eugenics had become clearly associated with naturalistic explanations in those settings (Blakey 1987, 1994a, 1994b). In an effort to construct alternative theory for the study of the health effects of social psychophysiological stress (beginning in 1978) in England and the United States, Marxist political economic and liberal human adaptability approaches were combined with an emphasis on racial discrimination.

The study's results showed that class and income differences brought about the conditions of anomie, frustrated social role and goal fulfillment, frequency and severity of stressful life events, sensed insecurity, low self-esteem, and hopelessness that produced the highest average rates of stress effects in the poorest segments of a population. There appeared to be no more comprehensive stressor than unemployment. Racial discrimination in Britain and the United States accounted for disproportionately low income among the Black British and African Americans. A host of affective moods and disorders were attributed to those stressors, as were differences in blood pressure, hypertension, and other stress-related organic diseases (Blakey 1985, 1994a).

This description of the problem (with the exception of the role of racial discrimination) is not much different from studies of socioeconomic status, social instability status, and stress-related disease being conducted by many epidemiologists at that time. Political economy, in my view, is operationalized in the analysis of how and why those social and economic differences were being perpetuated. An analysis of capitalism showed that these inequities functioned to maintain profit in the hands of a few at the expense of working (and unemployed) people.

These social and economic relations are intrinsic to capitalistic societies. And while some individuals and even ethnic groups can achieve social and economic mobility, the conditions under which blacks must seek mobility are weighted against their achievement by racist discrimination.

The alternative, liberal, biocultural approaches to stress research also seemed problematic (Blakey 1994b). Biological anthropologists were, during the 1970s and 1980s, beginning to return to Western industrial population studies using "modernization" theory. They were also using homeo-static models of physiological adaptation to explain biological differences among "modernizing" populations. Essentially, immigrant or industrializing populations were seen as moving through three stages (with my alternative classifications in parentheses): (1) traditional/homeostatic (rural agricultural economies); (2) transitional/heterostatic (unskilled and low-skilled wage laborers, migrant workers); and (3) modernized or accultur-ated/homeostatic (middle-class, skilled, managerial and professional workers, college students). Homeostatic and modernization models mask the observed socioeconomic stratification under the guise of organic func-tionalism and progressive evolutionism. Socioeconomic strata are inter-preted as a single population at various points along a (presumed inevitable) transition toward a "middle-class life-style."

Critical reformulation of theory went much further than these issues. A critique of the most fundamental, dogmatic assumptions of stress research was also undertaken. The "fight-or-flight" syndrome concept, which remains unquestioned in most stress research, was found to be based on erroneous and highly politicized notions about human evolution. The initial framers of "fight or flight" were imbued with the Hobbesian and Spencerian characterizations of human evolution as the result of vio-lent interspecific and intraspecific competition for survival and rank. These ideas were acceptable to mainstream evolutionary anthropology for most of the twentieth century. They began to be challenged during the 1960s as an emphasis on aggressive competition gave way to an emphasis on adaptation to other aspects of the biotic and abiotic environments. By the 1970s and 1980s, a new understanding of "gatherer-hunters" showed food sharing and cooperation were more common and essential to early human adaptation than were competition and violence. What is more, hominoid studies showed the importance of affective bonding and the rel-ative rarity of violent competition. The cogency of previous theory seems predicated mostly on the extrapolation of laissez-faire capitalist economic relations to human origins and, therefore, to human 'nature.'

The sociological, epidemiological, and psychological literature, how-ever, showed consistently that stress effects resulted mostly from perceived threats of social separation, loss, and alienation. Although psychophysio-logical stress seems to be a generalized response to fear, the most common and powerful anxieties in humans were those related to fears about one's status within and effective control of important social relationships, rela-tionships upon which the satisfaction of all biological needs depend in highly socially dependent hominoid species. Psychophysiological stress had been adapted, by my critical reformulation of theory, as a physiological component of the glue that held human society together, by constituting a visceral pain of alienation not unlike the sensations of hunger and thirst that motivated the adaptations of eating and drinking (Blakey 1985, 1994a). The sensation of stress motivated the seeking of social support, and that required the acquisition of cultural behaviors that engender social acceptance. Pathological distress in our society resulted from chronic frustration of these efforts to achieve a sense of social security and worth.

This critique and reformulation of theory pointed to a very different conceptualization of what the socioeconomic patterns of stress effects mean for our society. According to the "fight-or-flight" model, humans are increasingly stressed in the industrial world because their innate, formerly adaptive tendency to fight or flee in the face of danger could not be applied to the kinds of stresses that were prevalent in civilized life. Thus, those who were most stressed (least "modernized") were constructed as those who were least able to contend with civilization effectively. On the other hand, If suppressed hostility is shown to be in the etiology of essential hypertension in African-American men (Harburg et al. 1973), "is it that the beast within black men is unable to contend with a civil world; or is it that *all* humans are socially sensitive organisms, frustrated and enraged by the inaccessibility and unpredictability of social gratification and security in what, for *some,* must be a beastly world?" (Blakey 1994a, 160). Certainly, being a member of the African-American male population has contributed importantly to my ability to raise these questions, just as Franz Boas's Jewish ethnicity made the low racial evolutionary ranking of Jews seem counterintuitive to him at the turn of the twentieth century.

Bioarchaeology: Political Economy, Critique, Cultural Vantage, and Public Engagement.   Between 1985 and the present, my students and I have been engaged in research on nutritional and disease stresses evinced in skeletal remains from historical African-American archaeological sites. These studies demonstrated the importance of sociohistorical data for adequate interpretation of skeletal pathology. They also revealed the low physical quality of life of African-American children in both the plantation South and urban North during the early nineteenth century (Blakey et al. 1992, 1994).

One bioarchaeological project, however, coalesced all of the elements of humanistic and critical biology that evolved during earlier studies and the debates regarding repatriation and public engagement. The New York African Burial Ground, rediscovered in 1991, became a project of the Cobb Laboratory in 1992.

The African Burial Ground had been the main cemetery for Africans in colonial New York City, most of whom were enslaved, during much of the eighteenth century. A federal building project brought about archaeological excavation of 427 remains, as required by the National Historic Preservation Act. Like so many Cultural Resource Management consulting projects, the clients' main objective was the removal of skeletons which impeded construction of their building. The archaeologists and physical anthropologists who were initially engaged seemed to be both insensitive to the concerns of the descendant, living African-American community and lacking in academic preparation and previous experience in African and African-American studies (LaRoche and Blakey 1997).

Initially, millions of dollars were being spent on rapid archaeological documentation and removal of the skeletons by anthropologists who had been unable to produce an acceptable research design to guide them. Many African Americans became incensed by the behavior toward them of the GSA (the U.S. General Services Administration, which was responsible for the building project) and their anthropologists. There were accusations of racism as the community's demands to have a principal say in the disposition of the site were dismissed. Protests grew large, and public pressure was brought to bear on the GSA. Between July and September of 1992, as the GSA was found in violation of its own legal agreements (including the lack of an acceptable research design and response to public input), both the city's mayor and the U.S. Congress would call a halt to the archaeological excavation and bring about the preservation of part of the site for memorialization.

Here was a confrontation between the African-American community and American anthropology (as well as with the U.S. government). Although religious and spiritual sensibilities of the black community were important considerations, there were many intellectual concerns as well. The African-American public had a heightened critical awareness of the politics of anthropology, history, and their means of dissemination (education).

The kinds of criticisms of slavery times that this paper attributed to Frederick Douglass have continued within the African-American community. The Eurocentric distortion and omission of the African and African-American contributions to national and global society have been persistently analyzed as means of white social control and black disempowerment within a society, deeply imbued with the ideology of white supremacy. These understandings are not exclusive to the intelligentsia, but comprise a widespread discourse within the general African-American, African, and Diasporic public. The African Burial Ground became a profound example of the literal covering up of an extensive colonial African presence, their economic contributions, and brutal enslavement.

The original physical-forensic anthropologists on the site raised additional concerns because they sought to characterize the cemetery population principally on the basis of biological race (not having much knowledge of the population's social and cultural history). They also raised concerns because of their opposition to the collaborative proposals of African-American researchers at Howard University whose laboratory facilities and academic backgrounds were more appropriate to the study area (an assessment made for the GSA by a federal scientific review panel and the U.S. Congress).

If anthropological research presented a means for restoring an accurate understanding of the colonial predecessors of the African-American people, the government's initial anthropological consultants did not seem particularly well suited for the task. On the whole, the situation that African Americans encountered on the site was both metaphorical and symptomatic of the racism that they encountered in their daily lives. The African-American anthropologists who stepped in to help shared an understanding of racism's mode of operation with the broader descendant community—an understanding of the involvement of racism at the site which Euro-American anthropologists tended to deny.

Still, the attitudes of the forensics team were not unusual for American anthropology. Albeit convenient in the absence of credentials in Africana studies, their emphasis on racing was presented as more objective and scientific than biocultural approaches which relied significantly on nonbiological criteria (historical records and artifacts) and biological methods of population affiliation that were nonracial (Howard University and John Milner Associates 1993). Howard University's researchers contended that the characterization of the population in simplistic racial terms and without sophisticated attention to social and cultural history would construct an identity of the skeletal population that had neither culture nor a history. Thus, by reinforcing racist stereotypes (and the concept of race) the scientistic approach of forensics had political implications, despite its claims to neutrality.

Furthermore, the research team that we assembled agreed that African Americans should have a key involvement in the research on the epistemological grounds that they were more likely to bring a perspective that might help rectify the distorting effects of Eurocentric denial of the scope and conditions of African participation in the building of the nation. We saw an opportunity to interest more African Americans in the practice of anthropology and to enhance the sophistication of a study of humankind that had come to be overwhelmingly limited to the perspectives of a single, macro-ethnic group in the United States—an ethnic group that had established and maintained a particularly oppressive relationship with African America. The struggle then, "to tell our own story," resonated with African Americans in New York City and throughout the country. Yet we also insisted on an ethnically diverse research team on ethical, political, and practical grounds.

The contract for analysis of the site had not been let in 1992, leaving an open field for Howard's bid to direct that portion of the project (and initially seeking to retain the original anthropologists as collaborators). The fact that the level of involvement in previous Africana research, academic credentials, and facilities of the African Americans involved were all superior to those of GSA's initial anthropological consultants failed to dissuade many Euro-American colleagues from leveling accusations of "reverse racism" and opportunism at Howard's researchers. Moreover, 87 percent of the fifty physical anthropologists from whom the forensics team had requested support rallied to the defense of their emphasis on racing by writing letters on their behalf (see Epperson 1996, for one outsider's view). Some argued that both racial and nonracial approaches should be taken in neutrality. I preferred to take a position (recall Douglass) seeing no advantage in accommodating a politically and scientifically backward classification, without objection from the black community. Howard University would ultimately receive a contract for the project. Unwilling to concede to our nonracial and biocultural approaches to analysis, the original forensics team dropped out of the project.

Perhaps most important, my colleagues and I were able to institute a policy of public engagement when I became scientific director for the project in the fall of 1992, in the wake of GSA's realization of its political vulnerability. There would be two clients: a business client (the GSA) and an ethical client (the descendant community). A primary obligation would be shown to the ethical client under an interpretation of the ethical and professional guidelines of the American Anthropological Association and the World Archaeological Congress. There were also important legal and business obligations to the federal government.

The research project, as it was being newly constructed, acknowledged the right of the descendant community to determine the disposition of the site, including the choice of immediate reburial without research. As a participant in the progressive World Archaeological Congress since 1986, I had engaged in a dialogue with representatives of indigenous peoples (including the Native American Rights Fund) on issues of reburial and repatriation. These dialogues convinced me that anthropologists needed to relinquish the presumption of authority over other peoples' ancestral remains and sacred sites. Such community empowerment seemed to be the only realistic starting point for a negotiation for scientific research that would represent a climate of mutual respect between anthropologists and culturally affiliated groups.

Under an engaged approach, the anthropologists would need to demonstrate the value of their research plans to the descendant or culturally affiliated community. Our approach included providing copies of the 130-page research design to all interested persons and holding hearings in downtown Manhattan and Harlem to receive feedback. We were interested in receiving the kinds of questions that the black community and other concerned citizens wished to have answered by our research. These hearings became forums for mutual education. A revised research design would be written that included suggestions of the community that were appropriate for a scientific program. A federal steering committee, mainly representing the descendant community, reviewed and approved the revised research design. The Office of Public Education and Interpretation for the project was established in New York City to provide continuous information flow between the project at Howard and the public.

As a result of this engagement process with our ethical client, broad sectors of the African-American public came to "own" the project in which they now had a stake. A skeletal population that initially seemed destined for immediate reburial became part of a six-year program of research (prior to reburial), was transported to another city (Washington, DC), and would be subjected to invasive methods (cutting of bone and teeth for studies associated with the population's origins), all with the strong support of the African-American community. Having been brought under the stewardship of an African-American research institution with a tradition of scholar activism, the project became a centerpiece for cultural construction in addition to anthropological and cognate research. Cultural and spiritual observances were encouraged, as were scholarly symposia on broadly related issues concerning the African Diaspora.

By accommodating the varied ways, cultural and political, that African Americans and Africans wished to treat these ancestral remains, interest in the scientific aspects of the project grew tremendously. By 1996, nearly 50,000 visitors had been served by the Office of Public Education and Interpretation and more than 2,000 adults visited the Cobb Laboratory along with thousands of school children. More than 100,000 people signed a petition (rejected by the U.S. Postal Service) to create an African Burial Ground postal stamp. There are more than 500 news and magazine articles and five documentaries about the African Burial Ground. At the 1995 meetings of the American Anthropological Association in Washington, a two-day symposium on the project was opened to the general public (a first for the AAA), who joined anthropologists, filling a room with 750 seats.

The fostering of political and cultural activity around the African Burial Ground contributed to the scientific endeavor in a number of ways. The public's input on the research design was useful in providing new questions and more appropriate language (the term *African*, not *African-American*, was to be applied to colonial blacks, consistent with references to European colonials. The persons buried there would be referred to as *enslaved Africans* rather than as *slaves*, emphasizing a cultural identity and imposed status). The range of the project's multidisciplinary studies is broader than for other projects of its kind (extending from molecular genetics to African art history, colonial New York history to African archaeology and diasporic ethnology). Funding would be on the order of eight figures, a level of support consistent with the broad scope of research and public programs, and probably impossible to achieve without the government's accountability to a broad, supportive, and vocal public. This was only possible by relinquishing scientific and Euro-American authority over the disposition of the remains.

The results of the skeletal research are only now being analyzed, as additional data are still being collected. Thus far we have discovered important West African symbolism among the artifacts, potential evidence of African ethnic affiliations (dental modification), high child and infant mortality, nutritional and health problems (metabolic disease indicators and growth disruption and delay), and widespread evidence of traumatic work and load-bearing stresses in men, women, and children (muscle attachment hypertrophy, enthesopathy, vertebral fractures, and cranial base ring fractures).

It is hoped that the project's results will contribute to the development of bioarchaeological methods and to education for anyone's benefit. What is already clear is that our findings have taken on significance within national and international forums concerned with strengthening the ties between Africa and African America. Already a royal delegation from Ghana has visited the site and laboratory as part of a reunification effort, and we have met with African and other representatives of the United Nations in Geneva and New York in order to discuss their interest in the relation of our findings to human rights and to policies of "moral compensation" for past enslavement.

The project does not shy from these political aspects of our work, but we insist that our participation is as scientists who adhere to a methodology requiring the systematic collection and analysis of material evidence. At the same time, we try to remain aware of the social and political implications of our work: work that is lent to the cultural construction, political activism, and spiritual observances of a broader community's expert practitioners. Ours is a study of the people, by the people, and for the people principally concerned.

Conclusion

I have attempted, not to point to a particular theory as a solution to the limitations of biological anthropology, but to examine anthropology's epistemological limitations in a way that presents a more sweeping opposition to them. Some ideas about the problems of physical anthropology and ways of finding solutions to them have been presented, all of which point to the need for a humanistic, critical, and political-economic approach to the study of human biology. Positivistic notions of objectivity, extending from the Enlightenment to the modern era, foster an attempt at scientific disengagement from society that merely amounts to denial. The tendency toward excessive naturalism simply feeds the denial of sociocultural influences on ourselves and the human phenomena we study. I argue that it is better to acknowledge and accept the social embeddedness of our thoughts and actions as scientists, in order to better scrutinize, explicate, and control the societal influences of our work and our world. While one might not escape these influences, by acknowledging them one can better choose among them intelligently.

The argument for public engagement (or activist scholarship) stems from this acknowledgment. Should scientists alone have authority over the political, cultural, and economic uses of their work? In the engaged work of the New York African Burial Ground Project, the authority and responsibilities of critique, design, and application of science are shared with those most impacted by our project. Here values of participatory democracy and pluralism have an obvious bearing on our work (see Forman 1994 for an argument for inclusion of these values within anthropological research programs). This is a new brand of science, and often it is a more wrenchingly difficult undertaking than one that is clothed in denial and able to enjoy the ostensible seclusion of the ivory tower.

In its nascency, the divergence of science benefited greatly from religious heresy. I want to begin to think, here, of what it is that will benefit from scientific heresy. Will it be a new science or another epistemological species altogether? What material history tells us is that science, as we know it today, is someday likely to go the way of alchemy.

REFERENCES

Allen, G. E. 1975. Genetics, Eugenics, and Class Struggle. *Genetics* 79:29–45.

Babcock, W. H. 1899. The Nanticoke Indians of Indian River Delaware. *American Anthropologist* 1:277–87.

Bernal, Martin. 1987. *Black Athena: The Afro-Asiatic Roots of Classical Civilization.* New Brunswick: Rutgers University Press.

Blakey, M. L. 1983. Sociopolitical Bias and Ideological Production in Historical Archaeology. In *The Socio-Politics of Archaeology,* ed. J. M. Gero, D. Lacy, and M. L. Blakey. Research Report no. 23. Department of Anthropology, University of Massachusetts-Amherst.

Blakey, M. L. 1985. Stress, Social Inequality, and Culture Change: An Anthropological Approach to Human Psychophysiology. Ph.D. diss. University of Massachusetts-Amherst.

Blakey, M. L. 1987. Skull Doctors: Intrinsic Social and Political Bias in American Physical Anthropology, with special reference to the work of Aleš Hrdlička. *Critique of Anthropology* 7:7–35.

Blakey, M. L. 1988. Social Policy, Economics, and Demographic Change in Nanticoke-Moor Ethnohistory. *American Journal of Physical Anthropology* 75:493–503.

Blakey, M. L. 1990. American Nationality and Ethnicity in the Depicted Past. In *Politics of the Past,* ed. P. Gathercole and D. Lowenthal, 38–48. London: Allen and Unwin.

Blakey, M. L. 1991. Man and Nature, White and Other. In *Decolonizing Anthropology,* ed. F. V. Harrison, 15–23. Washington: Association of Black Anthropologists and American Anthropological Association.

Blakey, M. L. 1994a. Psychophysiological Stress as an Indicator of Disorder in

Industrial Society. In *Diagnosing America: Anthropology and Public Engagement,* ed. S. Forman, 149–92. Ann Arbor: University of Michigan Press.

Blakey, M. L. 1994b. Passing the Buck: Modernization and Individualism as Anthropological Expressions of Euro-American Denial. In *Race,* ed. S. Gregory and R. Sanjek, 270–84. New Brunswick: Rutgers University Press.

Blakey, M. L. 1996. Skull Doctors Revisited: Intrinsic Social and Political Bias in the History of American Physical Anthropology. In *Race and Other Misadventures,* ed. L. Reynolds and L. Lieberman, 64–95. Dix Hill, NY: General Hall, Inc.

Blakey, M. L. 1997. Past is Present: Comments on "In the Realm of Politics: Prospects for Public Participation in African-American Plantation Archaeology." *Historical Archaeology* 31:140–45.

Blakey, M. L., T. E. Leslie, and J. P. Reidy. 1992. Chronological Distribution of Dental Enamel Hypoplasia in African American Slaves: A Test of the Weaning Hypothesis. *American Journal of Physical Anthropology Supplement* 14:50 (Abstract).

Blakey, M. L., T. E. Leslie, and J. P. Reidy. 1994. Frequency and Chronological Distribution of Dental Enamel Defects in Enslaved African Americans: A Test of the Weaning Hypothesis. *American Journal of Physical Anthropology* 95:371–84.

Douglass, Frederick. [1854] 1950. The Claims of the Negro Ethnologically Considered. In *The Life and Writings of Frederick Douglass,* ed. P. S. Foner. New York: International Publishers.

Drake, St. Clair. 1980. Anthropology and the Black Experience. *Black Scholar* 11:2–31.

Epperson, Terrence W. 1996. The Politics of 'Race' and Cultural Identity at the African Burial Ground Excavations, New York City. *World Archaeological Bulletin* 7:108–17.

Feyerabend, Paul. 1978. *Science in a Free Society.* London: NLB Press.

Fisher, G. P. 1895. To So-Called Moors that Live in Delaware. *Milford Herald,* June 15.

Forman, S., ed. 1994. *Diagnosing America: Anthropology and Public Engagement.* Ann Arbor: University of Michigan Press.

Glick, L. B. 1982. Types Distinct from Our Own: Franz Boas on Jewish Identity and Assimilation. *American Anthropologist* 84:545–65.

Gould, Stephen Jay. 1981. *The Mismeasure of a Man.* New York: W. W. Norton.

Harburg, E., J. Erfurt, and L. Hausenstein. 1973. Socioecological Stress, Suppressed Hostility, Skin Color and Black-White Male Blood Pressure. *Psychosomatic Medicine* 35:276–96.

Herskovits, M. J. 1953. *Franz Boas.* New York: Charles Scribner's Sons.

Howard University and John Milner Associates. 1993. *Research Design for Archaeological, Historical and Bioanthropological Investigations of the African Burial Ground (Broadway Block), New York, New York.* New York: General Services Administration.

Kuhn, Thomas. 1970. *The Structure of Scientific Revolutions.* Chicago: University of Chicago Press.

LaRoche, Cherly, and Michael L. Blakey. 1997. Seizing Intellectual Power: Scientific and Public Discourse on New York's African Burial Ground. *Historical Archaeology* 31:84–106.

Leone, M. P., et al. 1986. Toward a Critical Archaeology. *Current Anthropology* 28:277–98.

Levins, Richard, and Richard Lewontin. 1993. Applied Biology in the Third World: The Struggle for Revolutionary Science. In *The Racial Economy of Science,* ed. S. Harding, 315–25. Bloomington: Indiana University Press.

Porter, F. W. 1978. Quest for Identity: The Formation of the Nanticoke Indian Community at Indian River Inlet, Sussex County, Delaware. Ph.D. diss. Department of Geography, University of Maryland.

Rankin-Hill, L., and M. L. Blakey. 1994. W. Montague Cobb (1904–1990): Physical Anthropologist, Anatomist, and Activist. *American Anthropologist* 96:74–96.

Stocking, George. 1976. Ideas and Institutions in American Anthropology: Towards a History of the Interwar Period. In *Selected Papers from the American Anthropologist, 1921–1945,* 1–54. Washington: American Anthropological Association.

Todes, Daniel P. 1989. *Darwin Without Malthus: The Struggle for Existence in Russian Evolutionary Thought.* New York: Oxford.

Tylor, Edward B. 1871. *Primitive Culture.* London: Murray.

Weslager, Clinton Alfred. 1943. *Delaware's Forgotten Folk: The Story of the Moors and Nanticokes.* Philadelphia: University of Pennsylvania.

Wilson, E. O. 1975. *Sociobiology: The New Synthesis.* Cambridge: Harvard University Press.

Chapter 17

Latin American Social Medicine and the Politics of Theory

Lynn M. Morgan

Other chapters in this volume address the applicability of political-economic theories to biological anthropology, arguing on empirical or theoretical grounds that political economy has much to contribute. This chapter takes a different approach by drawing attention to the sociopolitical and economic context within which a critical, political-economic theory might rise to prominence. I will use the example of the social medicine (*medicina social*) movement in Latin America to argue that the introduction of political economy into biological anthropology will have as much to do with circumstances outside the academy as with either its explanatory power or the eloquence and theoretical persuasiveness of its proponents.

Political economy has had an overwhelmingly positive impact on the overall direction of medical anthropology, but I do not want to imply that examples provided by social medicine or critical medical anthropology are the "correct" or "best" way to introduce these issues into *biological* anthropology. A social approach to medicine existed long before medical anthropologists arrived on the scene, and in the current era medical anthropologists are neither its best nor its only practitioners (see Krieger 1994; Singer, this vol., chap. 4; Turner 1995). As we attend to contributions from fields such as sociology and public health, we should also note variants of the political economy of health being elaborated outside of North American and European contexts. Where political-economic analysis emerges in response to a different set of epistemological and, especially, political, concerns, we find the theory and practice of social medicine more explicitly tied to popular social struggles. The comparison serves as a reminder that theoretical preoccupations and predilections emerge from specific historical, sociopolitical, occupational, and epistemological conditions. As some biological anthropologists strive to incorporate political economy into their field, we are well served to examine the historical reasons why some analytic models become unsatisfactory at particular historical junctures. What kind of sociopolitical contexts drive paradigm shifts or theoretical innovations? Why are some biological anthropologists arguing *now* for the incorporation of political-economic theories? The comparison of U.S.-style critical medical anthropology and Latin American social medicine highlights the social contexts that shape theoretical variation.

Before I discuss the Latin American social medicine movement, however, it will be helpful to explain briefly the ways in which the political economy of health has been used in theorizing by North Americans. This will set the stage for contrasting North American and Latin American variants of the political economy of health, which may, in turn, affect how biological anthropologists think about or utilize political-economic theories.

Political Economy of Health in North America

The political economy of health is a theoretical orientation which holds that health and disease processes are generated by and embedded in social and productive relations. Political economists of health reject explanations of disease etiology that focus solely on the identification and treatment of pathogens; they further reject the idea that social aspects of disease can be reduced to simple "risk factors" equivalent to other epidemiologic variables. Without rejecting biological mechanisms of disease, political economists hold that health and disease must be understood historically, in the context of a hierarchically organized society. For this reason, political economists emphasize historical and collective explanations over individualistic, cultural, or psychological explanations. Political-economic analysis highlights not only the social production of disease and distress, but the ideological obfuscation manufactured and perpetuated by biomedicine. In the words of Singer and Baer, "A primary task of critical medical anthropology . . . must be the unveiling of official ideologies masquerading as empirical realities" (1989, 100). Political economists reject the "natural-ness" of the environment within which disease is created, preferring instead to unmask the ideological fallacies which permit "constructed" environments to appear "natural" (see Singer 1992b). In sum, the political economy of health is "a macroanalytic, critical, and historical perspective for analyzing disease distribution and health services under a variety of economic systems, with particular emphasis on the effects of stratified social, political, and economic relations within the world economic system" (Morgan 1987, 132). In the United States, at least four distinct approaches can be grouped under the rubric of the political economy of health: orthodox Marxism, dependency theories, cultural critiques of medicine, and critical phenomenology.

Orthodox Marxist Political Economy of Health

Orthodox Marxists use the theory of historical materialism to analyze health and biomedicine as features of Western capitalism. (In fact, Morsy prefers the unwieldy construction "political economy of medical anthropology" to "critical medical anthropology" precisely because the former phrase makes explicit the links to Marx and Engels and to a tradition of sociomedical work in historical materialism [1990, 27].) Marxist historical materialists analyze social processes of health and disease in terms of historical relations of production, with special attention to the logic of capital accumulation, the labor process, and social class. In addition to the production of disease, Marxists also analyze the unequal distribution of medical care, both within capitalist countries and in the capitalist world system. This approach often takes a comparative international or cross-national look, for example, at the exportation of Western capitalism's biomedical models and products (e.g., Cueto 1994; Solórzano 1992). The major strength of this approach lies in its ability to look at structural causes, to connect specific social forms and expressions to underlying historical processes.

In spite of its analytic power, orthodox Marxism is used infrequently by medical anthropologists (exceptions include Susser 1985; Nash and Kirsch 1986; and others, like sociologist Ray Elling [1986], who examine labor processes). The thinness of the ranks may stand in direct proportion to the virulence of anti-Marxist rhetoric; the political repercussions of sustaining a Marxist analysis in the largely inhospitable academic and political climate of the United States can be devastating, as Vicente Navarro (1985) has often pointed out. Beyond that, however, anthropologists sympathetic to Marxist analysis in health are dissatisfied with its inability to explain the agency and resistance of local actors and the dynamic persistence of ethnomedicine after the intrusion of Western biomedicine. Furthermore, its macro-level abstractions cannot accommodate the nuances or detail so important to ethnographers. Rather than locating their analyses within the school of orthodox Marxism, medical anthropologists have borrowed from it selected features such as historical materialism, economic exploitation, and social stratification as factors underlying the social production of disease, the commodification of disease and healing, and an awareness of the ideological affinities between biomedicine and capitalism.

Dependency Theories

Dependency theories in the political economy of health (which I have elsewhere reviewed in greater detail [Morgan 1987]) are related to orthodox Marxist theories in that they are driven by an examination of the dynamics of capitalism. But while the Marxists emphasize the social relations of production and class formation, dependency theorists are preoccupied with the expansion of capitalism (and biomedicine) into the underdeveloped world. According to the dependency theorists, the introduction of capitalist biomedicine is synonymous with exacerbated poverty, inequality, and disease. Capitalist biomedicine extracts resources from the periphery (by way of money spent on biomedical necessities like hospitals, high-tech equipment, and drugs; products like pharmaceutical raw materials; and trained professionals), while it introduces new diseases such as malnutrition (caused by the substitution of cash crops for subsistence foods, or the promotion of infant formulas) and cancer (caused by the exportation of toxic industries, or of cigarettes, for example, as U.S.-based tobacco firms expand their markets to the Third World). Even more than classical Marxist approaches, the dependency approach is comparative and international, emphasizing the underdevelopment generated in the wake of capitalist expansion. This approach made sense to many of the medical anthropologists first experimenting with political economy, probably because the devastating effects of Western "development" (including biomedicine) were so obvious to anthropologists doing fieldwork in remote regions of the underdeveloped world. These days, however, it seems fair to say that the popularity of dependency theories has peaked, in medical anthropology as well as in other social sciences, because of widely acknowledged theoretical shortcomings such as a continued lack of concern for the actions of those in underdeveloped regions (Henfrey 1981; Roseberry 1989). Nonetheless, critical medical anthropologists continue to borrow from dependency theories the idea of a direct (if nonlinear and heavily mediated) relationship between underdevelopment in the periphery and (over-)development in the center. Contemporary examples might include the detrimental health effects of "export-for-development" strategies and the impact of Western health aid on the health status of people living in underdeveloped countries, as well as the global health effects of medical industries controlled by large private corporations.

Cultural Critiques of Medicine

When medical anthropologists began to broaden their traditional community studies to include political economy in the 1970s, many were attracted to the theoretical variant known as the cultural critique. The most important word characterizing this approach is "power," specifically the social organization of medical power. Appropriate objects of study include medical professionals and hospital hierarchies, institutionalized inequalities (race, ethnicity, gender, socioeconomic status), interest group politics and partisan battles, and processes of cooptation and social control. Cultural critics are quick to point out medicine's detrimental effects, including its iatrogenic, misogynistic, and racist manifestations and consequences. The cultural critics see in the health–disease process a reflection of an unjust social system, but many do not take the extra step of connecting social inequality to capitalism per se or to any historical process. Cultural critiques were a favorite idiom of left-liberals in the 1970s and 1980s, but anthropologists were also attracted, perhaps because it was easier to broaden a community study to include its immediate surroundings than to jump another level of abstraction to orthodox Marxism. Cultural critiques retain their popularity among medical anthropologists for a couple of reasons. First, there are solid reasons to criticize mid-range sociopolitical decisions (such as federal retrenchment from housing and health programs) that adversely affect the health of the poor (see Abraham 1993). Also, there may be a wider audience for cultural critiques than for Marxist approaches deemed "dogmatic" or "rhetorical"; in these days of relentless attack on all manner of leftist analysis, pragmatism can be a valuable tool of political reform.

Critical Phenomenology

A more recent theoretical innovation within critical medical anthropology is Scheper-Hughes and Lock's "critical phenomenology," which analyzes the day-to-day experience of suffering in the context of unjust political, economic, and gender relations (see Lock 1988; Scheper-Hughes 1992;

also Taussig 1980). Scheper-Hughes and Lock use their commitment to fieldwork to generate rich ethnography, to show the sufferers' eloquence and insight; the anthropologist-humanist's task is to make evident the metaphoric dimensions of illness and show the links between somaticized distress and societies within which such conditions are created. It is a compassionate and truly anthropological approach to the political economy of suffering which is generating considerable debate and interest from outside, as well as inside, the field of medical anthropology.

Summary

Each of the four approaches carries important messages used in the elaboration of critical medical anthropology. From classical Marxism comes a powerful indictment of the inequality, disease, and death forced by a particular mode of production and accompanying class relations. This perspective is all the more powerful today for what it reveals about the production of health and illness. Dependency theories examine the persistent structural inequalities between North and South, reminding us that developed areas benefit at the expense of underdeveloped areas (worth bearing in mind as we contemplate the effects of the North American Free Trade Agreement; see Frenk 1993; Laurell and Ortega 1992). Dependency theories illustrate the links between what transpires in financial and political capitals and what happens at the farthest reaches of an ever-more-destitute periphery (Leatherman 1994; Luerssen 1994). Cultural critiques offer a unique set of tools for analyzing complex societies, where power and professionalization may become the dominant variables in a sociological analysis of health. Finally, the perspective of critical phenomenology shows how real people, specifically situated, internalize, embody, and make "sense-full" the conditions under which they live. The political economy of health has contributed to medical anthropology an awareness and sensitivity that our choices of topics and theories are, invariably, political choices. The "choice" of theory (ecological, ethnomedical, hermeneutic, phenomenological) is virtually overdetermined by one's personal and professional positioning in a specific society with its unique historical constraints and contradictions (Breilh and Granda 1989; Morgan 1990).

Toward the Politics of Theory

Perhaps we must look to politics to explain why the "biocultural synthesis" so optimistically presaged by Johnson and Sargent (1990, 8) is still largely missing from critical medical anthropology. McElroy (1990) may have been closer to the mark when she said that medical anthropology is moving *away* from the biocultural pole. Whereas earlier theories linked medical anthropology explicitly to adaptation and evolution, the postmodern influence has turned contemporary theorizing from scientific toward deconstructionist realms (see Haraway 1989). McElroy thus feels justified in stating, "Clearly, there are conceptual canyons separating biocultural researchers and political economists" (1990, 383). The rift was spotlighted by Singer's accusation that ecological anthropology is inattentive to processes of social stratification and transformation (Singer 1989, 93, 96). But a larger political context also affects these debates. Leftists, I suspect, are turned off to biological analyses by the populace's willingness to interpret social issues—such as race, gender, homosexuality, and poverty—through reductionist biological lenses in the service of conservative social agendas. There is thus a theoretical backlash against biology; biology provides the wrong tools—the reasoning goes—for those of us interested in progressive social analysis, so let's trash it, or at best ignore it (exceptions include feminist critics of biological reductionism such as Evelyn Fox Keller [1995] and Levins and Lewontin [1985]). For all these reasons, biological topics have scarcely been admitted into critical medical anthropology. The assertion made by Armelagos et al. (1992, 38)— "There is nothing inherent in the biocultural model that prevents a consideration of political and economic spheres of influence. In fact, we consider political-economic factors crucial to the understanding of health and illness in human populations"—is moot unless people like Brooke Thomas, Alan Goodman, and Tom Leatherman can convince others to withdraw from the "backlash against biology" and join them in the enterprise of building a political economy of biological anthropology. Perhaps one of the goals of a political economy of biological anthropology should be to investigate critically the history of political economy in biological anthropology, a task which Michael Blakey (this vol., chap. 16) has begun.

Medicina Social en América Latina

> Calls for 'new values' and 'cultural revolutions' (without understanding the material structure on which bases those values are reproduced) will not do. (Navarro 1989, 201)

I admit to performing a minor sleight of hand by comparing Latin America's social medicine movement with critical medical anthropology, because the two are not exactly equivalent. Much of what passes for medical anthropology in Latin America is decidedly "acritical": descriptive ethnomedical and ethnopharmacological accounts of healing dimensions among minority (often indigenous) populations. The social medicine movement, in contrast, is more analogous to what North Americans call the political economy of health, specifically its Marxist variants. More of its practitioners come from medicine and public health (especially epidemiology) than from the social sciences, and they are more wedded to the scientific method than U.S. medical anthropologists tend to be. Nonetheless, I take up the example of Latin American social medicine to illustrate two points: first, that we should examine the particular historical and political conditions that give rise to theoretical innovation (and lack of same), to understand, as Navarro says, the "material conditions" affecting paradigm shifts; and second, to underscore the close relationship between theory and social change in the Latin American context in contrast to that of the United States.

Though social medicine has a long history in Latin America (see García 1986), the movement began to coalesce in the 1970s with a realization that economic growth was not resulting in improved health indices; rather, the health profiles of Latin America started to reflect what Laurell (1989, 1183) calls "the worst of both worlds," mixing the pathologies of affluence with those of poverty. Motivated by their direct, often personal involvement in student organizations and labor unions, a number of young Latin American intellectuals began using the theory of historical materialism to analyze public health issues.

Cristina Laurell, one of the founders and principal proponents of the social medicine movement in Mexico, explains that particular problems (including health) become "socially visible" at given historical moments because of the demands posed by social movements (1989, 1183). Indeed, even for heuristic purposes it is not easy to separate the social medicine movement from the popular political issues that galvanized the activists of the early 1970s. Events such as the Brazilian military coup of 1964, Mexico's Tlalteloco massacre of 1968, and the 1970 election of Chilean president Salvador Allende, coupled with widespread violent repression of political dissidents and demonstrators, spawned and fortified a multitude of Latin American social movements concerned with enhancing the accountability of politicians and clerics, improving economic and educational opportunities, resisting political repression and cooptation, and fostering community organizing and empowerment. Breilh and Granda

(1989) note that the heterogeneity of social, political, and economic circumstances in Latin America gave rise to different emphases and concerns within social medicine (similar to the theoretical variation described previously for the U.S. political economy of health). In spite of this diversity, however, there is no question that Latin American social medicine began not with an abstract interest in Marxist theory, but with an urgent concern for "social and labor rights, among which health occupies a relevant place" (Laurell and Ortega 1992, 331). This prototypically Latin American approach to participatory research-activism ("investigación-acción participativa" in the work of Fals-Borda [1985]), while not without its U.S. corollaries, took on a special urgency throughout the 1970s and 1980s in a context of ongoing governmental hostility, repression, and heightened levels of social and economic inequality.[1]

Today the social medicine movement maintains organizational coherence through the Asociación Latinoamericana de Medicina Social (ALAMES), headquartered in Venezuela. Major centers of research and theorizing are located in Brazil, Ecuador, and Mexico. The Mexican nucleus, centered in the Programa de Medicina Social at the Universidad Autónoma Metropolitana at Xochimilco, is known for its innovative work on workers' health and the labor process (Bay 1986; Laurell 1988; Laurell and Márquez 1983). Health systems research has dominated the social medicine field in Brazil, where investigators have been acutely aware of growing systemic inequities between the public and private health and social security sectors (Laurell 1989, 1183). In Ecuador, Dr. Juan César García emerged as a principal theorist of Latin American social medicine in the 1960s and 1970s. More recently, the Centro de Estudios y Asesoría en Salud (CEAS) has been noted for developing and refining a Marxist epidemiology, complete with sophisticated statistical techniques used to assess correlations between social class and health status (Campaña n.d.). Contributions to the social medicine movement have also come from Argentina, the Dominican Republic, Bolivia, Colombia, and Venezuela. (I should note Cuba's absence from this list. While North American political economists of health have been generally sympathetic to Cuba's health policies and priorities [see Feinsilver 1989], the Cubans have made minimal contributions to the theory or practice of social medicine in spite of their progressive rhetoric.)

Perhaps the most important theoretical innovations to emerge from the social medicine movement come to (and from) the field of epidemiology. Social epidemiologists at CEAS, under the direction of Jaime Breilh

(who received a master's degree in "Ciencias y salud" from the Universidad Autónoma Metropolitana, in Mexico), have developed an elaborate
critique of traditional epidemiologic methods and have conducted several
important and revealing studies using their own techniques. Their primary
focus has been a critique of the role of the state in promoting a particularly
narrow vision of what constitutes public health; public health, they say,
cannot be improved solely through the extension of medical or sanitary
services (Breilh 1982; Campaña 1986). They are extremely critical of mainstream governmental vital statistics, which, they say, are used to "lie with
precision" (Breilh et al. 1987, iii; see also Escudero 1980) while obscuring
the relationship between social class and the risks and realities of death
and disease. In the opinion of the CEAS team, mainstream epidemiologic
surveillance strategies emphasize national (or at best provincial) aggregates. All too frequently, data on occupation, education, migration or
work histories, or other class-relevant variables are not collected. Methods
of data collection enable governmental officials to assert, for example, that
their countries are undergoing a national transition from an "underdeveloped" to a "developed" health profile, without considering the bipolar
splits that may be emerging as health improves for some while deteriorating for others.

The CEAS group questions the use of indicators such as aggregate life
expectancy, causes of death, and infant mortality rates as measures of
national well-being. They have developed epidemiologic categories and
measures designed to show differential morbidity and mortality by social
class. Contrast, for example, CEAS's epidemiologic classifications with
those used in mainstream epidemiology: while CEAS approximates economic well-being by devising categories which get at social/economic *relationships* (including new petty bourgeois, bourgeoisie, traditional petty
bourgeois, typical and non-typical proletariat, subproletariat, and three
categories of peasantry), mainstream epidemiologists might be concerned
with mean household income as a measure of economic well-being. Rather
than tying their causal thinking to isolated factors such as ethnicity or
mothers' educational attainment, the Latin American social epidemiologists look to the "forms of social reproduction, that follow from the
specific manner in which the social groups are inserted in the capitalist
economy, and from the forms of domination to which they are subjected"
(Laurell 1989, 1186). Health and disease are not individual, but collective,
inherently social, phenomena. This theoretical approach justifies their
attention to social class and details of the labor process in analyzing dif-

ferential patterns of morbidity and mortality. As a consequence of their methods, the CEAS group has been able to explain the determinants and distribution of disease by historical moment (for example, with relation to Ecuador's oil boom of the late 1970s) and by "geographic ecology" (e.g., as recent migrants to Quito become inserted into the urban economy) (see Breilh et al. 1990).

The CEAS team is committed to the unity of theoretical and practical work (Breilh and Granda 1989, 1123). They engage in a kind of epidemiological praxis in the service of the poor. This entails a particular vision of epidemiology as the diagnostic branch of social medicine, as a set of theories and techniques that can identify contradictions, problems, and priorities which result in ill health. Their brand of epidemiological investigation creates a radically different way of conceptualizing and identifying health problems and the theories used to explain them. CEAS theorists posit an association between unicausal, germ-theory type models of epidemiology and the rise of monopoly capitalism, and between the crisis of imperialism and multicausal models of disease etiology (Breilh and Granda 1989, 1123); in other words, they argue that theory follows from, and corresponds to, economic changes. Their theory views epidemiology as a form of ideological struggle: their work, they say, "takes on historical authenticity only in the extent to which it is established as an instrument for democratic awareness and popular organization" (1989, 1126; my translation).

One site of struggle is the field of medical education and the training of health personnel. Beginning in the 1960s, analysts realized that there might be benefits to training physicians in the social sciences (García 1986, 24–28). With assistance from the Milbank Foundation and the Pan American Health Organization, attention was directed to the process of medical education in laying the foundations for health services structures equipped to handle the health problems of poor, underdeveloped countries. This emphasis on medical education and the preparation of health personnel continues today, as adherents of social medicine—including those at CEAS—sponsor training programs in schools of medicine and public health throughout Latin America.

One of the longest-standing centers of training in social medicine is the Universidad Autónoma Metropolitana in Xochimilco, Mexico. There, Laurell has focused on the process of capitalist production. She utilizes Marxist epidemiology to understand the social relations of labor and logic of capital appropriation in the workplace. In this context she has refined and delimited certain epidemiological categories; for example, it is necessary to know precisely what kind of work is performed by each factory worker, for how long, and how the health effects of each particular job will become manifest (Laurell 1988; Laurell and Márquez 1983). This detailed empirical work has implications for national health policy. For example, the health effects of certain kinds of work are evident in the workers' bodies, while others affect subsequent generations. "Biological process," says Laurell (1989, 1184), "takes on specific historical forms." Thus when national governments use aggregate infant mortality rates, for example, as indicators of national development, they obscure many historic, geographic, and socioeconomic intricacies (Laurell 1981; Laurell et al. 1977). Laurell's work contains an implicit critique of dependency theories, too, because dependency theories imply that health inequalities are a function of the poor distribution of benefits or simply of material poverty, rather than of the process of production itself (Campaña 1986, 128).

The theoretical orientation of social medicine is a strict and unified historical materialism, which, predictably, carries certain limitations. The single-minded Marxism has, until now, precluded issues that might be expected to dominate the cultural critiques, such as gender or ethnic inequalities. In Ecuador, for example, a number of social scientists have recently become interested in gender analysis, but even CEAS's extensive discussions of abortion and maternal-child health make no reference to the feminist literature on the subject. There are no personal voices in most reports emanating from the social medicine movement; this is not an ethnographic endeavor, or, if it is, the individual experience of suffering is squelched while the (Marxist) scientist speaks authoritatively. Nor has the social medicine movement been much concerned with the global dynamics so important to dependency theories, in spite of the fact that the international division of labor is critical to workers' health, for example, on the northern Mexican border. Rather, those involved in Latin American social medicine have focused their analytic gaze on health problems within their own borders, using, of course, a context which includes the internationalization of capital and demands imposed by multilateral lending agencies, but focusing largely on the domestic expressions and contradictions implied by capital accumulation and surplus extraction. Unlike dependency theorists, then, the social medicine literature does not devote much attention to lambasting U.S. medical imperialism, although Breilh (1990, 22) does point out that it would be sheer lunacy for Latin American countries to emulate U.S. medical models when the United States has the highest health expenditures per capita in the world and yet does not meet the health needs of a substantial portion of its population.

One of the similarities between Latin American social medicine and North American political economy has to do with the underwhelming reception given to the theories by mainstream theorists and practitioners. Like their North American counterparts, the proponents of Latin American social medicine have had to contend with ostracism and marginalization from the mainstream. But perhaps this is inevitable. I am reminded of the comment that the goal of critical medical anthropology is not to be assimilated or adopted by biomedicine, but to remain forever a thorn in its side. In a recent review of the "new public health," Frenk disingenuously misrepresents the nature of Latin American social medicine by stating that the term "social medicine" is "acceptable when studying only the social dimension of health" (1993, 476), but is of limited relevance otherwise. He reduces valid theoretical disagreements to mere disciplinary turf battles when he cautions that "biological reductionism of the past should not be replaced by a sociological reductionism" (1993, 477). Political-economic approaches inevitably represent a threat to power in both theoretical and applied realms. Careers, funding, prestige, and academic and political legitimacy are all threatened by political-economic analysis. Proponents of political economy can therefore always expect to be criticized, or worse. The enterprise of political economy is most satisfying, perhaps, when applied to practical sociopolitical problems.

Where's the Action?

Social medicine is not new. Laurell points out that the social nature of health has been periodically rediscovered over the past 150 years, yet its practical repercussions have been minimal. This "contradictory situation—recognition of the social character of disease which is negated in practice" (Laurell 1979, iii) should not be surprising, because the "conservatizing" features of biomedicine (and of the academy) have been thoroughly documented in the literature of political economy (Singer 1989). Yet whereas the social medicine movement obtains its raison d'être, as well as its controversies, from popular social struggles, much of what passes for critical medical anthropology in North America has been activist mainly at the level of rhetoric. There are, to be sure, a number of medical anthropologists who are committed to various forms of popular political activism: working outside academia, often with community organizations, coauthoring articles with research assistants and participants, writing grant proposals for progressive organizations, testifying on behalf of the poor at local and national levels, working in political campaigns, and so on. Nevertheless, medical anthropologists continue to be underrepresented in the important health policy discussions occurring today in the United States. With the exception of Faye Ginsburg's well-received book on abortion (1989), anthropologists—with their extensive cross-cultural knowledge—are not contributing much to national debates over abortion, for example, or the shockingly high rates of infant mortality among certain classes in the United States. Progressive biological and medical anthropologists *could* be working together to document and publicize what Alan Goodman, Tom Leatherman, and Brooke Thomas (this vol., chaps. 1 and 2) call the "biology of poverty," but we have not put this type of work high on our list of collective priorities. Even as we become more aware of the political nature of our work and thoughts, critical medical anthropologists do not contribute what we should to public debate.

What Singer (1992a, 2) calls "the new regard for theory" has meant another step away from social activism for many anthropologists. Rectifying this situation will require continued work on several simultaneous fronts: to resist the depoliticizing reward and prestige structures that characterize much anthropological work; to take teaching into the community and bring communities into the classroom; and to assail the paralyzing effects of heightened attention to "politically correct" (if ineffectual) radical interpretations of text and postmodernisms. Biological as well as medical anthropologists can learn from the example of social medicine that social change comes through deliberate, overt, and persistent efforts to problematize and politicize the contradictory, ill-health–producing features of our societies. Yet we also learn from social medicine that the popular social context of political struggle is an important motivator of theoretical innovation. In other words, we need to know our roots. For biological anthropologists to internalize and act upon progressive principles, it would be useful to have in hand an autobiography which spells out the social and historical nature of the subfield, its connections to the ideologies of biology and biomedicine, its theoretical sacred cows, and the likely political ramifications of attempting to transform dominant paradigms. The task of creating a political-economic biological anthropology can be made easier if biological anthropologists work together with others who seek the same goals.

NOTES

Thanks to Mario Bronfman, Alan Goodman, Nancy Krieger, Tom Leatherman, and Jim Trostle for helpful comments on earlier drafts of this chapter.
1. Saúl Franco Agudelo dedicated a paper to two of his teachers and friends "killed by the violence they were attempting to combat" (1992, 365).

REFERENCES

Abraham, Laurie Kaye. 1993. *Mama Might Be Better Off Dead: The Failure of Health Care in Urban America.* Chicago: University of Chicago Press.

Armelagos, George J., Thomas Leatherman, Mary Ryan, and Lynn Sibley. 1992. Biocultural Synthesis in Medical Anthropology. *Medical Anthropology* 14:35–52.

Bay, Ignacio Almada. 1986. Las ciencias sociales en salud en Mexico. In *Ciencia Sociales y Salud en América Latina: Tendencias y Perspectivas,* ed. Everardo Duarte Nunes, 133–41. Montevideo: Organización Panamericana de Salud and CIESU.

Breilh, Jaime. 1982. *Epidemiología: Economía, Medicina y Política.* 2d ed. Santo Domingo: Ministerio de Salud y Bienestar Social.

Breilh, Jaime. 1990. La salud enfermedad como hecho social: Un nuevo enfoque. In *Deterioro de la Vida,* ed. Jaime Breilh et al., 21–34. Quito: Corporación Editora Nacional.

Breilh, Jaime, and Edmundo Granda. 1989. Epidemiología y contrahegemonia. *Social Science and Medicine* 28 (11): 1121–27.

Breilh, Jaime, Edmundo Granda, Arturo Campaña, and Oscar Betancourt. 1987. *Ciudad y Muerte Infantil.* Quito: CEAS Ediciones.

Breilh, Jaime, et al. 1990. *Deterioro de la Vida.* Quito: Corporación Editora Nacional.

Campaña K., Arturo. n.d. *Desarrollo de la medicina social ecuatoriana y surgimiento del CEAS.* Quito: CEAS Documentos 10.

Campaña K., Arturo. 1986. Las ciencias sociales en salud en Ecuador. In *Ciencias Sociales y Salud en América Latina: Tendencias y Perspectivas,* ed. Everardo Duarte Nunes, 117–32. Montevideo: Organización Panamericana de Salud and CIESU.

Cueto, Marcos, ed. 1994. *Missionaries of Science: The Rockefeller Foundation and Latin America.* Bloomington: Indiana University Press.

Duarte Nunes, Everardo, ed. 1986. *Ciencias Sociales y Salud en América Latina: Tendencias y Perspectivas.* Montevideo: Organización Panamericana de Salud and CIESU.

Elling, Ray. 1986. *The Struggle for Workers' Health: A Study of Six Industrialized Countries.* Farmingdale, NY: Baywood.

Escudero, José Carlos. 1980. On Lies and Health Statistics: Some Latin American Examples. *International Journal of Health Services* 10 (3): 421–34.

Fals-Borda, Orlando. 1985. *Conocimiento y Poder Popular.* Mexico: Siglo Vein-tiuno Editores.

Feinsilver, Julie M. 1989. Cuba as a "World Medical Power": The Politics of Symbolism. *Latin American Research Research Review* 24 (2): 1–34.

Feinsilver, Julie M. 1993. *Healing the Masses: Cuban Politics at Home and Abroad.* Berkeley: University of California Press.

Franco Agudelo, Saúl. 1992. Violence and Health: Preliminary Elements for Thought and Action. *International Journal of Health Services* 22 (2): 365–76.

Frankenberg, Ronald. 1974. Functionalism and After: Theory and Developments in Social Science Applied to the Health Field. *International Journal of Health Services* 4 (3): 411–27.

Frankenberg, Ronald. 1980. Medical Anthropology and Development: A Theoretical Perspective. *Social Science and Medicine* 14B (4): 197–207.

Frankenberg, Ronald. 1988. "Your Time or Mine?" An Anthropological View of the Tragic Temporal Contradictions of Biomedical Practice. *International Journal of Health Services* 18 (1): 11–34.

Frankenberg, Ronald. 1992. The Other Who Is Also the Same: The Relevance of Epidemics in Space and Time for Prevention of HIV Infection. *International Journal of Health Services* 22 (1): 73–88.

Frenk, Julio. 1993. The New Public Health. *Annual Review of Public Health* 14:469–90.

García, Juan César. 1986. Juan C. García entrevista a Juan C. García. In *Ciencias Sociales y Salud en América Latina: Tendencias y Perspectivas,* ed. Everardo Duarte Nunes, 21–28. Montevideo: Organización Panamericana de Salud and CIESU.

Ginsburg, Faye D. 1989. *Contested Lives.* Berkeley: University of California Press.

Haraway, Donna. 1989. *Primate Visions: Gender, Race, and Nature in the World of Modern Science.* New York: Routledge.

Henfrey, Colin. 1981. Dependency, Modes of Production, and the Class Analysis of Latin America. *Latin American Perspectives* 8:17–54.

Johnson, Thomas M., and Carolyn F. Sargent, eds. 1990. *Medical Anthropology: A Handbook of Theory and Method.* New York: Greenwood Press.

Keller, Evelyn Fox. 1995. *Refiguring Life.* New York: Columbia University Press.

Krieger, Nancy. 1994. Epidemiology and the Web of Causation: Has Anyone Seen the Spider? *Social Science and Medicine* 39 (7): 887–903.

Laurell, Asa Cristina. 1979. Prologo. In *Epidemiología, economía, medicina y política,* by Jaime Breilh. Mexico City: Fontamara 19.

Laurell, Asa Cristina. 1981. Mortality and Working Conditions in Agriculture in Underdeveloped Countries. *International Journal of Health Services* 11 (1): 3–19.

Laurell, Asa Cristina. 1988. Proceso de trabajo y salud en el análisis demográfico. In *La Mortalidad en México: Niveles, Tendencias y Determinantes,* ed. Mario Bronfman and José Gómez de León, 401–18. Mexico City: El Colegio de México.

Laurell, Asa Cristina. 1989. Social Analysis of Collective Health in Latin America. *Social Science and Medicine* 28 (11): 1183–91.

Laurell, Asa Cristina, and M. Márquez. 1983. *El desgaste obrero en México.* Mexico City: ERA.

Laurell, Asa Cristina, and Maria Elena Ortega. 1992. The Free Trade Agreement and the Mexican Health Sector. *International Journal of Health Services* 22 (2): 331–37.

Laurell, Asa Cristina, et al. 1977. Disease and Rural Development: A Sociological Analysis of Morbidity in Two Mexican Villages. *International Journal of Health Services* 7 (3): 401–23.

Leatherman, Thomas L. 1994. Health Implications of Changing Agrarian Economies in the Southern Andes. *Human Organization* 53 (4): 371–80.

Levins, Richard, and Richard Lewontin. 1985. *The Dialectical Biologist.* Cambridge, MA: Harvard University Press

Lock, Margaret. 1988. New Japanese Mythologies: Faltering Discipline and the Ailing Housewife. *American Ethnologist* 15:43–61.

Luerssen, J. Susan. 1994. Landlessness, Health, and the Failures of Reform in the Peruvian Highlands. *Human Organization* 53 (4): 380–87.

McElroy, Ann. 1990. Rejoinder. *Medical Anthropology Quarterly* 4 (3): 379–87.

Morgan, Lynn M. 1987. Dependency Theory in the Political Economy of Health: An Anthropological Critique. *Medical Anthropology Quarterly,* n.s., 1 (2): 131–54.

Morgan, Lynn M. 1990. The Medicalization of Anthropology: A Critical Perspective on the Critical-Clinical Debate. *Social Science and Medicine* 30 (9): 945–50.

Morsy, Soheir. 1990. Political Economy in Medical Anthropology. In *Medical Anthropology: Contemporary Theory and Method,* ed. Thomas M. Johnson and Carolyn F. Sargent, 26–46. New York: Praeger.

Nash, June, and Marx Kirsch. 1986. Polychlorinated Biphenyls in the Electrical Machine Industry: An Ethnological Study of Community Action and Corporate Responsibility. *Social Science and Medicine* 23 (2): 131–38.

Navarro, Vicente. 1985. U.S. Marxist Scholarship in the Analysis of Health and Medicine. *International Journal of Health Services* 15 (4): 525–44.

Navarro, Vicente. 1989. Radicalism, Marxism, and Medicine. *Medical Anthropology* 11: 195–219.

Roseberry, William. 1989. *Anthropologies and Histories.* New Brunswick: Rutgers University Press.

Scheper-Hughes, Nancy. 1992. *Death Without Weeping: The Violence of Everyday Life in Brazil.* Berkeley: University of California Press.

Scheper-Hughes, Nancy, and Margaret Lock. 1986. Speaking "Truth" to Illness: Metaphors, Reification, and a Pedagogy for Patients. *Medical Anthropology Quarterly* 17 (5): 137–40.

Scheper-Hughes, Nancy, and Margaret Lock. 1987. The Mindful Body: A Prolegomenon to Future Work in Medical Anthropology. *Medical Anthropology Quarterly* 1 (1): 6–41.

Singer, Merrill. 1989. The Coming of Age of Critical Medical Anthropology. *Social Science and Medicine* 28 (11): 1193–1203.

Singer, Merrill. 1992a. The Application of Theory in Medical Anthropology: An Introduction. *Medical Anthropology* 14: 1–8.

Singer, Merrill. 1992b. Farewell to Adaptationism: Unnatural Selection and the Politics of Biology. Paper prepared in advance for participants in symposium no. 115, "Political-Economic Perspectives in Biological Anthropology: Building a Biocultural Synthesis," organized by the Wenner-Gren Foundation for Anthropological Research. Oct. 30–Nov. 7. Cabo San Lucas, Baja California Sur, Mexico.

Singer, Merrill, and Hans A. Baer. 1989. Toward an Understanding of Capitalist and Socialist Health. *Medical Anthropology* 11:91–107.

Solórzano, Armando. 1992. Sowing the Seeds of Neo-Imperialism: The Rockefeller Foundation's Yellow Fever Campaign in Mexico. *International Journal of Health Services* 22 (3): 529–54.

Susser, Ida. 1985. Union Carbide and the Community Surrounding It: The Case of a Community in Puerto Rico. *International Journal of Health Services* 15 (4): 561–83.

Taussig, Michael. 1980. Reification and the Consciousness of the Patient. *Social Science and Medicine* 14B:3–13.

Turner, Bryan S. 1995. *Medical Power and Social Knowledge.* 2d ed. London: Sage.

Chapter 18

Nature, Political Ecology, and Social Practice: Toward an Academic and Political Agenda

Søren Hvalkof and Arturo Escobar

Ecological approaches in the social sciences and the humanities are experiencing a renaissance in many parts of the world in the form of what is now frequently called "political ecology." Political ecology has been characterized as "an emerging agenda" in third world and environmental studies. Different disciplines and fields (e.g., geography, anthropology, history, sociology, feminist theory, ecological economics, environmental history, historical archaeology) seem to be engaged in a novel reformulation of the relationship between society and nature, humans and environment, biology and history, which could be encompassed under the generic term *political ecology* (Bryant 1992; Peet and Watts 1996).

This new interest in "ecology" and "nature" is evidently spurred by the increasing environmental crisis that societal development has inflicted upon human livelihood on a global scale. At the heart of this new interest lie important intellectual and political questions. On the one hand, the politicization of political ecology has been fostered by the introduction of the canon of sustainability in the third world development debate and by the emergence of social movements represented by a multiplicity of organizations and interests, ranging from environmental NGOs (nongovernmental organizations) to indigenous peoples' struggles—all staking claims over the production of nature and the control of natural resources. In the academic world, on the other hand, postmodern and poststructuralist deconstruction and critiques of essentialism have raised fundamental questions regarding the very constitution of the modern knowledge and cultural configuration—the modern "episteme"—governing our relations to "nature."[1]

The combination and ordering of the terms *political* and *ecological* suggest that nature's "housekeeping" needs to be recontextualized in a social field significantly larger and more complex than that of biological imperatives. Such a "socialization" of ecosystems and environmental relations is not new to anthropology, where approaches seeking to theorize the relationship between humans and the natural environment—such as cultural ecology, human ecology, and social ecology—have long been in existence. However productive these different conceptualizations might have been, they have almost without exception operated within a Cartesian universe, where the place and constitution of "nature" and its human/social adversary are already given, making impossible radical challenges to the underlying episteme. A dichotomized view of nature and society—also embedded in the separation of subject and object of knowledge—became a founding principle of modernist paradigms.

Political ecology tends to dissolve these boundaries. Defined as *the study of manifold constructions of nature in contexts of power,* political ecology scrutinizes the ecological in ways that incorporate into the inquiry human decision making, political strategies, preferences and choices, cognitive mapping of the social and the natural, as well as operating at various scales and domains. It also brings to the fore the question of the construction and identity of "nature" and "the natural," assuming that it can no longer be taken for granted; in doing so, political ecology makes visible the political implications that follow from a significant questioning of the underlying epistemic order. Contrary to most postmodern discourses, in which this questioning takes place with little regard for social and political accountability, political ecology intensifies anthropology's endemic tension between theory and practice. As we shall argue, it also provides novel elements toward re-imagining such a relation.

To anticipate our argument, political ecology highlights the fact that social movements in particular are becoming central to both struggles over nature and our attempts to theorize the natural. To the extent that social movements can be seen as defending local meanings and practices of nature—that is, as movements of ecological attachment to culturally defined territories—they can also be seen as mediating our practice as anthropologists and experts of the natural/cultural. Social movements and political ecology thus constitute a rich conceptual and political space for rethinking questions of reflexivity, writing, and intervention in ways that are theoretically sophisticated and consciously political. Political ecology can thus be seen as an appropriate space for articulating a new theory of practice and a new practice of theory for anthropology (Escobar 1996, n.d.; Hvalkof 1996).

In this chapter, we seek to provide the rudiments of an anthropological political ecology following the orientation sketched above. After providing a brief historical overview of the anthropological involvement with ecology in the first part of the chapter, we move on to discuss the "nature of nature's identity" today, by rethinking the natural as lying at the intersection of biology and history. In the final part, we discuss the political dimensions of such a reconceptualization in relation to third world development in general and rain forest communities in particular. By recentering the theoretical contributions of poststructuralism (particularly antiessentialism) onto the sphere of political activism, we hope to anticipate and overcome some of the reactions, justified or not, to our attempt at recontextualizing our human and biological reality by appealing to theories originating primarily in the human and the social sciences.

The Anthropological Affair with Ecology

The interest in the relationship between human culture and the physical environment in anthropology can be traced back to the last century's proto-anthropological initiatives in continental Northern Europe. Following a modernist paradigm, which for nearly a century stood unchallenged (at least in anthropology), nature was seen as the medium for the development of human society. It was the plasma of which human culture and civilization formed its space and molded its identity, the wild and uncontrolled cosmos, the domestication of which was intrinsic to any development, as expressed in Newtonian equations and the laws of thermodynamics. This conception was manifested in a simple geographical and environmental determinism, the most famous proponent of which was the German geographer Friedrich Ratzel (1889, 1896), who formulated his "antropo-geografie" as a explanatory scheme for cultural history—a precursor of both modern cultural geography and ethnology.

This interest in human/environment relations developed simultaneously in the United States but, contrary to the European tradition, it was linked to government policies of internal colonization, particularly the control of resources and of Native American populations.[2] Besides the inherent ecological dimension in these attempts, the potential for politicization and applicability of U.S. research was apparent in the mapping of contested spaces, natural resources, and peoples within the researcher's own society. These activities were fundamentally political in character, whether they were motivated by state control and expansion into Native American territories or by attempts to defend indigenous territorial rights. Thus the incipient ecological approach in anthropology provided instruments that could be brought to play in a variety of fields of interest.[3] Out of this geographical and ethnological hinterland evolved a new ecological anthropology—a purely American phenomenon.[4] It became manifest in the late 1930s as a *modern rationalist and materialist reaction* to the particularistic tradition introduced earlier by Franz Boas. This reaction was also shaped by the social crisis in U.S. society in the 1930s, Roosevelt's New Deal policy, and the Indian Reorganization Act, which together prompted (some) anthropologists to seek more practical and socially useful academic possibilities, and which added some structure to the former "planless hodge-podge" that characterized the anthropology of the preceding period (Lowie 1920, 1938).[5]

The first distinctly ecological program for a new anthropology, largely inspired by cultural geographer Carl Sauer, was launched by Julian Steward under the rubric of "Cultural Ecology" (Steward 1936, 1941, 1949, 1955, 1956, 1968). Steward's intent was to establish a science with greater social relevance. His cultural ecology searched for causal relationships between human society and culture and the biotic environment. Its focus was a techno-environmental "cultural core," defined as those activities most closely related to production and subsistence. Interested in recuperating evolutionist theory without falling back into simplistic social Darwinist schemes, Steward's cultural ecology highlighted multicausal relationships and concluded in a theory of multilinear cultural evolution. Despite its effort to diversify causal relationships, this cultural ecology was a rather reductionist and deterministic theory, and it has been widely criticized as such. But Steward succeeded in placing ecology permanently on the anthropological agenda and in fostering, beyond its outmoded theoretical model, a great deal of interesting and inspiring thinking that has continued until today. It should be noted that Maurice Godelier much later paraphrased Steward and recognized his theory of multilinear evolution as identical with the general theory of economic systems, which in his view is the ultimate object of economic anthropology (Godelier 1974). Many of the attempts by structural marxists at theorizing noncapitalist societies in the 1960s and 1970s could be seen as an unacknowledged replication of what Steward and White had tried to do two decades earlier (Terray 1972; Meillassoux 1964; Hindess and Hirst 1977).

During the same period, Leslie White was undertaking the task of rein-stating a grand theory of broad evolutionary schemes in anthropology with his cultural evolutionism. White's motivation was much more explicitly political in its orientation; he had derived his inspiration from L. H. Morgan, the Marxist classics, and a visit to the Soviet Union in 1927, a time when a mechanistic developmentalism of a modernist utopia was being fomented. He developed a unilineal and monocausal theory, focusing on levels of energy consumption as determinants of stages of cultural evolution (White 1943, 1947, 1949). Whatever can be said about the rigidity and mechanistic reductionism of his theory, White developed a systemic notion of culture as process, a view which in many respects was ahead of its time and which did not receive the attention it merited (White 1959). After World War II the ecological project in anthropology was continued by a new generation of anthropologists, who endeavored to overcome some of the weakness and contradiction of earlier approaches. Those who favored cultural evolution as an explanatory model tried to merge (or mediate between) Steward's multilineal specificity and White's broad evolutionary brush strokes by focusing on issues such as specific aspects of evolution, the emergence of the state, and differences in scope and scale.

These attempts were still haunted by the ghosts of environmental determinism but also opened the way for an inclusion of political processes in the ecological approach, particularly through the focus on the emergence of the state (e.g., Sahlins and Service 1960). Those who were more interested in functional relations of cause-and-effect in local contexts tried to explain social organization and culture as forms of adaptation of human populations to the local environment. This explanation was based on a model of homeostatic equilibrium and sustainability that borrowed most of its concepts from biological ecology and systems theory, focusing on organic feedback relationships (e.g., Vayda and Rappaport 1968). This neo-functionalism was as reductionist as earlier attempts and was restricted to closed (eco)systems. But the concept of adaptation to the environment became widespread and has dominated the ecological discourse in modern anthropology until recently. Inspired by the cultural materialism of Marvin Harris (1968, 1979), the new ecological approach eventually evolved into a research program on protein procurement widely criticized for its fixation on deterministic explanatory schemes devoid of any sociopolitical or historical considerations and leaning toward a new scientism (Gross 1975; E. Ross 1978, 1980; J. B. Ross 1980; Hill and Hawkes 1983).

A much more imaginative and productive route was chosen by less rigidly thinking scholars who shifted their analytic focus from social structure to social process. This new *processual ecological* approach may, in retrospect, be seen as a forerunner of some of the later poststructuralist approaches although it did not succeed in breaking from modernist epistemological constraints. Roy Rappaport in particular came to play a very prominent part in this development. Inspired by the works and inclusiveness of Gregory Bateson's ecology and cybernetics, Rappaport moved from a functionalist position at first presented in his famous *Pigs for the Ancestors* (1968, 1971a, 1971b) to a rather nonconventional consideration of an ecology merging God, reason, nature, and adaptation into a very dynamic approach profoundly critical of the maladies of civilization, even if still constrained by the belief in modern science as savior (e.g., Bateson 1979; Rappaport 1976, 1977a, 1977b, 1979; see Hvalkof 1982 for a discussion). This effort was soon echoed from outside anthropology by Anthony Wilden (1980, 1987), a communication and systems theorist with a passion for Jacques Lacan's reinterpretations of Freudian psychoanalysis inspired by Saussurean linguistics. This rather unexpected support for Rappaport's (and Bateson's) cybernetic ecologies of mind propitiated a new sensitivity toward psychological interests in ecological anthropology, represented by the cognitive approaches of ethnoecology and ethnoscience, previously regarded as peripheral to cultural ecology (Conklin 1957, 1961, 1972; Sturtevant 1964; Berlin 1973, 1976).

It is in this processual ecological anthropology, developed in the late 1970s and early 1980s, that we find the seeds of a politicization of the ecological approach, embodied in the critique of civilization and of earlier eco-anthropological practices, which also fostered a lively epistemological debate (Bergman 1975; Kelly and Rappaport 1975; Rappaport 1977b, 1979; Friedman 1974, 1979; Sahlins 1976; Vayda 1986; Vayda and McCay 1975, 1977). The creation of a *political ecology approach* proper took place in the late stages of this processual approach, animated by Marxist-based critiques of ecological functionalism (Cook 1973; Friedman and Rowlands 1977) and leading to the infusion of ecological anthropology with political economy and historical considerations (and vice versa, to a lesser degree). This intellectual ferment also led to important breakthroughs in the ecological approach in European social anthropology (Burnham and Ellen 1979; Ellen 1982).

In the 1980s, and continuing into the late 1990s, such political-economy–driven political ecology was in turn permeated with other elements from the growing postmodern and poststructuralist developments, particularly the poststructuralist analyses of meaning, knowledge, institutions, development, and social movements (Peet and Watts 1996), and the feminist insights into the gendered character of knowledge, environment, organizations, and social and economic relations (Rocheleau, Thomas-Slayter, and Wangari 1996). From these two recent works—purporting to guide research under the rubrics of "liberation ecology" and "feminist political ecology," respectively—a more complex and nuanced account of both nature–society relations and political ecology is emerging. It highlights the interwoven character of the discursive, material, social, and cultural dimensions of the relation between humans and nature. While empirical studies based on these frameworks have been taking place for some years, it is also recognized that "in a sense the theoretical work has just only begun" (Peet and Watts 1996, 39). Further fertilizing this critical and reconstructive process have been the poststructuralist critiques of the modernist epistemic order and of the essentializing tendencies that characterize it. We now turn to these critiques and attempt to apply notions of constructedness and anti-essentialism to the field of the natural. Our goals are simultaneously to make visible the political implications hidden in purely science-oriented views of nature, on the one hand—to debunk unexamined positions of naturalism—and to suggest new ways to account for the biological without bracketing the political.[6]

Nature: Constructed or Essential?

To ascertain that the meaning of nature has shifted throughout history according to cultural, socioeconomic, and political factors may sound trivial, yet it might be the source of novel insights into the nature of nature. As Raymond Williams succinctly put it in a remarkable text, "the idea of nature contains, though often unnoticed, an extraordinary amount of human history" (1980, 68). In rejecting essential statements about the nature of nature, he goes on to assert that in such statements, "the idea of nature is the idea of man . . . the idea of man in society, indeed the idea of kinds of societies" (70). That nature came to be thought of as separate from people, for instance, is related to the view of "man" brought about by capitalism and modernity. Nature came to be increasingly produced through labor, even if that labor is made invisible by ideology. Following in Williams's tradition, Barbara Bender writes that people's experience of landscapes "is based in large measure on the particularity of the social, political and economic relations within which they live out their lives" (1993, 246). There is a politics of landscapes, she argues, that belies the class myths of "untouched nature" that circumscribe it, and which has everything to do (in England at least) with gendered identities and the commodification of history as national heritage. As Lansing (1991) also showed in his study of the engineered landscapes of Bali—the beautiful system of agricultural terraces and canals usually portrayed as timeless and unchanging—landscapes are not only the product of human history, but they bear the marks of a particular cultural, social, and economic set of conditions. A sort of landscape ethnography emerges from these works, one that would read history back into the seemingly natural text of nature.

These analyses are important and perceptive. Yet nature, landscape, and our knowledge of them are confronted with a new challenge, besides those posed by the environmental crisis, one for which we might be neither culturally nor epistemologically prepared. As various authors have observed (Strathern 1992; Haraway 1991; Rabinow 1992; Soper 1996), we might be witnessing—in the wake of unprecedented intervention into nature at the molecular level—the final decline of the modern ideology of naturalism, that is, the belief in the existence of pristine Nature outside of history and human context. Let us be clear about what this ideology entails. We are talking here about nature as an essential principle and foundational category, a ground for both being and society, nature as "an independent domain of intrinsic value, truth and authenticity" (Soper 1996, 22). *To assert the disappearance of this notion is quite different from denying the existence of a biophysical reality* with structures and processes of its own, which the life sciences try to understand. It means to emphasize, on the one hand, that for us, humans (which also includes life scientists and ecologists!), nature is always constructed by our meaning-giving and discursive processes, so that what we perceive as natural is always already—at least in some sense—cultural and social. On the other hand, our own beliefs in nature as untouched and independent are giving way—with molecular technoscience, from recombinant DNA to gene mapping and nanotechnology—to a new view of nature as artificially produced. This entails an unprecedented ontological and epistemological transformation which we have hardly begun to understand, requiring an entirely different approach which we identify broadly with anti-essentialism.

It is true, however, that postmodern thinking has advocated somewhat hastily the idea that since there is no nature outside history, there is nothing natural about nature. As Kate Soper constructively discusses, this has placed cultural theorists at odds with environmentalists and life scientists who for the most part continue to espouse the belief in external, prediscursive nature (Soulé and Lease 1995). It is thus necessary to strive for a balanced position that acknowledges both the constructed nature of nature in human context and nature in the realist sense—that is, the existence of an independent order of nature, including a biological body, even as an a priori condition for culture—and the representations of which constructivists can legitimately query in terms of their history or political implications. Paraphrasing Soper (1996, 23), we can thus navigate between "'nature endorsing' and 'nature-skeptical' perspectives" in order "to incorporate a greater awareness of what their respective discourses on 'nature' may be ignoring and politically repressing."[7]

Worldwide, the inscription of the cultural onto the biological is yielding a great variety of forms of the natural. The question is what new combinations of nature and culture will become permissible and practicable and what kind of political practice these combinations will nourish. There is still a long way to go before a political theory of nature is formulated, but it seems that the present development of a political ecology approach is heading in this direction. If it is true, given the ineluctability of power, that the political "must be conceived as a dimension that is inherent to every human society and determines our very ontological condition" (Mouffe 1993, 3), it is revealing that such a political theory of nature itself has not been developed within the environmental movement or in ecological approaches of the social and human sciences.

Escobar (1999) has recently suggested that we consider "nature" as a product of the manifold and changing articulations of history and biology. For analytical purposes, Escobar identifies three types of such "nature regimes." The first is the organic nature regime, constituted by the inclusive and integral view of nature held by many nonmodern peoples and societies, which does not separate the cultural from the natural, the human from the nonhuman and the spiritual, and the organic from the physical. The second is the modern capitalist nature, identified as commoditized, disciplined, essentialized, simplified, dichotomized, and evolutionist (Smith 1984). The third are the techno-natures being produced by new technosciences, characterized by hybridizations of the organic and the artificial, even if perhaps opening toward some of the features of organicity found in the first regime. Political ecology could be seen as the study of the cultural, technoeconomic, and ecological processes through which each regime is produced, and the articulations and contradictions that characterize their increasing conflict and engagement in concrete situations.

To sum up, we suggest that it is possible to speak about "nature's identity" in the same way in which poststructuralist theorists talk about individual and collective identity as unfixed and always under construction, as opposed to something that progressively develops out of an unchanging core. This is what we mean by anti-essentialism. This identity, to be sure, is constructed out of biophysical, cultural, and technoeconomic elements and through a variety of biological and social processes. "Nature" can thus be seen as the result of the intersection of history and biology in concrete situations.

From Nature as Constructed to an Alternative Theory of Practice

Ethnographic research is essential for illuminating different nature regimes; said differently, ethnographic research can make visible discourses of cultural, social, and economic difference among third world communities in contexts of globalization and development. This analysis has perhaps advanced the most in connection with the rethinking of the relation between environment and development. As anthropologists, geographers, feminist researchers, ecologists, and others involved in third world situations have demonstrated with increasing clarity, it is very often the case that rural communities "construct" nature in strikingly different ways from the prevalent modern forms. In other words, many third world communities signify—and thus use—their natural environments in ways quite different from *modern* (dominant) attitudes and uses. This insight has led a growing group of scholars and others (including some "developers") to argue that precisely these different systems of meanings-uses of nature—and the social relations in which they exist—should be the basis for sustainable development proposals, instead of the managerial and rationalist recipes promoted by the ecodevelopment establishment. Let us briefly review the evidence for this type of ecological and cultural difference, and the political struggles to which it is giving rise, as an important and hopeful aspect of postdevelopment.

Ethnographic studies unveil a significantly different set of practices of thinking about, relating to, constructing, and experiencing the biological and the natural in many third world communities (Milton 1993; Hobart 1993; Dahl 1993; Descola 1994; Descola and Pálsson 1996; Restrepo and del Valle 1996; Gudeman and Rivera 1990, for peasant communities). In a classic article on the subject, Marilyn Strathern (1980) made the case that we cannot interpret native mappings of the social and the biological in terms of our concepts of nature, culture, and society. For many indigenous and rural groups, "'culture' does not provide a distinctive set of objects with which one manipulates 'nature' . . . nature is not 'manipulated'" (174–75). In contrast to modern constructions with their strict separation between biophysical, human, and spiritual worlds, the anthropology of local knowledge suggests that constructions of nature are often predicated on links of continuity between the three spheres. Continuity is culturally established through symbols, rituals, and practices and is embedded in particular social relations which also differ from the modern capitalist type (Hvalkof 1989).

A local model of nature could thus exhibit features such as the following (which may or may not correspond to the parameters of modern nature, or only partially): categorizations of human, social, and biological entities (for instance, of what is human and what is not, the domestic and the wild, what is produced by humans and what is produced by forest, what is innate and what emerges from human action, what pertains to spirits and what pertains to humans, etc.); boundary settings (differentiating say, man from animal, forest from settlement, men from women, or among various segments of the forest); systematic classification of animals, plants and spirits; and so forth. It may also contain mechanisms for maintaining the good order and balance of biophysical, human, and spiritual circuits; or a circular view of time and of biological and social life, ultimately validated by Providence, gods, or goddesses; or a theory of how all beings in the universe are "raised" or "nurtured" out of similar principles, since in many nonmodern cultures the entire universe is conceived of as a living being with no strict separation between humans and nature, individual and community, community and the gods (see Escobar n.d. for a review of this literature).

While specific formulas for arranging all of these factors vary greatly from group to group, they tend to have certain features in common, such as a complex image of social life that is not necessarily opposed to nature (in other words, one in which the natural world is integral to the social). This social life can be thought about in terms of relations such as kinship, extended kindred, and vernacular or analogic gender. Local models also evidence a particular attachment to a territory conceived of as a multidimensional entity that results from many types of practices and relations;

and they also establish relations between symbolic/cultural systems and productive relations that can be highly complex. What is most important about these models from the perspective of postdevelopment is that they could be said to constitute ensembles of meanings-uses that, while existing in contexts of power that increasingly include transnational forces, cannot be reduced to modern meaning and uses. The increasing emphasis and documentation of local knowledge (Hobart 1993; Warren, Slikkeveer, and Brokensha 1995) clearly suggest that it is possible to articulate a discourse of ecological difference of cultural origin.

This task is actually being advanced by two separate but increasingly interrelated social actors: social movement activists in a variety of communities and social settings, and political ecology theorists attempting to articulate an alternative theory of ecological rationality and sustainable development, a political theory of nature if you like. The main point on the agenda is finding ways to weave together the cultural, the ecological, and the technoeconomic into a different theory of production that is not subordinated to the economized production of commodities for profit and the rationality of managers and planners (Leff 1993, 1995; Escobar 1996). Although much remains to be done in this respect, this research already suggests ways in which discourses and practices of cultural and ecological difference could be used as the basis for alternative social and economic projects.

The articulation of these proposals is evidently not taking place in an isolationist academic structure but clearly in spaces of convergence and interaction between theorists and activists, and activists and communities; in both of these spaces, the development of political tools for action takes on a pragmatic and political character. The social movements representing such myriad alternative realities and futures are crucial for any such academic effort and hopefully the link between academics and activists will develop into a dynamic and symbiotic relationship. Political ecology offers a pertinent space for such a converging endeavor, which we outline in the remainder of the chapter.

The Politics of Political Ecology

Postmodern and poststructuralist approaches in anthropology and other fields have been criticized for retreating into academism, depoliticizing cultural analysis and restricting their scope to hermeneutic and deconstruction exercises with a concomitant absence of social, political, and ethical criteria and responsibility (Hvalkof 1990, 1996). Marxist scholars like David Harvey and Frederic Jameson have similarly chastised postmodern proponents for abandoning the attempt at theorizing social reality as a whole, without which, in their view, political praxis is impossible. Although these criticisms are certainly warranted in many instances, it is not given that anti-essentialism—as used here—will inevitably lead to a depoliticized aesthetics or to a "seductive poetics of fascism," to paraphrase Taussig (Hvalkof 1997). The same failings are often found within the modern paradigms. What seems crucial at this point in history is to develop a theory of practice and a practice of theory that enable both a pluralistic universe of multiple truths and a measure of ethics and political scrutiny.

For poststructuralist theory, truths are "statements within socially produced discourses, rather than 'facts' about reality" (Peet and Watts 1993, 228). "Truth" is anchored in specific sociocultural contexts and inextricably linked to power. Many authors have underscored the paradoxical nature of this position, since it seemingly results in the idea that responsibility can only be gauged in terms of the relative truth of each specific discourse. No overall political or ethical criterion can be generated without it being suspect—that is, seen as sheltering some kind of universal or essentialism linked to forms of domination. This puts an enormous responsibility on the individual researcher, requiring ethical and political criteria which are not at all explicitly developed in the practices of academic knowledge production. Poststructuralist critiques have undeniably liberated thought from the confinement of modern epistemic regimes and dissolved rigid dogmas, but unreconstructed politically they tend to leave us with a fragmented and particularistic universe, creating a serious political vacuum. How do we establish political responsibility within a universe of partial, situated truths? What are the criteria for political and ethical choices? How do we make ourselves accountable without falling back to essentialist and ahistorical arguments about the nature of things? How do we articulate, in a context without firm universals, an ethics of expert knowledge as political practice? We shall return to these questions in the conclusion of the chapter.

The political ecology sketched above suggests ways for the articulation of such a political dimension if "political" entails an integral social praxis. We contend that such a politics could very well be catalyzed by relating academic practice directly to social movements which are today's major articulators of "democratic" alternatives to the reproduction of hegemonic capitalist structures, and the agents of postdevelopment options and livelihoods. Because of the authors' personal involvement and experience with social movements of rain forest peoples, we will exemplify briefly such a nonessentialist political ecology approach by drawing on our respective work in Colombia and Peru.

"Rain Forest" Social Movements and Political Ecology

To refer to "social movements of the rain forest" is actually misleading and, in fact, contradicts much of the main argument we have put forward here. First of all, those social movements operating in, and out of, the "rain forest" that represent an alternative agenda of postdevelopment and nonmodern paradigms are nearly exclusively of indigenous peoples and similar local groups organized on ethnocultural identity platforms. Many poor peasants in the same areas are often (but not exclusively) identified with modern practices of colonization, farming, extraction, and so on. They rarely establish or relate to social movements in the same areas.[8] It is also not certain that all social movements represent alternatives to the status quo (Hvalkof 1989, 1994; Alvarez, Dagnino, and Escobar, 1998).

The "rain forest" is actually a construction intimately related to modernist paradigms. It implies the idea of a bounded and uncontrolled space, where Western civilization's dreams about otherness and its utopias and fantasies have been frequently projected. The "rain forest" as such is seen as one of the last remaining "naturally (wild) grown" and "noncontrolled" (savage) spaces on earth. According to the same ideology, rain forest peoples are similarly seen as the most "natural" people left on earth and as possessing the most natural knowledge for saving the rain forest, namely, "indigenous knowledge." This monolithic conception of an enormous natural biological system is an ideological construction which partly confirms an existing system of thought, and partly legitimizes paternalistic and technocratic intervention regarding its "rain forest" object. Furthermore, this focus has entailed a consistent and unfailing depoliticization of the discourse. It has also maintained a biological fixation in the debate, making it a question of threatened plant and animal species, rather than of political choices and strategies.

Environmental NGOs have benefited from this depoliticization. It allows concerned individuals to take part in the environmental movement and support a "cause" without getting squeezed in the traditional left–right dichotomy, which can risk embarrassing conflicts with colleagues or family. Nature conservation presents itself in mainstream discourses as politically uncontaminated. However, the following points unmask this discourse, and illustrate the political content of the rain forest image.

1. The "rain forest" does not exist as such in biological terms; as is well known, there are many different types of tropical forest and combinations of biotopes in the geographical areas where so-called rain forests are supposed to be situated, covering several continents. No such single empirical formation as "the rain forest" exists.

2. These forest areas are not instances of "untouched nature." If we take the Amazon as an example, the majority of the areas have been in use or impacted upon by humans during history and prehistory. Population estimates for the Amazon basin in 1492 range from 6 to 11 million inhabitants (Denevan 1966, 1976; Dobyns 1966). At this time around 2 million indigenous inhabitants reside in the same area (not counting the non-indigenous population). Long before the conquest the aboriginal population cut jungle, made horticultural swiddens, constructed major residential areas, established complex social organizations, hunted, fished, collected, made turtle hatcheries and fish farms, and engaged in long-distance trade with rain forest products. Thus, the rain forest systems in the Amazon cannot at all be regarded as untouched nature, but should rather be regarded as a cultural landscape, an integral part of human formation, like so many other landscapes/wildlands on this planet. Similarly, the Pacific Coast rain forest regions of Colombia have been commonly seen as "isolated," even if archaeological and historical evidence shows patterns of occupation dating back to many centuries before the arrival of the Spaniards to the region in the late sixteenth century, including possible contact with East Asian and Mesoamerican cultures well before 1492 (Escobar and Pedrosa 1996; Escobar 1997).

3. It is not biological factors which determine the ecological state of different rain forest areas today, but social and political processes. For example, the forest areas of the Amazon are unequally distributed within the boundaries of eight different national states and a French protectorate, each with their own legislation, with different policies, each with unique compositions of populations, each with unique histories. In the Colombian Pacific, it is large-scale development plans and the increasing presence of capital-intensive oper-

ations in recent years (shrimp farming, African oil palm planta-tions, timber extraction, industrial gold mining etc.) that are dras-tically transforming local human and biophysical ecologies.

4. These different tropical forest areas are not deserted biological reserves. They are inhabited by millions of people (close to one mil-lion in the Colombian Pacific, for instance, an area 600 miles long and 50 to 100 miles wide, with some of the world's richest biodi-versity) and have been so in some cases for millennia; this includes different indigenous and other population groups (90 percent of the Pacific Coast population is black), who are engaged in political demands for human, cultural, and territorial rights. They are reluc-tant, to say the least, to let themselves be defined as "wild nature." To this should be added several other types of non-indigenous pop-ulations, like settlers of a variety of origins, who are also striving to survive in these areas.

In short, rain forests should be seen as much more than ecological entities; they are first and foremost socially and politically determined systems. Conservation strategies (if this is what is wanted) have to take this realiza-tion as their point of departure. But this is not what is happening. Rather, there is a global tendency toward the reinforcement of the political status quo and of ruling power structures under the guise of ecologically sound ("sustainable") development policies and biodiversity conservation strate-gies. This is reflected in the techno-biological fixation of the debate and the proclivity toward decontextualized managerial practices. These tendencies have been characterized by terribly undemocratic methods, especially with regard to local populations. Issues that are of public interest and the con-comitant contested policies linked to them are thus removed from the sphere of political decision making and shifted to the domain of anony-mous and inaccessible expert languages; the results are faceless policies produced by organizations without accountability, thus reinforcing the centrality of bureaucratic and expert-based practices characteristic of modernity, to the exclusion of other modes of being, knowing, and doing.

Within modern versions of "nature," Amazonian Indians—as much as indigenous and black peoples of the Colombian Pacific Coast region—have always been classified and defined as an integral part of Nature. Even when the language indicates otherwise, as in terms such as "indigenous cultures," there is a binarism at play that suggests that these cultures are "nature grown," unlike non-indigenous or "Western" cultures. The resulting objectifization of indigenous peoples has had profound and far-reaching effects; this objectification is, indeed, one of the constitutive prerequisites for the permanence of slavery, the commodification of Indians as a natural resource (indentured labor), and the atrocities still committed against them by modern societies (Hvalkof 1995, 1997). This occidental-based conception of indigenous people as objectified "nature" is widespread and spans from multinational corporations and the big Northern environmental organizations to third world governments and the Shining Path revolutionary movement. This "naturalization" and "objectification" of indigenous people is constantly being reproduced, a process in which environmental agencies also play a part.

As long as indigenous populations are defined as an integral part of "nature," they are seen as controllable and can be confined to, or accepted in, natural "protected" areas. When, however, they begin to put forward political demands and to reassert control over their resources and future, their presence and legitimacy begins to be questioned. Nature—it is of course assumed—does not act politically; it has its own managerial hierarchy and self-appointed spokespersons. Strategies of biodiversity conservation and protection of "nature" based on modern structures of thought will invariably reflect and reproduce the very same hegemonic order and power structure in which they originate, for which nature conservation and conservation of the political status quo are two sides of the same coin (Escobar 1997; Hvalkof 1996, 1997; Johnson 1996).

The preceding analysis highlights the importance of a nonessentialist view of nature and political ecology as a powerful political instrument for moving away from these tendencies. Similarly, social movements have a central importance in the political ecology we envision because they enact a different politics of representation and practices of nature, which they see as existing in the local practices of their communities. The social movements that have grown out of "rain forest" settings find a common denominator in their articulation of four fundamental rights: to their identity, their territory, political autonomy, and their own vision of "development" or social practice. Most of these movements are explicitly conceived in terms of cultural difference, and on the ecological difference this difference makes. They are not movements for development and the satisfaction of needs, even if economic and material improvements are important for them. They are movements of cultural and ecological attachment to a territory. For them, the right to exist is a cultural, political, and economic question. They necessarily open up to certain forms of market exchange and technoscience (e.g., through critical engagement with biodiversity conservation strategies), while resisting a complete capitalist and scientific valorization of nature. They can thus be seen as advancing through their political strategy a tactic of postdevelopment, to the extent that they forcefully voice and defend discourses and practices of cultural, ecological, and economic differentiation and diversification (Hvalkof 1997; see Escobar 1997 and Grueso, Rosero, and Escobar, 1998, for the social movement of black communities of the Pacific Coast of Colombia).

It is incontrovertible that neither the renewal of political ecology—related to recent critiques of development—nor third world social movements predicated on a politics of difference will bring an end to modern ecocidal development practices. We can say, however, that together they adumbrate a postdevelopment era and the end of development as we have known it until now—that is, as an overpowering organizing principle of social life and the ultimate arbiter of thought and practice in what until now has been known as the Third World (Escobar 1995).

Conclusion

We have emphasized an open conception of political ecology as the study of the manifold articulations of history and biology, and of the inevitable cultural mediation through which such articulations are necessarily effected. We also suggested that such a political ecology practice could be an important tool for social movements striving to counteract impositions of modern development and conceptions of nature. An anti-essentialist political ecology of this type would recognize the plurality of natures that exist today and the contrasting roles that the social and biological play in these various regimes. This view of nature regimes might provide us with novel ways to release the political effectivity of those forms of the cultural and the biological we wish to defend. To bring local constructions and practices of nature to the terrain of social theory thus becomes an epistemological and political act. As Malaysian anthropologist Wazir Jahan Karim states, referring explicitly to the environmental arena, "whose definitions one may use becomes important," as does "uplifting indigenous knowledge to the level of social theory" (1996, 135). Anthropologists have an important contribution to make in projecting the global potential of local knowledge, a task which can be fraught with unexpected difficulties.[9]

Within the academic discipline of anthropology, such an approach would tenaciously encourage integrationist practices between its different and seemingly growing and fragmented subfields (cf. Goodman and Leatherman, this vol., chap. 1). Biological anthropology, medical anthropology, and archaeology are of key importance in anthropological political ecology for releasing the biophysical and interpretive potential of the "biological." Perhaps the best way to achieve this goal would be by integrating biological and sociocultural perspectives in concrete and project-oriented situations. Such an integration could help overcome preexisting conceptual and epistemological tensions between essentialist and nonessentialist thinking, and between rigid scientism and depoliticized deconstruction, to the extent that the articulation of a new plural approach would have to take place in a shared political and epistemological space. This space would not be defined by programmatic academic manifestos, but through pragmatic engagement, putting our academic potential at play in the fields of the world. It would force the discipline to develop new methodologies and approaches challenging the academic structure and its practices, from fieldwork to writing. Otherwise, anthropology might remain a largely irrelevant and provincial exercise couched in Western theoretical language and endorsing the social interests that keep this language in place.

This approach would require, in turn, that academic analyses and production be thought out with, and made accessible to, other political actors. In other words, to ensure that it is truly political, political ecology must avail itself of a lucid notion of social practice as an integral part of its theoretical and methodological toolkit. Such a strategy would help overcome the common view of postmodernism and poststructuralism as "narcissistic" (Hvalkof 1990, 1996). By articulating intellectual academic production with social movements and other social processes (including the politics of expert knowledge) the "political" would be endowed with the same centrality on the academic agenda that political theorists envision for society as a whole (Mouffe 1993; Laclau 1996). As natural and social scientists, we are called upon to fulfill this task by the events of the day, for they construct the cultural and the biological as ineluctably political. Political ecology today is a significant attempt to measure up to this task.

NOTES

1. The notion of "episteme" originates in the work of Michel Foucault (1973), who outlined the emergence of life, labor, and language as modern objects of knowledge in the sciences of biology, political economy, and linguistics. Those interested in the history of the development of a rational language of illness and life

might find particularly enlightening Foucault's study of the birth of modern medicine (1975).

2. We are referring particularly to the mapping projects of O. T. Mason (1896, 1901) for the Smithsonian Institution at the turn of the century based on geographical and linguistic correlations identifying twelve "ethnic" environments. This was followed by classificatory schemes such as that of Clark Wissler based on subsistence forms and published in *The American Indian* (1922), work that later led to the culture-area concept which haunted anthropology for years (Wissler 1912, 1922, 1926).

3. We limit our outlook to cultural anthropology, not including the human ecology of the Chicago School of Urbanists, which belongs to another tradition; also excluded from consideration here are sociobiology and evolutionary biology, which are dealt with in detail in other essays of this volume.

4. For a brief discussion of the reasons for this different development in American cultural anthropology and European social anthropology, see Hvalkof (1996).

5. As it is known, only some North American anthropologists opted for the "materialist" path in the search for new theoretical frameworks. Others got their theoretical inspiration from psychology, leading to the well-known culture and personality school. Although the motivation for restructuring anthropology into a scientific endeavor was the same for both tendencies, they soon came to be at odds with each other leading to a lot of unproductive and derisive accusations.

6. For those who are less familiar with the postmodern jargon, let us clarify that the term *modern* does not denote *contemporary* but refers to the specific episteme governing modernity as a historical formation, and anchored on certain ideas of objectivity and rationality. Generally speaking, it is unquestionable that the breakdown of the modernist paradigm and the increasing doubts regarding universal truths has put Western rationality under broad attack. Critiques of eurocentrism have come from all quarters, pinpointing hegemonic usurpation of Reason as a universal form controlled by the West and related to colonial expansion. As summarized by Peet and Watts (1993, 228–31), in the paradigm of modernity "truth" resides in the correspondence between an externalized "objective" reality (nature) and a mental representation of it (culture). Based on a universalistic premise that all minds are structurally similar, the scientific paradigm became the production of "facts" about "reality." The entire poststructuralist enterprise can be seen as a massive critique of this type of rationality, a deconstruction of Western culture as a universal norm, and—in recent years—an attempt at reconceptualizing the world from a plurality of perspectives.

7. Alan Goodman (pers. comm.) points out that a similar "problem" has plagued medical anthropology. So much effort has gone into deconstructing an "essentialized human body" that many medical anthropologists have grown increasingly unaware of basic physiology. There might not be anything "essential" about the body, there is surely something real about it. We shall make a similar argument for nature as whole.

8. An obvious exception is the extractive reserve peoples of the Brazilian Amazon (such as rubber tappers) who have been active in struggles for territorial rights and organized into unions and in other forms, resembling a social move-

ment. Contrary to this example stand the peasant settlers from the Andean region, who rarely have organized movements, with the exception of guerrilla movements in some rain forest areas; an example in this latter category is Peru's Shining Path, which at a certain time in history could be classified as a social movement, even if embedded in a modernist development paradigm. It should be pointed out, however, that innovative and important issues of collective identity are also emerging in some areas of colonization in Latin America.

9. For instance, see Brosius (1997) and Conklin and Graham (1995) for the paradoxical nature of anthropological critiques of the form that constructions of "local knowledge" may take at times by environmentalists or other social actors, including local leaders themselves.

REFERENCES

Alvarez, Sonia, Evelina Dagnino, and Arturo Escobar, eds. 1998. *Cultures of Politics/Politics of Culture: Revisioning Latin American Social Movements.* Boulder: Westview Press.

Bateson, Gregory. 1979. *Mind and Nature: A Necessary Unity.* London: Fontana.

Bender, Barbara. 1993. Stonehenge—Contested Landscapes. In *Landscape: Politics and Perspectives,* ed. Barbara Bender, 245–79. Oxford: Berg.

Bergman, Fritjof. 1975. On the Inadequacies of Functionalism. *Michigan Discussion in Anthropology* 1 (1): 2–23.

Berlin, Brent. 1973. Folk Systematics in Relation to Biological Classification and Nomenclature. *Annual Review of Ecology and Systematics* 4:259–71.

Berlin, Brent. 1976. The Concept of Rank in Ethnobiological Classification: Some Evidence from Aguaruna Folk Botany. *American Ethnologist* 3:381–99.

Brosius, Peter. 1997. Endangered Forests, Endangered People: Environmentalist Representation of Indigenous Knowledge. *Human Ecology* 25 (1): 47–69.

Bryant, Raymond. 1992. Political Ecology: An Emerging Research Agenda in Third World Studies. *Political Geography* 11 (1): 12–36.

Burnham, P., and R. F. Ellen, eds. 1979. *Association of Social Anthropologists Monograph 18.* London: Academic Press.

Conklin, Beth, and Laura Graham. 1995. The Shifting Middle Ground: Amazonian Indians and Eco-Politics. *American Anthropologist* 97 (4): 695–710.

Conklin, Harold C. 1957. Hanunóo Agriculture: A Report on an Integral System of Shifting Cultivation. FAO Forestry Development Paper Series, No. 12. Rome: FAO.

Conklin, Harold C. 1961. The Study of Shifting Cultivation. *Current Anthropology* 2 (1): 27–33.

Conklin, Harold C. 1972. *Folk Classification: A Topically-arranged Bibliography.* New Haven: Yale University Press.

Cook, Scott. 1973. Production, Ecology and Economic Anthropology: Notes Towards an Integrated Frame of Reference. *Social Science Information* 12:25–52.

Dahl, Gudrun, ed. 1993. *Green Arguments for Local Subsistance.* Stockholm: Stockholm University Press.

Denevan, W. M. 1966. Comment on Estimating Aboriginal American Population: An Appraisal of Techniques with a New Hemispheric Estimate by Henry F. Dobyns. *Current Anthropology* 7:429

Denevan, W. M. 1976. *The Native Populations of the Americas in 1492.* Madison: University of Wisconsin Press.

Descola, Philippe. 1994. *In the Society of Nature.* Cambridge: Cambridge University Press.

Descola, Philippe, and Gísli Pálsson, eds. 1996. *Nature and Society: Anthropological Perspectives.* London: Routledge.

Dobyns, H. F. 1966. Estimating Aboriginal American Population: An Appraisal of Techniques with a New Hemispheric Estimate. *Current Anthropology* 7:395–416.

Ellen, Roy. 1982. *Environment, Subsistence and System. The Ecology of Small-Scale Social Formations.* Cambridge: Cambridge University Press.

Escobar, Arturo. 1995. *Encountering Development: The Making and Unmaking of the Third World.* Princeton: Princeton University Press.

Escobar, Arturo. 1996. Constructing Nature: Elements for a Poststructuralist Political Ecology. In *Liberation Ecologies,* ed. R. Peet and M. Watts, 46–68. London: Routledge.

Escobar, Arturo. 1997. Cultural Politics and Biological Diversity: State, Capital and Social Movements in the Pacific Coast of Colombia. In *Between Resistance and Revolution: Culture and Social Protest,* ed. Orin Starn and Richard Fox, 40–64. New Brunswick: Rutgers University Press.

Escobar, Arturo. 1999. After Nature: Steps to an Anti-essentialist Political Ecology. *Current Anthropology* (in press).

Escobar, Arturo, and Alvaro Pedrosa, eds. 1996. *Pacífico: Desarrollo o Diversidad? Estado, Capital y Movimientos Sociales en el Pacífico Colombiano.* Bogotá: CEREC/Ecofondo.

Foucault, Michel. 1973. *The Order of Things.* New York: Vintage Press.

Foucault, Michel. 1975. *The Birth of the Clinic.* New York: Vintage Books.

Friedman, Jonathan. 1974. Marxism, Structuralism and Vulgar Materialism. *Man* 9:444–69.

Friedman, Jonathan. 1979. Hegelian Ecology: Between Rousseau and the World Spirit. In *Social and Ecological Systems,* ed. P. Burnham and R. F. Ellen. Association of Social Anthropologists Monograph 18. London: Academic Press.

Friedman, Jonathan, and M. J. Rowlands, eds. 1977. *The Evolution of Social Systems.* London: Duckworth.

Geertz, Clifford. 1963. Agricultural Involution. *The Process of Ecological Change in Indonesia.* Berkeley: University of California Press.

Godelier, Maurice. 1974. *Un Domain Contesté: L'Anthropologie Economique.* Paris: Mouton.

Gross, Daniel. 1975. Protein Capture and Culture Development in the Amazon Basin. *American Anthropologist* 77:526–49.

Grueso, Libia, Carlos Rosero, and Arturo Escobar. 1998. The Process of Black Community Organizing in the Southern Pacific Coast of Colombia. In *Cul-*

tures of Politics/Politics of Cultures: Revisioning Latin American Social Movements, ed. Sonia E. Alvarez, Evelina Dagnino, and Arturo Escobar, 196–219. Boulder: Westview Press.

Gudeman, Stephen, and Alberto Rivera. 1990. *Conversations in Colombia: The Domestic Economy in Life and Text.* Cambridge: Cambridge University Press.

Haraway, Donna. 1991. *Simians, Cyborgs and Women: The Reinvention of Nature.* New York: Routledge.

Harris, Marvin. 1968. *The Rise of Anthropological Theory.* London: Routledge and Kegan Paul.

Harris, Marvin. 1979. *Cultural Materialism: The Struggle for a Science of Culture.* New York: Random House.

Hill, Kim, and Kristen Hawkes. 1983. Neotropical Hunting among the Aché of Eastern Paraguay. In *Adaptive Responses of Native Amazonians,* ed. Raymond B. Hames and William T. Vickers, 139–88. New York: Academic Press.

Hindess, Barry, and Paul Hirst. 1977. *Mode of Production and Social Formation.* London: Macmillan.

Hobart, Mark, ed. 1993. *An Anthropological Critique of Development.* London: Routledge.

Hvalkof, Søren. 1982. Intet nyt under solen: Om kulturøkologiens civilisationskritiske indhold (Nothing New Under the Sun: On the cultural-ecological critique of civilization. Bateson's and Rappaport's contributions). Working Papers from the Institute of Ethnology and Anthropology, University of Copenhagen. To be published in "Marxistisk Antropologi," *Journal of IMRA (International Movement of Radical Anthropologists),* Aarhus University (English translation in preparation).

Hvalkof, Søren. 1989. The Nature of Development: Native and Settlers' views in Gran Pajonal, Peruvian Amazon. *Folk* 31:125–50. Copenhagen: Danish Ethnographic Society.

Hvalkof, Søren. 1990. Applied Anthropology and the Enigmatics of Post-Modernism—A Danish perspective. Paper presented at the XVI Congress of Nordic Anthropologists, Reykjavik, Iceland, June.

Hvalkof, Søren. 1994. Territorial Organization and Democracy in Peruvian Amazon. The Current Asháninka Struggle for Land, Autonomy and Recognition. Paper presented at Symposium on "Sacred Land, Threatened Territories—Contested Landscapes in Native South America," 48th International Congress of Americanists (ICA), Stockholm/Uppsala, July 4–9.

Hvalkof, Søren. 1995. Sustainable Development: Democratic improvement or conserving status quo? A perspective from the Amazon. Paper presented at Colloquium on "Sustainable Development and Indigenous Rights: Can development take place without compromising indigenous communities?" Sponsored by New York University Environmental Law Journal.

Hvalkof, Søren. 1996. Political Ecology in Retrospect: From Environmental Determinism to Participatory Interactionism. Paper presented at the panel on "Political Ecology and Social Practice: Rethinking the Anthropological Approach." AAA 95th Annual Meeting, San Francisco, Nov. 20–24.

Hvalkof, Søren. 1997. Outrage in Rubber and Oil. Extractivism, Indigenous Peoples and Justice in the Upper Amazon. In *Peoples, Plants and Justice: Resource Extraction and Conservation in Tropical Developing Countries,* ed. Charles Zerner and Rainforest Alliance. New York: Columbia University Press (forthcoming).

Johnson, Melissa A. 1996. The 'Nature' of Crooked Tree: Politics and the Meaning of Nature in Transnational Conservation Efforts. AAA 95th Annual Meeting, San Francisco, Nov. 20–24.

Karim, Wazar Jahan. 1996. Anthropology without Tears: How a 'Local' Sees the 'Local' and the 'Global.' In *The Future of Anthropological Knowledge,* ed. Henrietta Moore, 115–38. London: Routledge.

Kelly, Raymond, and Roy A. Rappaport. 1975. Function, Generality, and Explanatory Power: A Commentary and Response to Bergman's Arguments. *Michigan Discussion in Anthropology* 1:24–44.

Laclau, Ernesto. 1996. *Emancipation.* London: Verso.

Lansing, Stephen. 1991. *Priests and Programmers.* Princeton: Princeton University Press.

Leff, Enrique. 1993. Marxism and the Environmental Question. *Capitalism, Nature, Socialism* 4 (1): 44–66.

Leff, Enrique. 1995. *Green Production.* New York: Guilford Press.

Lowie, Robert. 1920. *Primitive Society.* New York: Harper Torchbook.

Lowie, Robert. 1938. Subsistence. In *General Anthropology,* ed. Franz Boas. New York: Heath.

Mason, Otis T. 1896. Influence of Environment upon Human Industries or Arts. Smithsonian Institution. Annual report for 1895, 639–65. Washington, DC.

Mason, Otis T. 1901. Environment. Handbook of American Indians North of Mexico. Part I. Bulletin 30, 427–30. Washington, DC: Bureau of American Ethnology.

Meillessoux, Claude. 1964. *Anthropologie Economique des Gouro de Cote d'Ivoire.* Paris: Mouton.

Milton, Kay, ed. 1993. *Environmentalism: The View from Anthropology.* London: Routledge.

Mouffe, Chantal. 1993. *The Return of the Political.* London: Verso.

Peet, Richard, and Michael Watts. 1993. Development Theory and Environment in an Age of Market Triumphalism. *Economic Geography* 69 (3): 227–54.

Peet, Richard, and Michael Watts, eds. 1996. *Liberation Ecologies.* London: Routledge.

Rabinow, Paul. 1992. Artificiality and Enlightenment: From Sociobiology to Biosociality. In *Incorporations,* ed. Jonathan Crary and Sanford Kwinter, 234–52. New York: Zone Books.

Rappaport, Roy A. 1968. *Pigs for the Ancestors: Ritual in the Ecology of a New Guinea People.* New Haven: Yale University Press.

Rappaport, Roy A. 1971a. The Flow of Energy in an Agricultural Society. *Scientific American* 225 (3): 116–32.

Rappaport, Roy A. 1971b. Ritual, Sanctity and Cybernetics. *American Anthropologist* 73:59–76.

Rappaport, Roy A. 1976. Adaptation and Maladaptation in Social Systems. In

The Ethical Basis of Economic Freedom, ed. Ivan Hill, 39–82. Chapel Hill, NC: American Viewpoint.

Rappaport, Roy A. 1977a. Maladaptation in Social Systems. In *The Evolution of Social Systems,* ed. J. Friedman and M. J. Rowlands, 49–71. London: Duckworth.

Rappaport, Roy A. 1977b. Ecology, Adaptation and the Ills of Functionalism. (Being, among other things, a response to Jonathan Friedman). *Michigan Discussions in Anthropology* 2:138–90.

Rappaport, Roy A. 1979. *Ecology, Meaning and Religion.* Richmond: North Atlantic Books.

Ratzel, Friedrich. 1889. Antropo-Geographie, oder Grundzüge der Anwendung der Erkunde auf die Geschichte vol.1 and Dei Geographische Verbreitung des Menschen. Stuttgart: J. Engelhorn (republished 1909–12).

Ratzel, Friedrich. 1896. *The History of Mankind.* London: Macmillan.

Restrepo, Eduardo, and Julio I. del Valle, eds. 1996. *Ranacientes del Guandal.* Bogota: Universidad Nacional and Proyecto Biopacífico.

Rocheleau, Dianne, Barbara Thomas-Slayter, and Esther Wangari, eds. 1996. *Feminist Political Ecology.* London: Routledge.

Ross, Eric. 1978. Food Taboos, Diet and Hunting Strategy: The Adaptation to Animals in Amazon Cultural Ecology. *Current Anthropology* 19:1–36.

Ross, Eric. 1980. Reply. *Current Anthropology* 21 (4): 544–46.

Ross, Janet B. 1980. Ecology and the Problem of Tribe: A Critique of the Hobbesian Model of Preindustrial Warfare. In *Beyond the Myth of Culture: Essays in Cultural Materialism,* ed. E. B. Ross, 33–60. New York: Academic Press.

Sahlins, Marshall D. 1976. *Culture and Practical Reason.* Chicago: University of Chicago Press.

Sahlins, Marshall D., and E. R. Service, eds. 1960. *Evolution and Culture.* Ann Arbor: University of Michigan Press.

Smith, Neil. 1984. *Uneven Development.* Oxford: Basil Blackwell.

Soper, Kate. 1996. Nature/'Nature.' In *FutureNatural,* ed. George Robertson et al., 22–34. London: Routledge.

Soulé, Michael, and Gary Lease, eds. 1995. *Reinventing Nature?* Washington, DC: Island Press.

Steward, Julian H. 1936. The Economic and Social Basis of Primitive Bands. In *Essays in Anthropology Presented to A. L. Kroeber,* ed. R. Lowie, 341–45. Berkeley: University of California Press.

Steward, Julian H. 1941. Determinism in Primitive Society? *Scientific Monthly* 53:491–501.

Steward, Julian H. 1949. Cultural Causality and Law: A Trial Formulation of the Development of Early Civilizations. *American Anthropologist* 51:1–27.

Steward, Julian H. 1955. *Theory of Culture Change.* Urbana: University of Illinois Press.

Steward, Julian H. 1956. The People of Puerto Rico (with Robert Manners, Eric Wolf, Elana Padilla, Sidney Mintz on R. Scheele). Urbana: University of Illinois Press.

Steward, Julian H. 1968. The Concepts and Methods of Cultural Ecology. In *Inter-*

national Encyclopedia of the Social Sciences, vol. 4, ed. David L. Stills, 337–44. New York: Macmillan.

Strathern, Marilyn. 1980. No Nature, No Culture: The Hagen Case. In *Nature, Culture and Gender,* ed. C. MacCormack and M. Strathern, 174–222. Cambridge: Cambridge University Press.

Strathern, Marilyn. 1992. *Reproducing the Future.* London: Routledge.

Sturtevant, William C. 1964. Studies in Ethnoscience. In *Transcultural Studies in Cognition,* ed. A. K. Romney and R. G. D'Andrade. American Anthropologist Special Publication 66:3, Menasha.

Terray, Emmanuel. 1972. *Marxism and "Primitive" Societies.* New York: Monthly Review.

Vayda, Andrew P. 1986. Holism and Individualism in Ecological Anthropology. *Reviews in Anthropology,* 295–313.

Vayda, Andrew P., and Bonnie J. McCay. 1975. New Directions in Ecology and Ecological Anthropology. *Annual Review of Anthropology,* 293–306.

Vayda, Andrew P., and Bonnie J. McCay. 1977. Problems in the Identification of Environmental Problems. In *Subsistence and Survival: Rural Ecology in the Pacific,* ed. T. P. Bayliss-Smith and R. G. A. Feachem. New York: Academic Press.

Vayda, Andrew P., and Roy A. Rappaport. 1968. Ecology, Cultural and Noncultural. In *Introduction to Cultural Anthropology,* ed. J. A. Clifton, 476–98. Boston: Houghton Mifflin Co.

Warren, D. Michael, L. Jan Slikkeveer, and David Brokensha, eds. 1995. The Cultural Dimension of Development. *Indigenous Knowledge Systems.* London: Intermediate Technology Publications.

White, Leslie A. 1943. Energy and the Evolution of Culture. *American Anthropologist,* 45:335–56.

White, Leslie A. 1947. Evolutionism in Cultural Anthropology: A Rejoinder. *American Anthropologist* 49:400–411.

White, Leslie A. 1949. *The Science of Culture.* New York: Grove Press.

White, Leslie A. 1959. *The Evolution of Culture.* New York: McGraw Hill.

Wilden, Anthony. 1980. *System and Structure: Essays in Communication and Exchange.* London: Tavistock.

Wilden, Anthony. 1987. *The Rules Are No Game: The Strategy of Communication.* London: Routledge and Kegan Paul.

Williams, Raymond. 1980. Ideas of Nature. In *Problems in Materialism and Culture,* ed. Raymond Williams, 67–85. London: Verso.

Wissler, Clark. 1912. The Psychological Aspects of the Culture-Environment Relation. *American Anthropologist* 14:217–25.

Wissler, Clark. 1922. *The American Indian.* New York: Oxford University Press.

Wissler, Clark. 1926. *The Relation of Nature to Man in Aboriginal America.* New York: Oxford University Press.

Chapter 19

What Could Be: Biocultural
Anthropology for the Next Generation

Gavin A. Smith and R. Brooke Thomas

Antecedents

The Wenner-Gren Conference that gave rise to this book was a remarkable academic experience. Not only were individual contributors striving,
in a variety of directions, for a new synthesis of biological and social perspectives, but they did so in a manner of extraordinary respect and support
for one another's work. The effort was an example of what could take
place in most departments of anthropology when interests are shared, and
the complementarity of approaches is acknowledged. Here, we would like
to impart some of the enthusiasm generated, and summarize the potential
for a new biocultural synthesis.

It is recalled that the purpose of the conference was to explore how
biological anthropologists who work in a variety of settings and time
frames could incorporate political-economic and critical perspectives into
their analyses. To facilitate this, advice was sought from social anthropologists and archaeologists who are at the forefront of applying these ideas
to diverse areas of research. The process of coming together, at first awk-
ward and guarded, grew over the course of a week into a dynamic interchange comparable to fording a dangerous river where concepts of adaptability and political economy lined opposite banks.

Biological anthropologists, unable to communicate over the roar of
the water to those on the far shore, cautiously waded in, entering at different points and taking different routes. By those on the other side they were
coaxed into the current, cautioned on avoiding treacherous holes, advised
against using flimsy boats, and assisted with paradigmatic poles and ropes.
But a point was reached where the drama of the endeavor took hold. No
longer comfortable just sitting on shore and yelling how to do it, the social

anthropologists and archaeologists also entered the water and helped negotiate the current. We emerged together on a new bank, having shared the experience of river crossing, how such assistance could enhance the perspectives of all involved, and how a bridge might be constructed.

Thus, a trek planned to explore how social relations influence human biology became expanded to include ways in which biological states affect social structure. As proposed by Lynn Morgan (this vol., chap. 17), amplifying the dynamics of this ongoing biocultural dialectic, where social relations mold aspects of people's bodies and the condition of those bodies in turn alters social phenomena, became the essence of the conference and the charge of this volume. Hopefully, it is a theme that has relevance to the work of most anthropologists and hence to the contributions our discipline can make in the future, if it is to hold together.

From Where We Stand

Coming from different sides of the metaphoric river, it might be useful at this point to situate our own work within the aforementioned biocultural dialectic and to contextualize a shared background that informs many of our conclusions. As a biological anthropologist (B.T.) with a human adaptability orientation and a sociocultural anthropologist (G.S.) with a political-economic perspective, we worked separately in the Andes of Peru for several decades during a period of rapid transformation. We watched as rural development and agrarian reform substantially reorganized Andean communities. The introduction of various commercial practices across the landscape virtually destroyed agricultural production dependent on the complementarity of ecozones, by driving a wedge into non-commodified configurations of social relationship. And these conditions—initiated at the national and international level—had a profound influence on the ability of poorer individuals to meet their basic needs. Not only was health adversely impacted, but such changes initiated large streams of migrants out of the Andes. By the 1980s the adaptive fabric of Andean peoples, however judged, had indeed worn thin, and rebellion spread across the highlands spilling into the cities and lowland areas (McClintock 1984). Once again lives were changed dramatically.

The Andes has long been a region where rich biological and social adaptations to a harsh and unpredictable environment have been juxtaposed against four centuries of exploitation by outsiders seeking to gain control over resources and labor, subsequently constraining people's efforts and compromising their biology. There might have been a time when these processes of adaptation and exploitation could have been studied separately as two faces of the Andes. Events of the 1980s, however, demanded that anthropologists of all sorts explain the reality that was unfolding in front of them. This was a reality where past strategies of complementarity, resilience, and reciprocity were disintegrating and pushing human biological plasticity beyond its ability to effectively respond (Leatherman 1996; this vol., chap. 10).

At the same time, out of this confusion and vulnerability, new historically based social relations sprang up. Confederations of households, for instance, which once complemented one another's production by distributing themselves in different ecozones, now located themselves in different sectors of the Peruvian economy. What one found was people in the shanty towns of Lima, and the people in the mines of La Oroya, and people in the market town of Huancayo, all having transformed vertical linkages along the Andean slopes in order to maximize their access, not to ecological diversity, but to sectors of the extremely unstable Peruvian economy, in order to play one sector off against the other (Smith 1989).

In a world where poor health, social disintegration, day by day coping with constantly changing political and economic conditions, and outright violence operated side by side, it was no longer feasible—or even honest— to keep adaptation and political economics separate. From a human adaptability perspective one had to explain adaptive disintegration where people attempted to adjust to changing conditions but found their adaptive repertoire to be insufficient—literally they were losing ground. Also in need of explanation was the interaction between adaptive disintegration and human agency. Here people, in assessing the hopelessness of adjusting to the social relations that structured their lives, actively tried to change these conditions, sometimes resisting and rebelling, and in doing so placing their biology and that of many others at risk (Thomas 1997). Similarly, from a political-economic orientation it was important to account for the new adaptive strategies being initiated across the land to circumvent or challenge shifting fields of power, and to document the biological costs of inequity as it influenced new social relations. It is this shared experience, viewed from different locations in the Andes and with different lenses, that has brought us together to try to make sense of how the two perspectives can better inform one another.

Situating Biological Anthropology

This concluding chapter is designed to build on Alan Goodman and Tom Leatherman's "Traversing the Chasm between Biology and Culture," which expresses concern over the fissioning of anthropology and justifies a biocultural synthesis as one starting point in binding it back together. Here, informed by the ideas of the contributors to this volume, we begin by looking to the future of what biological anthropology, within a more integrated anthropology, could become.

We have taken the liberty of commencing with some personal views that underlie our course of argument. More important, these views lay out the challenge this volume holds in broadening and possibly transforming inquiry in biological anthropology. Long overdue and much needed, a consideration of political-economic perspectives offers considerable promise, especially to a younger generation of biological anthropologists who seek more comprehensive explanations to human biology and health.

Over the past decade many biological anthropologists have read with interest the rich developments of political-economic and critical theory taking place in other areas of our discipline, and across the social sciences and humanities. We have been impressed by their relevance in addressing essential aspects of recent change, and by their broader scope that places contemporary conditions in historical context and links local change to external process. With an emphasis on social relations and the material conditions of life, it has required little imagination to realize the import such a perspective holds for interpreting human biological and environmental well-being.

Nevertheless, biological anthropology has resisted serious consideration of political-economic insights. Both methodological issues and the politicized tenor of theoretical arguments are frequently cited reasons for incompatibility between adaptive and political-economic approaches. Clearly, ideological and epistemological barriers divide the paradigms. Thus, for some, complementarity seems an impossibility. Critiques of a functionalist, empiricist, positivist, reductionist, and ultimately alienating science are countered with a disdain for a nonscientific, ideologically explicit, advocacy approach to information generation which frequently lacks and denies either objectivity or testability. The debate has unmasked many of the weaker assumptions and analytical biases of the adaptive approach, and it has challenged the limitations of adaptive perspective and method (Singer 1996).

To continually rehash such debate with the purpose of concluding that one of these perspectives is most appropriate may be counterproductive. The extent to which it has forced one to decide between human adaptability or political economy as best expressing a materialist reality is unfortunate (Leatherman, Goodman, and Thomas 1993). First, the concept of adaptation in various forms will undoubtedly remain central to biology, and hence biological anthropology, because of its ability to explain biobehavioral change. More important, biological anthropologists remain convinced that the adaptive perspective, which examines in detail environmental and human interactions, has much to offer. This is particularly the case in a rapidly changing world that is challenging the capacity of many groups to adjust, and where biological adjustment frequently suggests eroded social and behavioral strategies. Indeed, to dismiss the importance of biocultural adjustments to such conditions, and the consequences they have on social relations, seriously diminishes the scope of anthropological interpretation.

Second, while it is exciting to envision a political economics of biological anthropology (e.g., Marxist anthropometrics or critical craniometrics), its acceptance will be greatly facilitated by a demonstration that it can enhance or complement adaptive inquiry. It, therefore, seems that if the approach is to serve biological anthropology, its goal should be to expand the scope of inquiry and analysis, increase the relevancy of findings, and advise on how best to present data and concepts in order that they be more accessible.

Over the years, most of the biological anthropologists contributing to this volume have been urging colleagues to go beyond the accepted use of socioeconomic status indicators and explore the social relations that shape human biology and environment. While they share a common concern in emphasizing the importance of social inequalities in forming adaptive opportunity, their efforts have been dispersed in different areas of the subdiscipline. Thus, they have by and large failed to present their ideas in a succinct or coherent enough manner to persuade their colleagues to adopt a new theoretical orientation.

It is, therefore, with considerable gratitude to the Wenner-Gren Foundation for Anthropological Research and the University of Michigan Press that we have been given the opportunity to present—in unison—how acceptance of a political-economic perspective has influenced other subdisciplines, and how it might lead to new lines of inquiry in biological anthropology. While some of our ideas and words—our adopted jargon—

may sound naive and tangled in exploring the potential of these new approaches, it is our opinion that achieving this end will be indispensable for the future of the subdiscipline. Fortunately, there is a strong research emphasis in the subdiscipline on the consequences of psychosocial stress, undernutrition, and disease, and on their contributing conditions. Similarly, biological anthropologists readily acknowledge—although not frequently in print—the importance of social conditions and the broader sociopolitical context within which they operate. Thus, the challenge is to encourage a broadening of scope in data collection into a richer array of social variables, and to interpret these data with regard to the biological and social consequences of inequity.

In summary, because of the pervasiveness of conditions of marginality and impoverishment, and the obvious consequences these have on human biology and subsequent human action, political-economic perspectives are urgently needed in biological studies. The distance from research presently being carried out to a more comprehensive biology of poverty or inequality does not entail a large conceptual or methodological leap. Most of the pieces are in place, and adaptive analysis, in expanded scope, can provide valuable insights into how people attempt to adjust to rapid change. Furthermore, this would serve to link adaptive concepts to the rich array of critical theory currently used in the discipline.

Of Things to Come: Anthropology Beyond 2001

While it might be possible to keep anthropology in such segmented disrepair a bit longer without exploding into separatist spheres, the events of the near future will demand a discipline such as ours to generate the comprehensive and disparate explanations of the rapid changes that are bound to engulf us all. And a holistic perspective, that concept with which we lure students to our introductory courses, and then—in good reductionistic tradition—denounce as naive, passé, and unfundable in graduate seminars, is bound to reassert itself whether we grasp the opportunity or not. As we are reminded on so many occasions with the coming of the twenty-first century, this will be a time of significant transformation and dislocation from previous ways of doing things and how we have come to understand ourselves.

Anthropology, one of the only disciplines to have avoided academic vivisection, is therefore in an exceptional position to bring together the disparate aspects of an interconnected and increasingly tangled world—

one where human biology, society, ideology, and ecology are bound together, yet in multiple states of renegotiation by different peoples. In offices up and down the corridors of anthropology departments, and especially in the students graduating from these institutions, it would seem that we have much of the combined theory and experience to start addressing the complex issues of rapid change. Furthermore, a discipline which entertains pluralistic approaches, considers the range of biocultural human diversity, and accepts as valid non-Western systems of knowledge is desperately needed at this time. Said more modestly, we are probably better prepared than most to lead this inquiry.

This is apt to be a world—for the remainder of our lives and those of our children—where security, order, and sense of "control-over" will be substantially uprooted, even for the well-off. Because of the inevitable interconnectivity of people and places, things long kept separate will come together: sometimes gently with unanticipated consequences, sometimes with great force and chaos. New peoples and cultures will encounter one another and have to negotiate their combined needs, sometimes in peace and sometimes in rebellion and war. And global economic integration will be resisted by attempts to maintain local control and cultural identity that provide meaning in a world becoming hypnotized by consumerism.

As the world population doubles by the middle of the next century, growing numbers of people will have to push their environments still further. In many places individuals will exhaust critical needs and join the migratory streams to urban slums. The one in six of humanity living in severe poverty, whose very health is at high risk, will undoubtedly grow to one in four. Yet, there will be places where people can find ways to renegotiate their place in nature and learn to sustain themselves ecologically and socially. It will be important to know how both processes work in different cultural, human biological, and ecological contexts.

The humanities will need to work with the sciences toward ends which truly serve humanity. And transdisciplinary sciences, such as political ecology, will have to expand to address complex issues where ecology, economics, health, and satisfaction intersect in a manner not well comprehended by reductionistic approaches. The redefinition of nature by biotechnological innovations, global communications, the growing consumption aspirations of the Third World, expanding inequities everywhere, and environmental regulations and management will sow their own contradictions. Global economic progress and local ecological sustainability may well be placed in a dire ideological contest comparable to the capitalism-versus-communism of an era past. Growing public recognition that the well-being of mind, body, and soul are dependent upon the health of food systems, the environment, and social relationships will generate a need for greater spirituality, challenging dominant systems of knowledge and ways of knowing and acting. Science and the academy, therefore, will be particularly tested to reevaluate its construction of truth and who it serves. And we will need to link theory and knowledge with practice and engagement, listening to and working closely with peoples negotiating these changes (Hvalkof and Escobar, this vol., chap. 18).

As a discipline, our hope in engaging these issues lies particularly in a younger generation of anthropologists moving through and just emerging from graduate school. They have been exposed to considerable theoretical breadth: evolutionary theory, human adaptability, ecological anthropology, political economy, critical theory, feminist approaches, and post-structural perspectives. These constitute different lenses with which to view and critique the multiple realities of our times. While the discipline, especially in recent decades, has encouraged one to traverse within the confines of one of these orientations (and argue tenaciously for its legitimacy above all others), to continue in this mode would seem to deny us the integrative potential that complementary perspectives provide in addressing the future.

In this volume, our task has been to argue for the coming together of human adaptability/ecology with political-economic and critical thinking, as a means of linking two predominant materialist theories. In a sense these perspectives represent an important dialectic operating throughout much of anthropological inquiry where dominant groups constrain the options (adaptive flexibility) of others in order to extract surplus, and subordinated peoples in turn attempt to find ways around these constraints, using what they have at their disposal (social organization, technology, their bodies).

Despite claims of being "the integrative discipline" there are, of course, limits to the theoretical and methodological repertoire one can control. In addition, past experience has warned us that patched-together anthropological theory can become too inclusive—too vacuous in leading to deeper insights. Nevertheless, if one approaches problems with a knowledge of how different perspectives can augment our interpretive scope, it seems possible not only to present data in a form that is relevant and accessible to experts in other areas but to challenge our own categories of inquiry. Ongoing investigation of the biological and social consequences of tourism on Maya communities of Mexico's Yucatan Peninsula is a case in point (Daltabuit and Leatherman, this vol., chap. 13; Pi-Sunyer and Thomas 1997). Scientific funding sources such as the Wenner-Gren Foundation are beginning to encourage such biocultural efforts which heretofore were not favorably reviewed by subdiscipline boards (Schell 1997).

In the end our challenge will lie in explaining how the rapidly changing conditions of the next century are to affect humankind. Said differently, will the conditions already in place override the ability of many groups and individuals to adjust, even in a species that specializes in adapting to rapid change? It would seem that a synthesis of human adaptability and political-economic theory can help here. While political-economic analysis best addresses the realities of social change and power relations, it frequently overlooks explanations of how human biological dysfunction and environmental degradation feed back on social conditions.

Human adaptability in its emphasis on "modernization" and seasonal change has built up considerable expertise in understanding the complexities of biobehavioral adjustment to unpredictable and fluctuating conditions. These are conditions in which multiple constraints and solutions converge, sometimes overloading the capacity to adjust in what is referred to as the limits of adaptation (Baker 1984). As Rebecca Huss-Ashmore has laid out in discussing these limits, much of adaptiveness and adaptability centers around a perceived and actual control of appropriate responses (Huss-Ashmore and Thomas 1997). Thus, adaptive attributes such as autonomy of action, multiple solutions, flexibility to change, storage, avoidance of irreversible actions, anticipation of disruptive events, creativity in initiating novel solutions, and altruism to support others become appropriate in periods of rapid change. Thus, measuring the enhancement or erosion of these attributes can serve us well in evaluating the consequences of social change.

The main point, however, is that political-economic analysis can lead us to a reformulation of human adaptability/ecology, and this, in turn, could expand the scope of inquiry into the consequences of power inequity. The rich theories contributing to this synthesis need not be threatened or diluted; rather each is challenged by incorporating different ways of viewing and explaining shared problems. It is out of such an interchange that a new set of anthropological problems will be forged. Our ability to accurately integrate the social, cognitive, biological, and environmental dimensions of these complex problems—that is, to encompass this new reality—

and to offer relevant solutions based on a more comprehensive understanding, will test our anthropological abilities and imagination.

Emerging from the Biological Cocoon: A Biocultural Metamorphosis

In a previous section ("From Where We Stand") we presented reasons as
to why a political-economic perspective should be introduced into biological anthropology and suggested that given its orientation toward human
health the conceptual leap need not be great. Left unexplained, however, is
why there has been such a uniform resistance to this way of viewing the
world, a resistance that embraces Darwinian medicine but finds Marxist
medicine suspicious. Since this is hard to justify on the basis of lacking
interesting research problems or their relevance to understanding the
human condition—and there is ample guidance on how to proceed from
the other subdisciplines—we suggest that an allegiance to evolutionary
theory has precluded other equally interesting possibilities. In short it has
formed, tracked, even railroaded the conceptual tools we use, and the
meanings we associate with these concepts, in a manner hardly realized.
And while colleagues in the biological sciences are left reassured that
human organisms operate much like other species, those in other areas of
anthropology are often miffed at what gets ignored or trivialized. Some
are openly hostile to persistent attempts to uncover the genetic basis of the
body and mind when problems dealing with more social aspects of human
biology remain unaddressed (Blakey, this vol., chap. 16).

It must seem to many social anthropologists that their biological colleagues operate as some strange species, perhaps an empirically oriented
inchworm that courses across bodies, measuring as it goes. They peer into
orifices, take samples of blood, spit, and urine, and occasionally bore out
a biopsy hoping to find this piece of biology correlating with that, or at
least with some nearby environmental variable. On occasion they will look
up, bleary-eyed, scanning the world beyond for close-range behavior or
social attributes that affect the body. Here, time or energy spent on various activities is recorded, as is the food consumed or the value of material
things around the house (socioeconomic indices). Replicable quantitative
measures seem to be their sustenance, and thus they pay little attention to
what people think or say about their lives—their feelings, anxieties, or
aspirations—or to the murkier socioeconomic realities which may
influence these. Self-reflection—as to underlying assumptions of the

research, whom the findings really serve, or the difficulties of empiricizing the world of the field and then presenting it as *the* reality—seems to generate little discourse.

Over two decades ago social anthropologist Daniel Gross (1976, 90) remarked in a *Yearbook of Physical Anthropology* article entitled "Reintegrating Anthropology" that biological anthropologists interested in contemporary problems are "hampered by the lack of a theoretical paradigm to orient their research. Thus studies tend to be uncoordinated and to remain at a relatively low descriptive level. One symptom of this malady is the substitution of research methodologies for theory." We maintain that this critique applies equally well to the present day in large part because neo-Darwinian evolutionary theory is simply not adequate.

Evolutionary theory (and its variants, including human adaptability) is *the* theoretical paradigm of biological anthropology. And while the theory has proven most successful in explaining general processes of biological change over generational time, it is but one way of looking at the world. In focusing on individuals and populations as competing units of analysis, and genetic adaptation as the ultimate process of directed change, one is set up with categories of analysis that have cause-and-effect expectations. This is an analysis where the natural environment and organism assume an independent and dependent variable relationship, and where finding out how the parts work is expected to lead us to the dynamics of the whole. Thus the organism is seen mostly as a passive adjuster to environmental conditions it cannot really control. No wonder Levins and Lewontin (1985) refer to this type of inquiry as an *"alienating science"* where agency and dialectics lie beyond analytical limits.

Such a view of reality is bound to overlook important biological phenomena, especially when these are affected by rapid changes taking place in one's lifetime, where environments are primarily socially constructed by nonlocal political forces, where socially constructed satisfaction norms frequently conflict with health, and where reproductive fitness and directed genetic adaptation seem largely irrelevant when trying to adjust to immediate challenges. This is not to discredit evolutionary theory or human adaptation approaches, for their contributions have been substantial, but to point out why social anthropologists find much of the work both lacking in its attention to the challenges of everyday life and dismissive of the social and cognitive phenomena that impinge on human biology.

This is what we refer to as the *human biological cocoon*—where biological analysis results in biological categories which give biological expectations and conclusions. As a consequence, biological research agendas come to take precedence over biosocial inquiry, and identification with the more "precise" sciences gradually leads to an orientation outside of anthropology, sometimes even to splitting off from anthropology departments. Such a critique is undoubtedly a bit harsh, and there are plenty of exceptions (e.g., Crooks 1996 and the series edited by Leatherman and Goodman [1997]). But, to scan the bulk of the articles in the professional journals of physical anthropology, where there is a reluctance to discuss any social theory or action, where voiceless subjects are lined up by sex-age groups, seems a bit odd in a discipline such as ours. Odder still is the enthusiastic embrace of new molecular genetic approaches to track human history into the distant past at a time when so many contemporary biosocial problems are in need of urgent attention. Maybe the next generation will demand answers to these omissions.

Why is it that the subdiscipline has been so quiet regarding biological and social insights on the conflicts in Central America, Central Africa, or the former Yugoslavia? Why are there so few reports on the biocultural dynamics of apartheid, rebellion, refugee camps, migrant laborers, domestic abuse, and the homeless? And why is it that phrases like "the biology of poverty," "the biology of tourism," or "the biology of environmental destruction," which provide such powerful examples of the consequences of unequal power relations, have such a strange ring? Is it not remarkable that such problems have been overlooked by biological anthropologists for so long? How is it that the subdiscipline has managed to keep itself so socially, politically, and cognitively neutral when it is widely acknowledged that these things really matter? A critical human biology which challenges and attempts to deconstruct the conceptual assumptions and tools of biological anthropology would be of immense service, however painful.

Theoretical constructs, of course, are designed to ignore irrelevant aspects of reality. Although human adaptability has grown out of evolutionary theory, we maintain that a political-economic perspective that informs how people bioculturally adjust will increase the likelihood of capturing the kind of social, economic, and environmental challenges human groups will encounter in the foreseeable future. In articulating with the rest of anthropology it seems critical to show how biologies are enmeshed in webs of social relations at the local level, which is intricately tied to the global. Dewalt (this vol., chap. 12) and Santos and Coimbra (this vol., chap. 11), who address the origins and consequences of environmental destruction on people's adaptive options and biology, are illustrative of what this approach can offer.

At the moment, we see two paths developing in biological anthropology which lie at different ends of a conceptual spectrum. One is primarily methodological and looks inward—far inward to our genes—and far backward as a way of further understanding our evolutionary selves. A second path is that proposed in this volume; it points toward a more socially relevant and socially rich biological perspective. It is one that looks outward—far outward—at social constructions of our environment and biology, and forward to the issues we are bound to confront in coping with rapid change in the forthcoming decades.

The *biocultural metamorphosis* we speak of takes us beyond functional complementarity where behavioral and biological responses operate together to avoid stressors or acquire resources, and attempts to embrace more fully the complexity of this interaction. A political-economic perspective is but one route to get there, albeit a seemingly robust and relevant one. In the words of Tom Leatherman, "It provides biological anthropology a way to link our long-term interest and expertise in analyzing environments as prime movers in human evolution and contemporary groups with historically, politically, and socially contextualized human–environment interactions. Moreover, it provides an opportunity of making more relevant one of the most relevant aspects of the human condition, people's biology" (Leatherman and Thomas, n.d.).

A Political-Economic Perspective

A political-economic perspective has meant many things to many people, and today it certainly is interpreted differently on either side of the Atlantic. While in Europe it has a rather conservative ring, in the United States it has come to act as a code word for "Marxist sympathies." But even in each discipline political economy has taken on different hues, and in this summary we have tried to suggest what might be a peculiarly anthropological perspective on this school of thought.

Not being formally trained in "political economy," we have found ourselves drawn into the paradigm in order to give a broader historical and geographical orientation to local conditions. Like many of the contributors to this volume, our advocacy for a political-economic perspective is not out of loyalty to some theoretical position, but because it is useful in helping resolve certain problems. In opening the book the editors comment, "although it has become relatively common to associate biological variation to some aspect of socioeconomic variation, it is rare that the context or roots of the socioeconomic variation are addressed (32–33)." This provides a good starting point in describing the specific way that political economy addresses the question of socioeconomic variation.

The first thing political economy teaches us is that we cannot stand back from ourselves or our social processes and master them the way we would like to. And just as we cannot separate out thinking about the world from the coded language we use, political economy also tells us that the link between particular words and their referents, or between concepts and reality, is a *historically driven process.* It is quite unhelpful, for example, to think that *locality* or *region* is a term superimposed by the inquirer while *community* or *household* is not. Rather, we have to understand how both sets of terms have their own historical specificity. Regions are not naturally given to us, but arise out of the conjuncture of specific political-economic forces (Harvey 1982; and Smith 1988).

What goes for regions goes equally well for communities or households, which are more the units of biological anthropologists. One of the ways of illustrating this is by taking seriously and generalizing Roseberry's ideas about (this vol., chap. 3) households as needing to be very carefully placed into historical context if they are to have meaning. As Tom Leatherman (this vol., chap. 10) shows, Andean communities with different historical backgrounds in the same locale end up having quite different health risks and outcomes. And these are best explained by their social relations rather than the altitudes at which they reside.

Inquiring further into the nature of social relations obliges us to be quite careful in our use of self-sufficiency versus surplus extraction, and subsistence versus market exchange. If the *self* in the term *self-sufficiency* refers to some kind of collection of domestic agents (father, mother, a few children), then it quickly becomes obvious that it is obscuring a whole series of very important mechanisms for extracting surpluses (i.e., setting up risks) *within* the domestic group. If, on the other hand, we prefer the term *subsistence* and then contrast it with products sold to the market for cash, we face another area of fuzziness—since we artificially separate out things that in reality are closely connected. Could a political-economic perspective help sort this out? Well, yes, we think it can, since it encourages us to be very careful about the dimensions along which we characterize social relationships, making strong distinctions between *production relationships* and *exchange relationships.* These, in turn, allow us to locate specific sources of exploitation and surplus extraction which impinge on exposure to stress or access to resources and, hence, shape biological exposure.

We might at this stage ask what is characteristic about political-economic approaches. What do these approaches have in common? In our view, they are all to a greater or lesser extent infused with a metaphor of society that uses the idea in terms of production and understands all forms of *production* to include relationships of *power.* This metaphor is often interpreted too narrowly by those wishing to criticize Marxists for their irredeemable economism and materialism, but by twisting the lens of common sense for a moment, we can quickly get a good idea of what the metaphor does for political, economic, and social inquiry. From this view *society* is a configuration of certain social relationships which are reproduced through history in the course of which certain physical goods are generated. Said differently, social relationships of a factory, a plantation, or a peasant community not only result in material outputs but spew out human biology as well.

What especially concerns political economists are the *processes that produce difference*—what Norbert Elias would call "the socio-genesis" of social and cultural differentiations under specific historic conditions: this is the linchpin of a political-economic analysis. In our view these differentiations don't just have to be class distinctions or the consequence of capitalism. Like feminism and a number of other endeavors addressing inequity, we want to argue that if political-economy cannot tackle the social production of ethnicity and gender variation, then it is not sufficiently sophisticated. What political economy attempts to do is to go to the heart of the forces that produce precisely the subjects, agents, concepts, and categories that as scientists we would like to hold independent from the historicity of our data. Like any social theory worthy of the name, political economy has to be able to explain itself. It has to be able to explain not just how the people we study become formed from historical processes, but how we too are a product of these forces: that is, how the problems we choose to study and the "solutions" we see to be possible are part of a larger historical process—and how we, as responsible scientists, must make it our task to understand and to build these questions into our analyses, not at the end when it is all over, but from the very beginning when the very nature of the problem is being formulated.

Methodological Issues

An important factor in having biological anthropologists accept this new perspective lies in challenging currently used concepts which either trivialize or distort social reality, in laying out alternate lines of inquiry, and in providing a set of methods whereby measures of biological well-being and environmental description can be expanded upon. For instance, the conventional use of socioeconomic status as a correlate of biological well-being needs to be shown as but a first step in uncovering the complexities of social relationships. And the so-called sociocultural environment constitutes a static trivialization of social processes. Understanding these social processes is important to biological anthropologists because they constitute fields of power that drive processes of social production and reproduction, and thus the actions, options, and biocultural responses of individuals.

Once having accepted that environments and responses—and thus the biology of people—are largely human constructions derived from history and social relations, the task is to explore a means of measuring *fields of power* as they change over time and space. Of particular interest is how power inequities influence the material conditions of people's lives, and how their biology responds to these conditions as part of a nested series of behavioral, social, and cognitive solutions. Operationalizing this concept in spatial and temporal measures seems essential if we are to develop a sophisticated notion of bioculturalism, for it asks under what circumstances biological responses (adaptive and maladaptive) will be initiated.

By broadening the perspective of biocultural inquiry we start uncovering the dynamics of adaptive dilemmas, as opposed to adaptive success stories where biology and culture (mostly behavior) functionally support one another. This leads us to uncovering the array of *contradictions* in maintaining biological well-being and cultural satisfaction levels, where the two in modern times frequently are not complementary. It also asks us to understand the *dialectic* between human adaptability and exploitation where social relations compromise people's options and *extract surplus* as they, in turn, try to escape or change these relations. We need to clarify what the overlap is between adaptability and agency, and whether the latter could lead us to consider an "adaptation of resistance." This is genuinely exciting stuff in which all anthropologists should take interest, and into which biological anthropologists can provide special insights.

Once again, in emphasizing studies of adaptive success (assuming people do worry about their biological well-being), *processes of adaptive retrenchment and disintegration* have been overlooked. Instead, we are left with bland failure records of morbidity and mortality or out-migration records where people disappear from our local stages of analysis. How do people fall apart and fail, and what are the social processes that drive this? What aspect of the nested adaptive repertoire (social support, household technology, biological responses, cognitive solutions) fails first, and at what point in the disintegration process are irreversible biological or social *thresholds of dysfunction* reached? Finally, how do we look at adaptive responses that attempt to reform or transform human conditions as opposed to simply reproducing them? This respects not just local peoples' interpretations of the world, but also their desire and ability to change it—and our potential to contribute to this enterprise.

Methods that can measure fields of power, extraction of surplus, thresholds of dysfunction, the saturation of conflict and contradictions, the limitation of options and responses, and the relative irreversibility of certain actions are essential if we are to understand how social relations compromise or enhance health. Clearly many of these measures are difficult to capture through the quantification of a single variable, and qualitative techniques will need to be introduced that allow people to talk out their aspirations and frustrations. As mentioned, either naively or arrogantly, biological anthropologists have generally sought to collect data and present results without human speech or emotion. It is doubtful that the preceding issues can be adequately explored without this input: ultimately the material conditions of life need be understood within their mental and emotional context. We are after all humans, not empirical representations.

Likewise, a set of methodological guidelines is needed to help expand our scope without diluting our expertise. *Historical precedence* that influences the construction of our measures and units of comparison (households, communities, regions) needs to be traced in a manner that does not turn biological anthropologists into historians. Critical social relations, likewise, need to be captured without us becoming sociocultural anthropologists. And the micro-conditions to which people are exposed need to be linked to macro-processes that so frequently structure the local (DeWalt, this vol., chap. 12). Such a dilemma would seem to encourage subdisciplinary collaboration. The idea would be to get together a biological anthropologist, a social anthropologist trained in political economy, possibly other scientists and activists, and members of the local population

who are addressing a particular issue, and from that point of view generate the problematic. Merrill Singer's group at the Hispanic Health Council in Hartford, which studies and provides health care to inner city
minorities and relies on both political-economic and adaptive perspectives, is exemplary in this regard.

Different Approaches

In exploring the potential of a more political-economic and critical biological anthropology, various approaches to this new bioculturalism are
considered. While the chapters in this volume uniformly agree that bioanthropological research requires expansion, and that political-economic
perspectives are of great utility in clarifying these contexts, there is less
consensus on the directions that a political economy of biological anthropology might take. Some researchers likely will not radically alter their
human adaptability research, but may conduct future work with a heightened awareness of the political-economic contexts in framing their investigations. Others will seek new paths for integrating political-economic and
adaptability perspectives. In the next sections we develop three directions
by which this might be achieved following Leatherman et al. (1993).

Dialectical Adaptation. Richard Levins and Richard Lewontin in their
influential book *The Dialectical Biologist* (1985) laid the groundwork for
this important concept, and many of the chapters in this volume have
attempted to develop what might be called a "dialectics of human adaptability." This perspective continues to utilize the concept of adaptation but
with a radical reformulation. In most human adaptation/ecological
approaches, the environment includes social and cultural milieus as well as
the biophysical environment. Having no ontological priority, these components of the environment are heuristic categories from which conditions
challenging the adaptive units (individuals, households, communities)
might be ranked and measured. As opposed to simple cause-and-effect
relationships where environmental constraints mold adaptive responses, a
dialectical relationship places emphasis on understanding adjustments as
they change the initial conditions, thereby creating new problems that lead
to further responses. Thus, a dialectical perspective on human adaptability focuses attention on the cost of adaptation, and emphasizes conflict
and contradiction in responses as entry points to the study of change. Fur-

thermore, it diverts attention from adaptive success to equally interesting aspects of adaptive failure.

In operationalizing this approach four types of information contribute to understanding the dialectical adaptive process: causation, impact, response, and consequence (Thomas, this vol., chap. 2). Causation inquires into the historical precedents of immediate social relations which structure specific stressors and limiting resources. In a similar sense, impact, response, and consequence are assessed as to how social forces limit action and ultimately feed back on the conditions of causation helping to shape their subsequent characteristics. Here, processes of social differentiation—poverty, inequality, and exploitation—which lead to differential control over resources are linked to processes of biocultural adjustment/adaptation. This complementarity of perspectives offers potentially rich insights into adaptive constraints.

Political Economy of Human Biology. The most common thread running through all of the chapters is an intensified focus on the social, political, and economic forces affecting health (this vol., chaps. 5–14). Within this common thread is an explicit attempt by some to make these forces the starting point of research (rather than to start with proximate links such as the biophysical environment). Here, unequal power and its underlying social relationships create differentiation in social production and reproduction, and this becomes reflected in health. Illness, in serving as a consequence of and a catalyst for deteriorating conditions, provides a sensitive lens with which to understand production and exchange relationships.

This path brings biological anthropology into alignment with a political-economic focus within critical medical anthropology (Singer, this vol., chap. 4) and with similar orientations outside of anthropology in the political economy of health (Doyal 1979) and nutrition (Sen 1981; Watts and Bohle 1993). With their abilities to provide detailed information on the biological consequences of inequality and related processes, the inclusion of more work from biological anthropologists should strengthen this approach. Problems applicable to the political economy of human biology are abundant, but for reasons stated previously this potential has been almost completely neglected.

Deere and de Janvry (1979) provide an empirical starting point for examining patterns of surplus extraction as a means to analyze the relations of production into which peasants enter. They propose seven different mechanisms through which such surplus extraction occurs. Three operate through rents that result from private appropriation of land and consist of rents in labor services (corvée), rents in kind (sharecropping), and rents in cash. Three more operate through markets by extraction of surplus value via low wages, unfavorable prices paid for items sold, and usury. A final mechanism is through the state in the form of taxes. The value of measuring these forms of extraction is that they identify areas of exploitation around which more detailed biosocial analysis can be conducted. As such, this approach provides a means of accessing key social relations in a manner accessible to biological anthropologists.

Critical Biological Anthropology. In addition to a more explicit political-economic perspective and a rethinking of adaptation, Michael Blakey (this vol., chap. 16) and Debra Martin (this vol., chap. 7) are leading the way to a reflexive, critical biological anthropology. Such an approach endeavors to expose the underlying assumptions and ideological dimensions of our work, and the sociopolitical and economic use of ideology in biological anthropology. In this vein, Morgan (this vol., chap. 17) comments that all biological anthropologists should make clear their agendas, in part by locating "researchers" as well as "subjects" in the research process. Once again, biological anthropologists have long resisted holding up the mirror to both themselves and their work. An exception is the provocative papers by Armelagos and Goodman (this vol., chap. 15; also see Goodman 1997) on race that are taken as inappropriately critical (in both senses of the word).

In moving toward a more critical stance, biological anthropologists will need to deconstruct the assumptions and system of knowledge they work within, and which they take for granted. At the Wenner-Gren Conference, Singer suggested the following nested arenas as a way to begin this inquiry. We need to first situate ourselves personally as producers of knowledge, and to come to an understanding of both the ends we would like this knowledge to accomplish and whom we want it to serve. Knowledge, of course, is not neutral, however objectively we try to collect our data. Self-reflection leads to a similar examination of the assumptions underlying biological anthropology. It warrants explanations as to why social issues of exploitation are relatively ignored while the quest to understand human genes remains so reified, and why the subdiscipline has been so empirically essentialized and cognitively neutral, not wishing to listen to people's aspirations beyond their aggregated responses to structured questionnaires.

In this vein we need to assess what the reality is that we seek to construct. Is it a biology which explains biology, or is it an anthropological endeavor acknowledging the interaction between environment, biology, culture, and broader socioeconomic processes? If we are not clear on this, we will produce segmented parts of a picture and expect someone else to paste them together. Similarly, whether we see adaptation as a passive phenomenon or rather as an active engagement in changing conditions will influence the problems selected, the selection of data, and the linkages we make with other areas of research to establish our models of reality. It will also influence how we present our results, in what journals, and whether we attempt a format that makes them truly accessible to the people we study. Once again, we are in the process of information construction, which is a form of power, and to ignore our complicity in this process does a disservice to our accomplishments.

In summary, there is considerable overlap among these paths, and they are not meant as the only directions toward more integrative biocultural approaches in anthropology. Rather, they are offered as possible starting points for future rapprochement of adaptability/ecological and critical anthropological perspectives. The point is to open up this arena for greater participation and together move forward in directions we all see as beneficial.

Conclusion

Biological anthropologists defend an adaptive perspective because they find utility in an approach that focuses directly on the immediate conditions of human action, and especially on responses to adverse conditions. Said differently, to eliminate adaptive inquiry would be a serious mistake in that it would trivialize human action and response to the conditions that are constantly forming who we are. Yet, because the adaptive perspective fails to inquire beyond these immediate constraint-causing conditions, the processes influencing their perpetuation and exacerbation are ignored. In contrast, a political-economic perspective highlights historical precedence, external political-economic relationships, and their impact not only on the structure of local social relations but on how individual actors use and lose their resources and environment. Emphasis is placed on processes of social differentiation and conflict—as opposed to social cohesion—and thus on different capacities to cope with constraints.

As a sociocultural anthropologist and a biological anthropologist with shared interests in the Andes, we see great utility in attempting to integrate these perspectives, and in striving for new biocultural syntheses. The urgency in achieving integrative perspectives is foreshadowed by the seriousness of problems of environmental quality, and the problems of human and social justice that we are likely to face in the future. In this volume the participants have begun a bridge across a river that has long kept human adaptability and political-economic perspectives separate. In so many ways, the potential of such complementarity seems most fruitful and relevant. We, therefore, invite a new generation of biological anthropologists to help shore up this bridge and build new ones in creating a human biology that can address the biocultural challenges of the forthcoming century.

REFERENCES

Baker, P. T. 1984 The Adaptive Limits of Human Populations. *Man* 19:1–14.

Crooks, D. L. 1996. American Children at Risk: Poverty and Its Consequences for Children's Health, Growth, and School Performance. *Yearbook of Physical Anthropology* 38:57–86.

Deere, C. D., and A. de Janvry. 1979. A Conceptual Framework for the Empirical Analysis of Peasants. *Amer. J. of Agricultural Economics* 61 (4): 601–11.

Doyal, L. 1979. *The Political Economy of Health.* Boston: Southend Press.

Goodman, A. H. 1997. Bred in the Bone? *Sciences* (March/April): 20–25.

Gross, D. R. 1976. Reintegrating Anthropology. *Yearbook Phys. Anthro.* 19:89–94.

Harvey, D. 1982. *The Limits of Capital.* Chicago: University of Chicago Press.

Huss-Ashmore, R., and R. B. Thomas. 1997. The Future of Human Adaptability Research. In *Human Adaptability Past, Present, and Future,* ed. S. J. Ulijaszek and R. Huss-Ashmore, 295–319. Oxford: Oxford University Press.

Leatherman, T. L. 1996. A Biocultural Perspective on Health and Household Economy in Southern Peru. *Med. Anthro. Quarterly* 10:476–95.

Leatherman, T. L., and A. H. Goodman. 1997. Expanding the Biocultural Synthesis toward a Biology of Poverty. *Amer. J. Phys. Anthropol.* 102:1–3.

Leatherman, T. L., A. H. Goodman, and R. B. Thomas. 1993. On Seeking Common Ground Between Medical Ecology and Critical Medical Anthropology. *Med. Anthro. Quart.* 7:202–7.

Leatherman, T. L., and R. B. Thomas. n.d. Political Ecology and Constructions of the Environment in Biological Anthropology.

Levins, R., and R. Lewontin. 1985. *The Dialectical Biologist.* Cambridge: Harvard University Press.

McClintock, C. 1984. Why Peasants Rebel: The Case for Peru's Sendero Luminoso. *World Politics* 27 (1): 48–84.

Pi-Sunyer, O., and R. B. Thomas. 1997. Tourism, Environmentalism and Cultural Survival in Quintana Roo, Mexico. In *Life and Death Matters: Human Rights and the Environment at the End of the Millennium,* ed. B. R. Johnston, 187–212. Walnut Creek, CA: Altamira Press.

Schell, L. M. 1997. The Evolution of Human Adaptability: Society, Funding, and the Conduct of Science. In *Human Adaptability Past, Present, and Future,* ed. S. J. Ulijaszek and R. Huss-Ashmore. Oxford: Oxford University Press.

Sen, A. K. 1981. *Poverty and Famines: An Essay on Entitlement and Famines.* Oxford: Clarendon.

Singer, M. 1996. Farewell to Adaptationism: Unnatural Selection and the Politics of Biology. *Med. Anthro. Quarterly* 10:496–515.

Smith, G. 1989. *Livelihood and Resistance: Peasants and the Politics of Land in Peru.* Berkeley: University of California Press.

Smith, G. 1998. *Confronting the Present: Towards a Politically Engaged Anthropology.* Oxford: Berg.

Thomas, R. B. 1997. Wandering toward the Edge of Adaptation: Adjustments of Andean Peoples to Change. In *Human Adaptability Past, Present, and Future,* ed. S. J. Ulijaszek and R. Huss-Ashmore, 183–232. Oxford: Oxford University Press.

Watts, M. J., and H. G. Bohle. 1993. The Space of Vulnerability: The Causal Structure of Hunger and Famine. *Prog. in Hum. Geog.* 17:43–67.

Contributors

George J. Armelagos is Professor of Anthropology at Emory University, Atlanta. His interests include diet in prehistory, the use of racial models in bioarchaeology, and the evolution of emergent diseases. He is the past president of the American Association of Physical Anthropologists.

Helen Ball is a lecturer in the Anthropology Department of the University of Durham, England. Her research interests cover parenting practices and infant well-being in historical and contemporary contexts. She is Project Director for the North Tees parent-infant sleep project, which is investigating the relationships between infants' sleeping environments and sudden infant death.

Michael L. Blakey is Professor of Anthropology and Curator of the W. Montague Cobb Human Skeleton Collection at Howard University, where he also serves as Director of the New York African Burial Ground Project.

Carlos E. A. Coimbra Jr. is a professor at the National School of Public Health, Rio de Janiero, Brazil. His major research interests include medical anthropology and the epidemiology of infectious and parasitic diseases. He is the editor-in-chief of *Cadernos de Saude Publica /Reports in Public Health.*

Deborah L. Crooks is Assistant Professor of Anthropology at the University of Kentucky. She has conducted fieldwork in Belize and eastern Kentucky. Future fieldwork will take place in the Philippines, where she and Filipino colleagues will research the household production of nutrition in a community undergoing rapid socioeconomic change.

Magalí Daltabuit is a full-time researcher at the Centro Regional de Investigaciones Multidisciplinarias of the Universidad Nacional Autonoma de

México. She has conducted fieldwork in southern Mexico, Belize, and Guatemala on biocultural adaptation to change.

Billie R. DeWalt is Director of the Center for Latin American Studies and Professor of International Affairs and Professor of Anthropology at the University of Pittsburgh. He has worked on natural resource, agricultural, land tenure, and food policies in Latin America and is editor of the *Pitt Latin American Series,* published by the University of Pittsburgh Press.

Arturo Escobar is Professor of Anthropology at the University of Massachusetts, Amherst. During the past five years, he has been doing research in the Pacific rain forest region of Colombia on the interrelations among state, capital, and social movements in the context of biodiversity and conservation.

Alan H. Goodman is Professor of Biological Anthropology and former Dean of the School of Natural Science at Hampshire College. He has conducted fieldwork in central and southern Mexico, Egypt, and the southwestern United States. During 1998–99, he will be a Weatherhead Resident Fellow, School of American Research, Santa Fe.

Søren Hvalkof is a senior social anthropologist at the Nordic Agency for Development and Ecology (NORDECO), Copenhagen, Denmark. He has worked extensively in the Peruvian Amazon on indigenous development and land titling projects. From 1994 to 1997 he was a visiting researcher and is currently an adjunct faculty member in the Anthropology Department, University of Massachusetts, Amherst.

Thomas L. Leatherman is Associate Professor of Anthropology at the University of South Carolina, Columbia. He has conducted fieldwork on the political ecology of diet, health, and nutrition in the Andes, Mexico, and in coastal South Carolina. His recent work, with Goodman, focuses on dietary commoditization and the penetration of junk foods (coca-colonization) in Mayan communities of the Yucatan.

Richard Levins is John Rock Professor of Population Science at the Harvard School of Public Health. He works in theoretical, agricultural, and epidemiological ecology and in the mathematics and philosophy of complex systems. He is coauthor (with Richard Lewontin) of *The Dialectical Biologist.*

Richard Lewontin is Alexander Agassiz Professor of Zoology and Professor of Biology at Harvard University. He is a population geneticist and statistician whose research is concerned with genetic variation within and between species and the relationships among gene, environment, and development. He is the author of *Biology as Ideology*.

Debra L. Martin is Professor of Biological Anthropology and Director of the Southwest Field Studies Program at Hampshire College. She has recently coedited *Troubled Times: Violence and Warfare in the Past*. Her research includes health in ancient groups with a focus on women and children in marginal desert environments.

Lourdes Márquez Morfín is Professor of Physical Anthropology and Subdirector of Research at the National School of Anthropology and History, Mexico and the former Director of Physical Anthropology of the Instituto Nacional de Antropología, México. Her research focuses on biocultural adaptation of ancient and postcontact Mesoamerican populations.

Lynn M. Morgan is Associate Professor of Anthropology at Mount Holyoke College. She is the author of *Community Participation in Health: The Politics of Primary Care in Costa Rica* and coeditor, with Meredith Michaels, of the forthcoming volume, *The Fetal Imperative: Feminist Positions*. She has conducted fieldwork in Central America and Ecuador.

William Roseberry is Professor of History at New York University. He has written extensively on anthropological political economy, including *Anthropologies and Histories*. He has conducted research on coffee and class formation in nineteenth century Venezuela, and is coeditor of *Coffee, Society, and Power in Latin America*. He is presently at work on liberalism and indigenous politics in nineteenth century Patzcuaro, Michoacan, Mexico.

Dean J. Saitta is Associate Professor and Chair of the Department of Anthropology at the University of Denver. He is writing a book on the political economy of ancient North America and conducting research on the archaeology of the Colorado Coal Field War, 1913–14.

Ricardo Ventura Santos is Associate Professor and Curator of Biological Anthropology at the National Museum and Associate Researcher at the

National School of Public Health, Rio de Janiero, Brazil. His major research interests are public health and biological anthropology of Amazonian Amerindian populations. From 1992 to 1995, he was a Fellow of the MacArthur Foundation in Brazil.

Merrill Singer is Executive Director of Research at the Hispanic Health Council in Hartford, Connecticut. He has written extensively on critical medical anthropology. Recent books in this vein include *Medical Anthropology and the World System* (with Baer and Susser), and *Critical Medical Anthropology* (with Baer).

Gavin A. Smith is Professor of Anthropology at the University of Toronto and President Elect of the Canadian Anthropological Society/Société canadienne d'anthropologie. Author of *Livelihood and Resistance,* he has conducted fieldwork in the Andes, Spain, and Italy. He recently coedited *Between History and Histories* (1998) and his *Confronting the Present: A Politically Engaged Anthropology* is in press.

Alan C. Swedlund is Professor of Anthropology at the University of Massachusetts, Amherst. His research interests are in historical demography and epidemiology of the American Southwest and New England. Current projects include an inquiry into the nineteenth-century U.S. mortality transition and population reconstruction of prehistoric Puebloan peoples.

R. Brooke Thomas is Professor of Anthropology at the University of Massachusetts, Amherst. Since the 1960s he has conducted research on biocultural adaptations of the high Andean Quechua and on the impact of mass tourism on the lowland Maya of the Yucatan Peninsula, Mexico.

Index

adaptation, xi, 9–12, 16–23, 48–70, 110, 112–15, 163, 245–49, 271, 395, 413, 429–30, 453–55, 459–61, 466, 468–71; and coping, 20, 22, 127, 246, 249–51, 254, 262, 264, 453, 463. *See also* human adaptability

African American, 365; and African diaspora, 401

agriculture, 271, 284–85, 296–98, 301–3, 305, 310–13, 321–23, 342–44; and agrarian reform, 64, 247–48, 253, 297, 452; and agribusiness, 278, 297, 392; and archaeology, 133–39, 151–65, 180–86; and development, 313

AIDS, 11, 30, 109, 197, 199

Alland, Alexander, 93

ambiguity, 128, 131, 139, 141–42

American Anthropological Association (AAA), 8, 103, 387, 400–401

American Association of Physical Anthropologists (AAPA), 8, 34, 214, 362

Anasazi, 128, 133, 137–39, 173, 180

Andes, 27, 63, 65, 88–89, 115, 177, 245–47, 251, 254, 264, 452–53, 472

anemia, 6, 51, 159, 161, 176, 282–83, 285, 329, 366

anthropometry, 345. *See also* nutritional status

antiscience perspective, 14, 94

Appalachia, 341, 343–45

archaeology, 14, 17, 19, 26, 29, 93–94, 127–28, 142, 147–48, 150–51, 154, 162–64, 171–74, 176–79, 186, 390, 401; and bioarchaeology, 15, 26,

127, 140, 147–48, 150, 165, 171–72, 176–77, 186, 390, 396

Armelagos, George, 33, 54, 150, 165, 373

Arroyo Hondo, 138

Baker, Paul, 245, 247, 265, 367, 373

Ball, Helen, 27, 191

Benedict, Ruth, 174

biocultural anthropology, 19, 25, 29, 114, 245, 360, 451; and split, 4, 6–7, 363

biocultural perspective, 264; and synthesis, xv–xvi, 4–35, 43–70

biological anthropology, xv–xvi, 5–6, 8, 11, 15, 17, 19, 21–22, 27, 29, 32–35, 43, 48, 53, 93–94, 97, 110, 117, 119–20, 171–75, 177, 186, 192–94, 214–15, 219, 238, 248, 265, 269, 288–89, 308, 357, 379, 384–86, 390, 402–4, 407, 413, 420, 443, 454–55, 460–63, 468–70, 472

biological explanation, 218

biology of poverty, 19, 26, 38, 43, 51, 53, 59, 68–69, 351, 420, 456, 462, 472

biomedicine, 32, 100, 103, 105–7, 116, 408–10, 419–20

Black Mesa, 138, 157, 179–80, 182, 184–85

Blakey, Michael, 29, 33, 372, 413, 470

blood groups, 366

blood pressure, 56, 70, 109, 340, 394

Boas, Franz, 362, 384, 388, 396, 428; and Boasian perspective, 77, 384

body mass index (BMI), 286–87, 340, 345–47, 352